Joe D. Goldstrich, M.D., F.A.C.C.

THE CARDIOLOGIST'S PAINLESS PRESCRIPTION FOR A HEALTHY HEART AND A LONGER LIFE

Also by Joe D. Goldstrich, M.D., F.A.C.C.

The Best Chance Diet

The 1-Day-At-A-Time Diet

Joe D. Goldstrich, M.D., F.A.C.C.

THE CARDIOLOGIST'S PAINLESS PRESCRIPTION FOR A HEALTHY HEART AND A LONGER LIFE

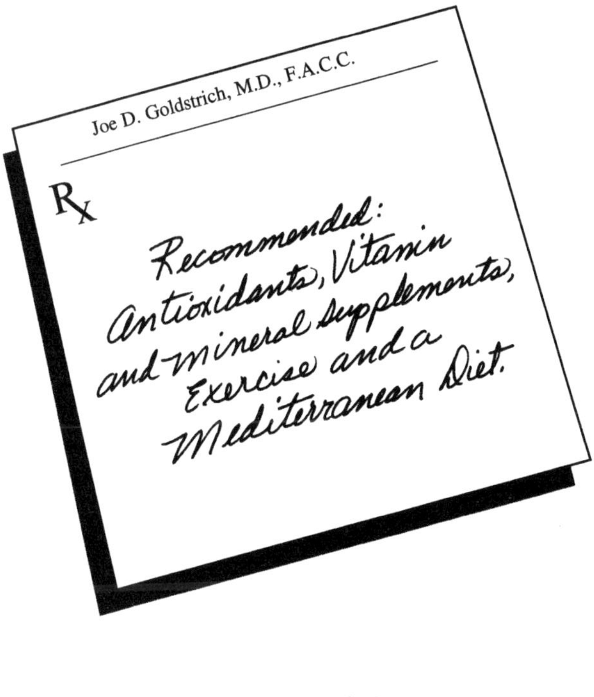

9-HEART-9 Publishing
Dallas, Texas

Printed in the United States of America

Library of Congress Catalog Card Number: 93-92831

ISBN: 0-9639877-0-4

Book design by Mary Jane Quandt Kelley

Cover design and graphics by Maxwell/Sandoz Advertising & Design

9-HEART-9 Publishing
8215 Westchester Drive
Suite 307
Dallas, Texas 75225

Dedicated

to my wife, Barbara Lipshy,
and to my parents, Edythe and Sydney Goldstrich,
with all my love

and to the memories of

Irving Goldstrich
Jennie Kahn
Leon Kahn
Elizabeth Ann Lewis
Scott A. Lewis
Ben A. Lipshy
Melinda Sue Marcus
Dick Price
Nathan Pritikin
Alan Reisman

Contents

Acknowledgments

A special thanks to Udys W. Lipshy, the best mother-in-law a man could have.

A much deserved thank you to my close friends, Harvey and Diana Lerer, for all their advice and assistance during the preparation of this manuscript.

I can't begin to tell you how delighted I was to have a chance to once again work with Shelly Usen, the editor of my second book, *The 1-Day-at-a-Time Diet.* Without her clarity of vision and insight, the final form of this book would not have emerged. Thank you, Shelly, and I look forward to working with you on book #4.

A very special thanks to Mary Jane Quandt Kelley for her help, guidance, diligence, and attention to detail in making the manuscript ready for publication. She was with me from the beginning of this project to its delivery at the printer. Thank you, Mary Jane.

My sincere thanks to Susan Jacobs, who went way beyond her duties in public relations to help me make many of the important decisions about the design of this book. Thanks again, Susan.

Finally, I want to thank all of my patients, who have put their faith in my ability to decipher this new medical literature on vitamin and mineral supplements, and who encouraged me to learn more and to share with them this exciting adventure.

Preface

The American Heart Association (AHA) predicts that as many as 1,500,000 Americans will have a heart attack this year and about 500,000 of them will die. Sixty percent of these deaths will occur before the person reaches a hospital and about half of them will be the very first indication of heart disease. Let me say that in a different way so you will be sure to appreciate the full magnitude of this last statistic: about one in three people with heart disease will not even know that they have heart disease. The first thing that will happen to them is that they will die! No problems, no warning, and an instant later they are dead. I personally would like to minimize the chances of this happening to me. That's only one of the reasons that I have been searching for realistic and nontoxic methods to prevent and reverse coronary heart disease.

Just about the time I was finishing my cardiology training, I lost two uncles to coronary heart disease. They had the best care that cardiology had to offer, but they still died. Those two tragic deaths set the stage for my career in cardiology. In my opinion, if half the money and energy spent on technological advances in cardiology were spent on prevention, we would have the disease whipped by now.

If you visit your doctor and say, "Doc, I want you to check me over and see if there is anything we can do to prevent coronary heart disease," chances are your insurance company won't even pay for the visit—even though heart disease is the nation's number one killer! The insurance company will pay $30,000 for a coronary bypass operation, but not one penny for prevention. There are, however, a few progressive insurance companies that are beginning to realize that a few dollars spent on prevention may actually cut costs and add up to higher profits.

Angiograms and bypass surgery are not the routes that I have chosen to follow in cardiology. I wanted to find a natural, safe way to prevent and reverse the whole process of atherosclerosis (the build-up of cholesterol deposits in the arteries). I have been prepared to go wherever the search might lead me.

I have had a unique career as a cardiologist: I have served on medical school faculty, in private practice, as national director of education and community programs for the American Heart Association (AHA), and as chief cardiologist and medical director at the Pritikin Longevity Center in California. During all this time, I have been searching for those elusive answers to the problems of cardiovascular disease. Some of my friends and colleagues say that I have been courageous in my search. My response is that I have had no choice. I have been driven to find the answers. Over the past twenty years, I have rarely missed a national meeting of the AHA or the American College of Cardiology. I have attended meetings of the American College for the Advancement in Medicine, the organization of the doctors who do chelation. I have gone to hypnosis, guided imagery, and stress reduction meetings. I have studied homeopathy and herbal medicine.

On my journey, I stopped off for a few years to study with Nathan Pritikin, who pioneered the prevention and reversal of coronary heart disease using diet alone. In my opinion, nothing new has been added to this dietary approach that Pritikin introduced almost twenty years ago. Every year or so a new book comes out reiterating the Pritikin principle—that a very lowfat, vegetarian, or extremely low-cholesterol diet is what it takes to prevent or reverse coronary heart disease. My first book, *The Best Chance Diet,* which was published in 1981, was also a reiteration of that concept. I, too, have learned that Pritikin's approach definitely works, but unfortunately only a few people can manage this kind of diet over the long haul, because it's so difficult.

It has been a long journey, and now for the first time I see a very bright light at the end of the tunnel. Coronary heart disease is both preventable and reversible. It is easier to prevent than it is to reverse, but both are definitely possible. I base these conclusions on the fact that THE MOST IMPORTANT BREAKTHROUGHS IN CARDIOVASCULAR DISEASE IN THIS CENTURY HAVE OCCURRED IN THE PAST THREE YEARS! These breakthroughs are in the area of nutritional supplements and drugs that can prevent and reverse coronary heart disease. You'll need your doctor and your insurance company for the drug part, but there are a tremendous number of things that you can do on your own with nutritional supplements to both prevent and arrest the progression of coronary heart disease.

In this book, I'll guide you through this nutritional maze and help you make sense of this otherwise confusing information. My recommendations are in no way a substitute for your physician's expert advice. If you are under the care of a physician and you are taking medication, you should always consult your physician before adding any supplement. I will detail the drug interactions with the nutritional supplements and describe any potential side effects as best as I can. However, your physician is always your best source of information about your medicine and your medicine's potential for adverse interactions with the supplements.

My desire is to give you tools that can help you take better care of yourself. Not just dietary guidelines that are very difficult or nearly impossible to follow, but real help. Don't get me wrong—diet is extremely important and if I had coronary heart disease, I would become a vegetarian overnight. However, most people can't or won't make all the sacrifices that are necessary to maximize diet therapy. If you are willing to make a few changes in your diet and to add nutritional supplements to your regimen, you can make a big difference.

I'll tell you which supplements are the best proven and the most likely to reduce your risk of cardiovascular disease. I'll tell you why the supplement works and how it might accomplish its desired effect. I'll tell you about any side effects and contraindications.

Some of the more technical research information, quoted from the medical literature, is set off in a box and is easily identifiable. Some of you may enjoy reading these findings by the top medical researchers in their fields; others may want to skip over the research details and get to the bottom line on whether you should take the supplement or not and how much to take. Some of you may even want to refer to the original research article listed in the Clinical Reference section at the back of the book, where you will find references for just about every claim I make. As I go along, I'll try to explain each medical term and concept I use.

It has taken me over ten years to integrate the nutritional information I first learned from Nathan Pritikin with the material that you will find in this book. I kept on searching because I knew that there had to be a better way than conventional medical and surgical methods. This book is my sharing with you the answers that I have found on my journey.

Joe D. Goldstrich, M.D., F.A.C.C.
Dallas, Texas, 1994

Introduction

The central theme of this book is that coronary heart disease can be prevented and its progression stopped through the use of antioxidant supplements. Antioxidants are compounds that neutralize, deactivate, decimate, demolish, and destroy free radicals.

Free radicals are molecules that are unstable due to an unpaired or uneven number of electrons in their outer orbit. These free radicals, in an effort to balance and stabilize their own outer orbit, will wrench or tear electrons from the outer orbits of other molecules that were previously stable. This electron-yanking action creates new free radicals, molecular instability, and may even initiate a chain reaction of free radical formation. Each time an electron is torn out, molecular damage is done.

This violent, destructive, electron-yanking process is called *oxidation*. Antioxidants can combine with and deactivate free radicals without themselves becoming unstable. They can stop this molecular devastation dead in its tracks.

As we will see, LDL-cholesterol (the bad cholesterol) can only participate in the blockage of the coronary arteries after it is attacked by free radicals and oxidized. Antioxidants protect against free radicals.

The Cardiologist's Painless Prescription for a Healthy Heart and a Longer Life is a book about antioxidants and other nutrients, vitamins, minerals, and foods that protect against the development and progression of coronary heart disease. It is a plan I prescribe for my patients that has proven results.

Some of the concepts about the protection of the heart by nutrients, vitamins, minerals, and foods might be considered radical by those unfamiliar with the medical literature. However, if it weren't for the documentation of each and every one of these revolutionary concepts in the extensive Clinical References section which is based on extremely current medical literature—the concepts might be considered radical.

Since it **is** all documented and based on good scientific evidence, the only thing radical would be **not** to use these concepts to protect your own heart.

Part I

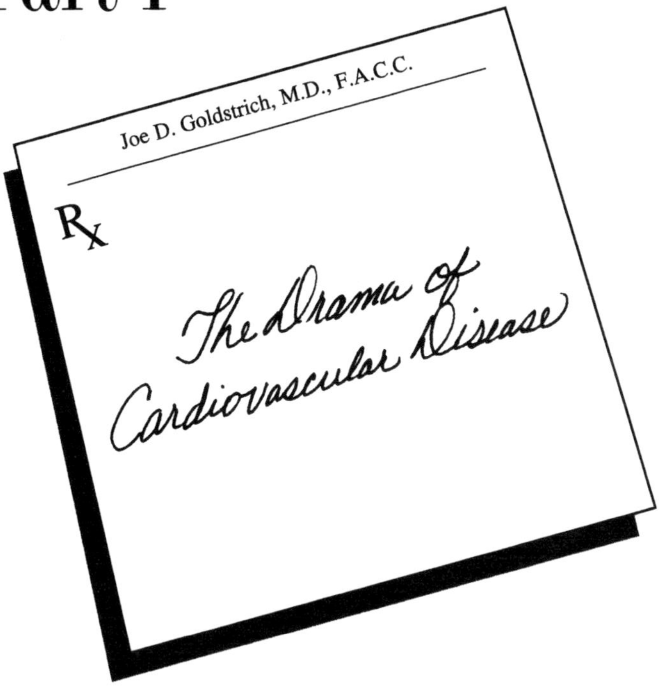

Heart disease is a national tragedy. According to the American Heart Association, about 50 percent of American deaths each year are due to cardiovascular disease. About half of these deaths are sudden and unexpected. Often, sudden death is the very first sign or symptom of heart disease. There is no warning. You thought you were OK and the next thing that happens is you die. *The Cardiologist's Painless Prescription for a Healthy Heart and a Longer Life* will give you tools to make this sudden disaster a lot less likely to happen.

In a perfect world, you could eat a perfect diet and breathe only clean, unpolluted air. Unfortunately that world doesn't exist. We can't eat every meal at home to be sure that it is as healthy as we would like. We can't always eat a 10 percent fat diet à la Nathan Pritikin or Dr. Dean Ornish. We can't always stop smoking or even get away from the tobacco smoke of the person sitting next to us. However, there are many things we can do when we can't do what we should do. This book is about those things—things that each and every one of us can do to have a healthier heart and a longer life.

Before I give you my *Painless Prescription for a Healthy Heart and a Longer Life*, let's first take a close look at the nature of cardiovascular disease and the risks involved. As the curtain rises on this information, you will understand the unique role my painless prescription will play in your life.

1 *Setting the Stage*

WHAT IS CHOLESTEROL?

Cholesterol is a waxy substance that is essential to our bodies. It is the backbone of many of our hormones, and it is required for the stability of all of our cell membranes. The body is able to make all the cholesterol it needs.

Many scientists believe that we were meant to be vegetarians and that all the cholesterol we eat in our diet is simply excess baggage. The reason for this belief is that cholesterol is indestructible in the body. It cannot be broken down or burned. It can only go out of the body through the bowel movement or modified and stored in the body. Unfortunately, one of the prime storage areas is in the plaque that blocks our arteries.

The National Cholesterol Education Program (NCEP) is a federally funded program that has established the normal or healthy blood levels of cholesterol for individuals in this country. According to the NCEP, an LDL-cholesterol level below 130 is desirable and a level above 160 is considered high-risk. Levels between 130 and 160 are borderline.

TOTAL CHOLESTEROL

When you go to the laboratory and have blood drawn to check your cholesterol, you will get several values on the lab report. Cholesterol, HDL, LDL, triglycerides, and sometimes Lp(a) will be reported. Below, we will examine the role of each of these major players in the coronary heart disease drama.

The cholesterol or total cholesterol value on the lab report is the sum of the LDL, HDL, Lp(a), and the cholesterol carried with the triglycerides, which is called VLDL. LDL, Lp(a), and VLDL are the villains in our drama and HDL is the hero.

Initially, much of the work on the relationship of cholesterol to coronary heart disease was done before researchers had worked out the precise role of each of the players. Consequently, you will still see articles written about "cholesterol" and how you should lower it, or not worry about it, or know its value, or whatever. These pronouncements are totally meaningless. LDL-cholesterol is directly related to cardiovascular disease, and the higher the LDL, the greater the risk of coronary heart disease. On the other hand, the higher the HDL-cholesterol, the lower the risk of coronary heart disease. It just doesn't make any sense to talk about "cholesterol" without specifying which component of the total cholesterol you are talking about.

I have seen a fair number of patients who were referred for treatment of their high "cholesterol" values when, in fact, their cholesterol level was elevated because their HDL-cholesterol was very high. These patients needed absolutely no treatment at all! They fall in the very low-risk category and often experience great longevity and total freedom from cardiovascular disease. When the HDL is too low, however, the risk of coronary heart disease is very high.

On the other hand, I have seen other patients with so-called "normal" values of total cholesterol who were at a very high risk. In these cases, the HDL level was extremely low and the LDL was high, but the total cholesterol level was well within the normal range. I recently treated such a patient with diet and vitamin and mineral supplements and was delighted to see the HDL level double. This took the person from a very high risk to a very acceptable and desirable level of risk.

2 *Players in Key Roles*

LDL-CHOLESTEROL

As we discussed, the higher the level of LDL (low-density lipoprotein), the greater the risk of coronary heart disease. For over twenty-five years, it was my firm belief that the **only** important thing a person could do to prevent blockages from building up in his or her coronary arteries was to control the LDL-cholesterol level. I held this belief for so long because it was and still is true that the higher the LDL level, the greater the risk of developing these blockages. In addition, it has been proven that intensive lowering of LDL slows the progression of coronary heart disease and reduces the number of heart attacks. In some cases, lowering LDL can even reverse these obstructions.

OXIDIZED LDL—THE REAL VILLAIN

Each day, evidence mounts supporting the theory that **only oxidized LDL is incorporated into the arterial obstructions.** The higher the LDL level, the greater the amount of LDL that is available for oxidation. The lower the LDL level, the less that is available for oxidation. As far as LDL is concerned, it appears that the best of all possible worlds for preventing and/or reversing the arterial obstructions is to have a low LDL **and** to prevent its oxidation.

HDL-CHOLESTEROL—OUR HERO

HDL (high-density lipoprotein)-cholesterol plays a protective role in our scenario by carrying the LDL away from the arterial wall before it becomes irreversibly trapped in and incorporated into the plaque. This ability is one reason why the higher the levels of HDL, the lower the risk of heart disease. The process of carrying away the LDL is called *reverse cholesterol transport*. The HDL carries the LDL back to the liver so it can be dumped into the bile and subsequently removed from the body in the bowel movement.

In addition to its protective role, HDL may also play a significant part in the regression of early fatty streaks, which I explain below.

One final note: HDL has been shown to protect against coronary disease by actually functioning as an antioxidant and preventing LDL oxidation!

Lp(a)

Lp(a) is a molecule that is half-LDL and half-clotting factor. Lp(a) can be oxidized just like LDL and it will also facilitate clotting of the blood, making it a doubly dangerous villain.

TRIGLYCERIDES

Triglycerides are fats that circulate in our bloodstream. The liver produces triglycerides, and the fat that we absorb from our diet also travels through the bloodstream in the form of triglycerides. Triglycerides are packaged with LDL in the liver, and this fatty-cholesterol package is known as VLDL. It appears that VLDL is toxic to the artery wall, but the exact nature of this toxicity, as well as how triglycerides accelerate atherosclerosis, is still unknown.

3 *The Drama Unfolds*

PLAQUE BUILD-UP

The very earliest findings of plaque build-up that are seen in the artery wall are called fatty streaks. We know a lot about the genesis of these fatty streaks and we also know that, if not treated, they will progress into full-blown cholesterol blockages. Let's see how this works.

Some of the LDL-cholesterol that is traveling around in the bloodstream filters through the wall of the artery in the course of its journey through the body. If this LDL happens to be oxidized, it attracts white blood cells called *monocytes*. These monocytes, which are also traveling in the bloodstream, force their way through the artery wall because of their very strong attraction to the oxidized LDL. LDL that is not oxidized will not attract the monocytes. The best explanation for this "fatal attraction" is that the monocytes see the modified, oxidized LDL as a foreign substance. It is the job of white blood cells, including the monocytes, to track down foreign substances and ingest them. This is one way that our body isolates and removes potentially toxic substances.

FROM MONOCYTES TO HEART DISEASE

Once the monocytes start their meal of oxidized LDL, they become insatiable. They eat and eat and eat until they become fat and laden with the oxidized LDL. They become so fat, in fact, that they get stuck in the tissue of the artery wall.

Monocytes that lose their mobility and become fixed in the tissue are called *macrophages*. Macrophages stuffed with LDL are called *foam cells*.

As these foam cells accumulate in the artery wall, the fatty streak begins to grow. Other factors come into play that stimulate the growth of the fatty streak and eventually turn it into a well-developed arterial plaque. These plaques then go on to block and obstruct the arteries. When the process takes place in the coronary arteries, coronary heart disease results. **This whole sequence can be markedly curtailed if levels of LDL are lowered and LDL is protected from oxidation.**

This process of plaque build-up takes place in almost everyone. If the build-up is fast, as in people born with very high LDL levels, a heart attack or myocardial infarction could occur even before age twenty. If the build-up is slow, there might be very little plaque in the coronary arteries after fifty or sixty or more years of life. This was the case when my friend and teacher Nathan Pritikin died. Although he had been diagnosed with high cholesterol levels, when his coronary arteries were examined at his autopsy, they were virtually free of plaque. He had significantly reduced his LDL level over many years. He did not take any supplements at all.

If the LDL is kept low enough over a long period of time, there will not be enough LDL present to yield much oxidized LDL, and plaque build-up will be minimized. By the same token, if the LDL is low enough, there won't be much LDL for the HDL to carry back to the liver and the risk will still remain low even in the face of lower HDL levels.

In some cases where the plaque build-up takes place over many years, there may be as much as 70 percent blockage of a coronary artery without any symptoms whatsoever. When there is enough obstruction to limit the flow of oxygen-rich blood to the heart muscle, angina can occur. Angina is chest and/or arm pain brought on by an oxygen deficiency to the heart muscle.

4 *The Plot Thickens: Clotting, the Ultimate Killer*

Clotting is the way the body stops bleeding. Without clotting, we would all bleed to death from the slightest injury. It is a necessary function of the body to stop bleeding. In heart disease, clotting takes on the form of a villain.

Clotting contributes to the process of plaque build-up, and it is the precipitating event in heart attacks. In order to better understand the role of clotting in atherosclerosis, we have to get a clearer picture of what the plaque looks like.

You remember the fatty streak. As it continues to grow into a full-blown blockage, it can take on one of two appearances. It either becomes a primarily fat/cholesterol-filled plaque, or it will have a little bit of fat and cholesterol and a lot of fibrous tissue. It's the former that is so dangerous. If a fat/cholesterol-filled plaque develops a tear or a fissure and the fatty material inside is exposed to the bloodstream, a blood clot will form. If this clot grows to completely block the coronary artery, a heart attack will occur. Our bodies' natural anticoagulants, aspirin, vitamin E, anticoagulant drugs, clot-busters, and other factors can all work to try and halt or reverse this process. If the heart attack is survived, the clot will resolve to a greater or lesser degree. The part of the clot that is not resolved will become added to the plaque and will contribute to the obstruction of the artery. This explains why some survivors of a heart attack will be left with angina when no angina was present before the heart attack.

About three out of four heart attacks occur in this way. The scary part is that the fatty plaques that give rise to most heart attacks are not even very big. They may not block more than 20 to 30 percent of the artery, and yet they are potentially the most lethal. There are several ways to defend against this treachery. The **first** is to minimize plaque growth by maintaining a low level of LDL. The **second** is by using antioxidants to prevent the LDL from oxidation. The **third** is to ensure that the risk factors that cause clotting are minimized. And the **fourth** is to control other factors that are known to contribute to heart disease and the clotting phenomenon. We have already touched on the LDL and its protection by the antioxidants, and we will address the use of antioxidants in detail in Chapter 7. Let's now examine the clotting factors; then we will go back and look at the heart attacks that are due to fibrous plaques.

CLOTTING RISK FACTORS

Platelet Stickiness

Platelet stickiness (or adhesiveness) has been one of the most studied clotting risk factors. Platelet stickiness is when the platelets (tiny disk-shaped elements circulating in the blood stream) come together and stick to each other. As they gather together, they form a platelet mass. This is the first step in the clotting mechanism, so if we can reduce platelet stickiness, we can stop the whole process before it even gets started. As we will see, lowering LDL levels, stopping smoking, using aspirin, vitamin E and the other antioxidants, magnesium, fish oils, alcohol, wine, bioflavonoids, nitroglycerine, and garlic will all reduce platelet stickiness.

The next step in the clotting sequence involves the transformation of fibrinogen to fibrin. Fibrin is the main constituent of the clot. It has now been shown that the more fibrinogen that circulates in the bloodstream, the greater the risk of heart attack. While the list of things that can be done to **inhibit** platelet stickiness is relatively long, the list of things that will definitely **lower** fibrinogen levels is all too short. Only exercise and cessation of smoking has been shown with certainty to reduce fibrinogen levels. Interestingly, even passive or environmental smoke will raise fibrinogen levels.

The more platelets that are circulating in the bloodstream, the greater the likelihood that platelet stickiness will be activated. At the present time, there is no easy treatment for a high platelet count. Also, the higher the blood viscosity (or thickness), the more likely the blood is to clot. Regular exercise can lower blood viscosity.

We have a natural mechanism in our bodies called *fibrinolysis* that is constantly dissolving clots that form. This system is activated whenever clotting occurs. It is part of the natural system of checks and balances so prevalent in our body. Exercise is one of the most powerful activators of this fibrinolytic system.

Much research has been done recently on dissolving clots in acute heart attacks. Clot-busters are now given routinely at the onset of a heart attack to try and dissolve the clot as quickly as possible. The more complete the obstruction of the artery, and the longer the clot blocks the artery, the more irreversible damage will be done to the heart muscle that receives its oxygen and nutrition from that artery.

TPA (Tissue Plasminogen Activator) is one of the most common drugs given to dissolve clots. Exercise activates our own natural TPA. We are probably developing small fissures in plaques all the time, and our natural fibrinolytic system is constantly halting clot formation. Regular exercise is just one more way that we can protect against clotting. If you are in the process of having a heart attack, don't try to activate your fibrinolytic system with exercise. It's too late for that now. Call 911 and get to the hospital for treatment immediately. If there is no strong reason not to, chew and swallow an adult-size aspirin tablet while awaiting the paramedics. This simple maneuver will begin to reduce platelet stickiness, even if you are on maintenance aspirin therapy.

Lp(a)

Lp(a), called "L, p, little a," was discovered in 1963, but its significance as a risk factor has only recently been appreciated. Lp(a) is perhaps the most villainous of all the risk factors because it is half-LDL, which can be oxidized and incorporated into plaque, and half-clot promoter. The clot-promoter part closely resembles plasminogen, as in Tissue Plasminogen Activator (TPA). Because of this structural similarity, the Lp(a) blocks the action of circulating TPA and clots are not broken down as readily in the presence of elevated Lp(a) levels. Testing for Lp(a) is difficult, and it is still primarily a research procedure. However, more and more laboratories are making the Lp(a) test available.

Dr. Linus Pauling and his associate, Matthias Rath, M.D., believe that Lp(a) is the most important of all the risk factors. They first noted that Lp(a) is present only in those species that don't manufacture their own vitamin C. Vitamin C deficiency leads to scurvy, a disease that causes weakened blood vessels. Pauling and Rath speculated that Lp(a) developed as the body's way to adapt to the weakened blood vessels caused by a chronic vitamin C deficiency. According to their theory, the Lp(a) acts somewhat like a patch on the weakened area of the artery wall. The patch is, in reality, the atherosclerotic plaque. They further postulate that by maintaining sufficient vitamin C levels, the effects of Lp(a) will be completely blocked (see Chapter 7).

There is no question that Lp(a) is a powerful risk factor for coronary heart disease. The question of how to treat it is not so easy to answer. Because of the enormous respect that I hold for Dr. Pauling, I list vitamin C as one of the therapies for Lp(a), although definitive research establishing vitamin C as a treatment for Lp(a) has not been done. At the present time, there is no really good treatment for elevated levels of Lp(a). Niacin is the only agent that has shown some consistency in lowering Lp(a) levels. Estrogen replacement in post-menopausal women and anabolic steroids have also shown some benefit in the treatment of Lp(a).

Homocysteine

If I only needed one reason to take B-vitamin supplements, it would be to protect against homocysteine. Homocysteine is an amino acid that is normally present in the bloodstream in very low concentrations. The higher the homocysteine levels, the easier the blood clots. Enzymes that control the level of homocysteine in the bloodstream are hereditarily determined. If a person gets a double dose of enzyme deficiency, i.e., from both parents, the homocysteine levels will be very high and the blood will readily clot. In this situation, heart attacks before age twenty are quite common.

In the past two years, there have been several studies published in the medical literature showing higher levels of homocysteine in patients with well-documented coronary artery disease, peripheral vascular disease, and cerebral vascular disease. Many researchers now classify elevated homocysteine levels as a confirmed coronary risk factor. The good news is that homocysteine levels can be easily reduced to normal using relatively small amounts of vitamins B_6, B_{12}, and folic acid.

Like the Lp(a) blood test, homocysteine testing is not readily available, so I put all my patients on these B-vitamins because they have numerous other benefits as well. I'll give you all the details on how to do it in Chapter 9.

Triglycerides

Some of the most severe and widespread vascular disease problems I have seen have been in patients with high triglyceride levels. Recent studies have confirmed that the higher the triglyceride levels, the greater the tendency for the blood to clot and the weaker the clot-clearing fibrinolytic system. Studies may eventually prove that triglycerides actually facilitate clotting. As we discussed, clots are constantly forming at the sites of fissures in the plaques in our arteries. The part of the clot that is not completely reabsorbed is left there to be incorporated into the plaque. High levels of triglycerides circulating in our bloodstream continually promote clotting and compromise our clot-clearing mechanism. Perhaps more clots are formed and just a little bit more of the clot is left over each time. Over the long haul, this will add up to more plaque and explain why high triglyceride levels are toxic to our arteries.

Just as some folks are blessed with low levels of LDL and high levels of HDL, others can thank the good Lord for low triglyceride levels. Drugs, niacin, L-carnitine, weight loss, fish oils, exercise, and lowfat and low-sugar diets are the treatments for high triglycerides.

CLOTTING AND HEART ATTACKS NOT DUE TO PLAQUE FISSURES

Other heart attacks are due to fibrous plaques. This occurs when clots form over plaques that are rich in fibrous tissue. Fibrous tissue is like scar tissue that builds up. It contains only small amounts of macrophages filled with oxidized LDL.

These fibrous-rich plaques probably grow from repeated clotting and the inability of the clots to become reabsorbed into the body due to injury to the cells covering the upper layer of the plaque. The injury can occur from turbulent blood flow, high blood pressure, smoking, or other mechanisms that are still unknown. If the clot grows to completely occlude (or block) the artery, a heart attack will occur, just as it does after plaque fissuring. Although these fibrous plaques cause only about 25 percent of the heart attacks, they probably cause about 75 percent of the angina.

5 *Behind the Scenes: Other Risk Factors*

HIGH BLOOD PRESSURE (HYPERTENSION)

There is no question that high blood pressure contributes to injury and atherosclerosis in the arteries. It not only increases the risk of coronary heart disease, it also makes a stroke much more likely. Elevated blood pressure causes injury to the artery wall and sets the stage for the development of more atherosclerotic plaque and subsequent blockage.

The bottom line on hypertension is that elevated blood pressure—both systolic pressure (the top number) and diastolic pressure (the bottom number)—needs to be lowered. If hygienic measures and nondrug therapy can do the job, terrific. If these natural measures don't work, then you must use drugs to lower the blood pressure and reduce the risk of heart disease.

Weight loss, if you are overweight, and exercise are the two proven hygienic measures. Some people are sensitive to salt and alcohol, and restricting these will also help. Magnesium, calcium, potassium, CoQ10, garlic, and a lowfat diet may also be helpful.

SMOKING AND PASSIVE ENVIRONMENTAL SMOKE

Tobacco smoke contains carbon monoxide. Sometimes, people who commit suicide do so by using carbon monoxide. The poison blocks the ability of the red blood cells to deliver life-giving oxygen to the cells of the body. In my opinion, smoking is a form of covert suicide, a failure to take in all the life-giving oxygen that is available.

Smoking raises, or is associated with an increase in, blood cholesterol level. For every three cigarettes smoked in men aged eighteen to sixty years, the total cholesterol is one point higher. The HDL-cholesterol is lowered by smoking. The more cigarettes a person smokes, the earlier his or her first nonfatal heart attack. Continuing to smoke after a heart attack puts a person at higher risk of death and recurrent myocardial infarction, compared to those who stop smoking after their heart attack.

If you are a nonsmoker and your spouse smokes, you have a 30 percent higher risk of coronary heart disease. The greater the exposure to environmental smoke, the higher the risk.

Smoking increases platelet stickiness and contributes to clotting of the blood. The oxygen deficiency that results from smoking injures the lining of the artery wall, making it more susceptible to injury, clots, and plaque formation. Smoking results in increased oxidation of the LDL and increased plaque formation.

I can't think of even one reason for smoking. I will admit, however, that of the French women and Japanese men who are big smokers, the risk of coronary heart disease is much lower than would be expected. I attribute this to their doing so many other things right—i.e., diet—that the adverse effects of smoking get canceled out.

If you smoke, stop! Your increased risk of coronary heart disease will begin to decrease right away.

If you can't or won't stop, you must take antioxidants (Vitamins E and C, beta-carotene, and selenium) to block the oxidation of LDL.

Almost every individual will gain weight when they stop smoking. If you are overweight and a smoker, I recommend that you go on a diet first. Start losing weight and use the vitamins, antioxidants, garlic, and aspirin to block the effects of the smoking for now. When you have gotten the diet routine down and have lost some weight, **then** stop smoking.

The Japanese are heavy smokers but they are skinny, eat a lowfat, high fish oil diet with lots of complex carbohydrates (rice), and they have a very low rate of coronary heart disease. I believe that one of the lessons we can learn from the Japanese is that the causes of coronary heart disease are multiple. The more things you do right, the lower your risk. There is room for some imperfection and we shouldn't be too hard on ourselves.

DIABETES AND ELEVATED BLOOD SUGAR

Diabetes is a strong risk factor for coronary heart disease and myocardial infarction. Type I diabetes has its onset at an early age and requires insulin to maintain life. Type II diabetes comes on later in life and can be treated with diet and exercise in many people. I would not have believed this if I had not seen it firsthand literally hundreds of times at the Pritikin Longevity Center in California. Time and time again, overweight Type II diabetics on oral drugs or insulin came to the Pritikin center for help. After a month of diet therapy plus plenty of exercise, they very often had blood sugar values in the normal or near-normal range, with no medication whatsoever. Diet and exercise can work miracles for the diabetic.

I remember a patient I saw in my private practice several years ago who was taking 90 units of insulin a day. After three months of a diet and a walking program, she lost about 30 pounds of excess weight and had a normal blood sugar value—without any medicine at all.

Even Type I diabetics can greatly improve their diabetic control with diet and exercise. It's not easy to do. You will need professional help and guidance to accomplish this end. I encourage you to seek out a diabetic specialist to help you. Or, if you can afford it, go spend some time at the Pritikin center. What you learn about diet and exercise will pay healthy, lifelong, and life-prolonging benefits.

There are steps that diabetics can take to lower their risk of coronary heart disease and heart attack. Both high and low levels of insulin have an adverse effect. Insulin levels should be optimum. Diet and exercise will help, as will a high-fiber diet. The high blood sugar levels of diabetes contribute to vascular diseases by binding to proteins and attaching to the artery wall, which adds to the plaque. Also, triglycerides are frequently elevated in diabetes and this contributes to the plaque and to clotting. Often the triglycerides will go down when the blood sugar is better controlled. Chromium supplementation can sometimes help improve the blood sugar and insulin levels. Fish oils may help lower the triglycerides and raise the HDL (see Chapter 12). Nutrients that may be helpful in diabetes include: magnesium, vitamin C, garlic, B-vitamins, vitamin E, and zinc.

The role of dietary fat and carbohydrate in diabetes is controversial. Some diabetics do best with a lowfat, high complex-carbohydrate diet. Others will gain weight on the high carbohydrate diet, making the diabetes worse. These people do better if they are allowed more fat and protein in their diet. Olive oil is the best dietary fat for the diabetic diet.

In my opinion, the best book to read about managing diabetes and diabetic diet is: *Diabetes: A Practical New Guide to Healthy Living* by James W. Anderson, M.D. All of the Pritikin books and the McDougall books are also helpful. Dr. Julian M. Whitaker has a book called *Reversing Diabetes*, which may also be helpful.

OBESITY

Dealing with obesity is no easy matter. I have studied it, fought it, and written two books about it: *The Best Chance Diet* (Humanics, 1981) and *The One-Day-at-a-Time Diet* (Knightsbridge, 1990). At age twenty, I weighed 205 pounds. Today, I weigh 175 pounds. I can tell you what it has taken me thirty-five years to learn in just one sentence: **drastically reduce your fat intake so your body can preferentially burn the stored fat and exercise for at least thirty minutes everyday (minimum total of 3.5 hours per week) to increase the rate at which your body will burn the stored fat.**

Obesity is a risk factor for heart disease. Losing weight will lower blood pressure, lower cholesterol, and raise HDL. If you have Type II diabetes, weight loss may be all the therapy you need to treat the diabetes. Weight loss for overweight people can be life-saving.

STRESS AND PSYCHOLOGICAL FACTORS

Everybody knows that stress is a risk factor for coronary heart disease, but what to do about it is a real problem.

In the spring of 1992, a brochure came across my desk announcing a symposium in Houston, Texas, on stress and cardiovascular disease. Many of the major experts in the field were going to be there. It was being sponsored by the Texas Heart Institute and Saint Luke's Episcopal Hospital—institutions well known for their Texas-sized heart programs. I thought this would be fantastic. I could spend the weekend in Houston and get all the material I would need to write a big, informative chapter on stress—and I would be getting my information from the real experts in the field.

I'm sorry to report that I was truly disappointed. In my opinion, research has only begun to scratch the surface of the whole stress/heart disease connection. I found going to Houston and not getting all the answers I wanted to be quite stressful.

There are some important things I **can** tell you about stress, however.

(1) The old concept of type A and type B behavior has not solved all the problems regarding stress and coronary heart disease. Type A personalities are supposed to be aggressive, bottom-line, hurry up-type people. Type B supposedly characterizes the more laid back, passive types.

Recent work suggests that if type A personality does increase risk of coronary disease, it may in part do so by lowering HDL levels. One implication here is that if you do enough other things to raise your HDL, you may be able to partially compensate for the type A behavior.

(2) Isolation, loneliness, and the lack of a confidant all contribute to a decreased survival in patients with coronary heart disease. Living alone after a heart attack more than doubles the risk of dying in the first year after that heart attack. Several years ago, it was shown that just having a pet improved survival. Someone to talk to, someone to share with, someone

to care for—even a pet—will improve the risk of survival after a heart attack.

(3) Depression amplifies the bad effects of all the risk factors.

(4) Mental stress will cause those arteries that are already obstructed to narrow even more. Trying to solve a problem that can't be readily solved could cause an episode of angina. Normal arteries will widen under mental stress.

(5) Aggression is associated with higher triglyceride levels.

(6) Job stress does not appear to be predictive of coronary artery disease.

(7) Commonly occurring stressful situations do not cause significant changes in blood cholesterol levels.

(8) Exercise is a great way to neutralize stress.

LACK OF EXERCISE

When I turned forty, I threw away my tobacco and began to exercise. This was one of the most beneficial things that I have ever done for myself. Lack of exercise increases the risk of many health problems, including coronary heart disease, hypertension, diabetes, osteoporosis, stroke, and stress. The American Heart Association has recently declared lack of exercise to be a bona fide risk factor for coronary heart disease. Surprisingly small amounts of exercise can make a huge difference. Just taking a brisk walk three or four times a week for twenty to thirty minutes may be extremely helpful.

Exercise is also an effective way to reduce the clotting tendency. Exercise will increase fibrinolysis, decrease platelet stickiness, decrease fibrinogen levels, and increase TPA. It is also one of the few proven ways to raise HDL. I could go on and on about the benefits of exercise.

A few weeks ago, I couldn't sleep. I was flipping through the late night channels when I came upon a "showmercial" for a piece of exercise equipment. The announcer was saying that nearly everyone would benefit from the device because exercise was as close to a panacea as we could get. This got me to thinking about all the benefits of exercise, and I decided that the announcer was in a large measure correct. Exercise is a panacea.

Our bodies were built for exercise. We were made to walk and run long before we adapted to driving cars. Modern times are not synchronized with the nature of our bodies. It is the denial of our basic nature that promotes disease. We all need exercise throughout our lives. Recent studies have shown that not only aerobic exercise is beneficial. Weight training and resistance exercise also provide cardiovascular benefits when performed properly. Training effects and cardiovascular benefits have even been demonstrated in individuals in their seventies and eighties. It's never too late to start an exercise program and begin deriving some of the benefits of exercise.

Most people can start a walking program on their own. However, if you are over thirty-five years old, or if you have any risk factors for coronary heart disease, the safe thing to do is to get an exercise treadmill test from a physician before starting your exercise program. I can't emphasize enough how important exercise is in an overall cardiovascular health program.

LOW VITAMIN E BLOOD LEVELS

If you search through the thousands of articles in the medical literature dealing with risk factors for coronary heart disease, you will not find low blood levels of vitamin E listed. Although

I can't take credit for doing the research that proves that low blood levels of vitamin E are a risk factor, I would like to be one of the first to go on record declaring its status as a major risk factor. Based on what I have learned in my research for this book, I would put low levels of vitamin E ahead of smoking and obesity in terms of its importance as a risk factor. Fortunately, it's a whole heck of a lot easier to treat low blood levels of vitamin E than either smoking or obesity.

THE LOW CHOLESTEROL CONTROVERSY

Can your total cholesterol level be too low? If you have documented coronary artery disease, you are more likely to die of your coronary artery disease than anything else. In this situation, the lower your LDL-cholesterol, the greater your protection from the coronary artery disease and the greater your chances of survival. As I mentioned above, it is relatively meaningless to talk about "cholesterol" or total cholesterol alone because the HDL-cholesterol is beneficial and the more you have the better.

Nonetheless, the research that has been reported is based on total cholesterol. If you don't have coronary artery disease, the total cholesterol level that gives you the best chance of survival across the board is between 160 and 200. Six percent of all middle-aged adults who have a total cholesterol value below 160 are at increased risk of fatal lung disease, intestinal disease, stroke, certain cancers, and traumatic mortality. As the cholesterol value increases over 200, the risk of coronary heart disease rises proportionately. Since 94 percent of middle-aged adults have cholesterol values above 160, high cholesterol is definitely a bigger problem than low cholesterol.

The way I put all this into perspective has changed over the past three years. I am no longer as paranoid about total cholesterol levels in the 200 to 240 level as I used to be. I get more concerned when the HDL level is below 40. I figure that the antioxidants will protect and render about half of the LDL harmless. I'll tell you about a study that found that low blood levels of vitamin E were more predictive of coronary heart disease than high blood levels of cholesterol (see Chapter 7).

OTHER NONTRADITIONAL RISK FACTORS

A decrease in the amount of estrogen produced in postmenopausal women may be a factor in the development of heart disease. Using estrogen-replacement therapy in women after the menopause, taking one or two alcoholic drinks a day (especially red wine), and using low-dose aspirin are all strategies that show a reduction in risk of coronary heart disease from 25 to 45 percent! We will explore all of these in detail in their respective chapters.

6 *Rewriting the Script: Reducing and Reversing the Blockages*

In September, 1989, Thomas J. Moore attracted national attention when an excerpt from his book, *Heart Failure*, appeared in *The Atlantic Monthly*. The headline read: "Diet has hardly any effect on your cholesterol level; the drugs that can lower it often have serious or fatal side effects; and there is no evidence at all that lowering your cholesterol level will lengthen your life." Some of what Mr. Moore says is true, and some is false.

Diet can definitely lower the cholesterol level. I learned this firsthand from Nathan Pritikin. The real question is: who is willing to make all the sacrifices necessary to accomplish this end? Yes, the drugs have serious and sometimes fatal side effects, but so do the problems for which they are prescribed. The important question is, is the risk of serious disability and death greater from the side effects of the drugs or from the condition left untreated? When the drugs are prescribed properly, their benefits will outweigh the risk of the side effects.

When Thomas Moore published his book, the data supporting prolonging life with lowering cholesterol was slim. Since that time, studies have been published showing that lowering LDL-cholesterol **can** save lives. The important point here is that when LDL-cholesterol lowering is targeted toward people with definite, established coronary artery disease, the lifesaving benefits are unequivocal. This would include people who have angina, or have had a heart attack, or bypass surgery, or angioplasty.

LDL-cholesterol lowering prevents heart attacks and death through plaque stabilization: lowering the LDL in individuals who have plaques that are loaded with fat and cholesterol will make these plaques less likely to tear or fissure. This, in turn, makes clotting and subsequent heart attack less likely to occur.

REDUCING LDL-CHOLESTEROL

In my first book, *The Best Chance Diet*, I reviewed the research done on animals in the 1970's, and I concluded that coronary artery disease was reversible. I deduced from the animal studies that if a person could get their total cholesterol down in the range of 160, they had a good chance of reversing the obstructions in their arteries. In 1987, Dr. David Blankenhorn of the University of Southern California at Los Angeles published the first controlled, randomized study documenting reversal of atherosclerotic plaque in human beings. In the cholesterol-lowering atherosclerosis study (CLAS), not only did a significant number of patients treated with the cholesterol-lowering drugs colestipol and niacin have reversal of some of the obstructions in their arteries, there was lack of progression in their other blockages as well. Since 1987, there have been at least nine additional published studies showing well-documented reversal of blockages in the coronary arteries.

A whole array of treatments has been used. In addition to cholesterol-lowering drugs, diet, exercise, stress management, intestinal bypass surgery to block cholesterol reabsorption, and extracorporeal LDL apheresis (a technique similar to kidney dialysis, except LDL cholesterol is removed instead of the kidney waste products) have all been shown to reverse obstructions in the coronary arteries. In several of these studies, the greater the reduction in LDL-cholesterol, the greater the magnitude of reversal of the obstructions.

Dr. Blankenhorn studied the patients who did not receive the drug therapy in the CLAS. He found that the greater the consumption of total fat—including polyunsaturated fat and olive oil—the greater the increase in new blockages in the arteries. Subjects who did not develop new blockages reduced their total fat intake and increased their protein and carbohydrate intake to replace the fat calories. Dr. Blankenhorn proved what Nathan Pritikin postulated but was unable to prove during his lifetime.

The most widely publicized of all the coronary reversal studies was that of Dr. Dean Ornish. Dr. Ornish used a lowfat, vegetarian diet along with stress management (meditation, yoga, group therapy) and mild exercise. Dr. Ornish has made a major contribution to our armamentarium for fighting heart disease. Like the nondrug patients in Dr. Blankenhorn's study, those patients who followed Dr. Ornish's diet showed improvement in coronary heart disease.

Almost everyone will benefit from a lowfat/low-cholesterol diet, antioxidants, clot-reducing strategies, and exercise. If coronary heart disease is already present, then all the tools available, including drugs, may be helpful in inducing regression of the coronary disease. Rarely intestinal bypass surgery or LDL apheresis may be needed to halt or regress the disease. **The common factor in all the studies that have shown reversal of blockages in the coronary arteries is a reduction of LDL.**

REVERSING THE BLOCKAGES: NATHAN PRITIKIN

Nathan Pritikin said that diet and exercise would cause reversal of the obstructions in the coronary arteries. Unfortunately, he wasn't able to prove it like the others. That was because Pritikin thought the angiogram was potentially dangerous and he didn't want to subject his clients to this procedure. Angiograms are the main way that the reversals have been demonstrated. As I review the wealth of medical literature that proves that heart disease can be reversed, I am amazed to find that virtually no one mentions or credits Nathan Pritikin for his extraordinary vision. He knew that lowering LDL-cholesterol would result in reversal of coronary heart disease, and he practiced what he preached.

Pritikin was an inventor, a brilliant man who used his intellect to solve his own problems and then shared the results with the rest of the world. In 1955, at age thirty-nine, he had a total cholesterol level of 280 and angina. He reviewed the medical literature and determined that a lowfat, low-cholesterol diet and exercise would reverse his condition. He embarked on what would evolve into the Pritikin Diet and a regimen of almost daily exercise. He monitored his own cholesterol over the next thirty years. In February, 1958, it was 210; in July, 1958, it was 162; and by September, 1958, it was 122. In 1963, it was 102 and in November, 1984, three months before his death, it was 94. At his autopsy, his coronary arteries were completely free of all plaque and cholesterol deposits. I guess he did prove that his diet would reverse coronary disease, at least in his own case.

In 1977, I joined Pritikin in Santa Barbara, California, as his chief of cardiology. One day, while going over the laboratory reports, I saw Pritikin's own lab work. His cholesterol was impressively low, but so was his hemoglobin (red blood cells). I asked him about this and he told me he had had a radiation exposure twenty years earlier (he was given radiation treatments to the skin for a superficial fungal infection) and that as a result of that radiation he had damage to his bone marrow. According to his biography, *Pritikin: The Man Who Healed America's Heart,* by Tom Monte and Ilene Pritikin (Rodale Press, 1988), he was diagnosed as having lymphocytic leukemia in 1976 and was given two to three years to live. He lived eight more years before his death in February, 1985.

Nathan Pritikin was a pioneer who taught me much about diet and heart disease. I miss you, Nathan, and thank you.

THE ROLE OF ANTIOXIDANTS

There is no question about it: antioxidants can definitely help halt the progression of coronary heart disease. How much they can do by themselves to reverse it is still under study. Researchers at the University of Mississippi have shown reversal of blockages in the arteries of monkeys who were given vitamin E supplementation.

According to a new and very exciting report from Japanese investigators, HDL-cholesterol can also be oxidized, and when it is oxidized its ability to transport LDL back to the liver is markedly decreased. Oxidation not only makes the LDL toxic, it also renders our protection from this noxious substance ineffective—just one more reason to be certain that we have adequate and abundant antioxidant protection in our bloodstreams at all times. In my opinion, antioxidants are the real protection that we all need in order to be healthy.

In fact, a study is in progress at the present time in human beings using cholesterol-lowering drugs in conjunction with the antioxidant prescription drug probucol. My guess is that those who take the probucol will fare much better and have more regression of their obstructions than those who only take the cholesterol-lowering drugs.

As we discussed at the beginning of Part I, according to the National Cholesterol Education Program, an LDL level below 130 is desirable and a level above 160 is considered high-risk. Levels between 130 and 160 are borderline. Now, let's say the LDL is 180 and antioxidants are used and are able to prevent 50 percent of this LDL from oxidizing. This would effectively lower the LDL to a very desirable level of 90. Fifty percent protection from oxidation has been achieved in several of the studies that have used antioxidants to block LDL oxidation. To me, this is the most exciting concept ever to emerge from cardiovascular research! It explains why a low blood level of the antioxidant vitamin E is a better predictor of coronary heart disease than is the cholesterol level. The concept of antioxidants protecting against coronary heart disease is so awesome that it is hard to put it aside.

In the chapters that follow, I will show you how to use antioxidants, vitamin and mineral supplements, and a healthy diet to win the fight with the heart disease villain. The prescription is painless because it is not based on deprivation. The emphasis is on positive things that you can do to help yourself. You won't have to feel guilty about not doing what you should do.

Part II

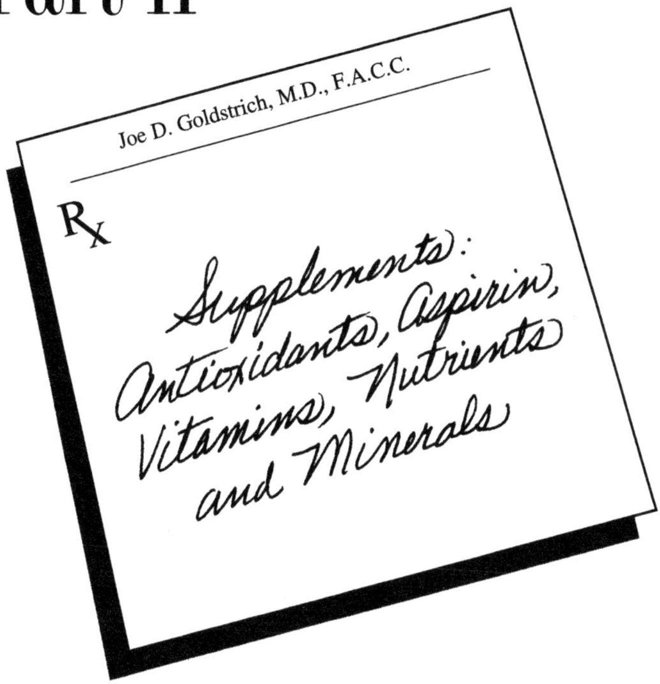

Optimum nutrition requires supplementation! It is virtually impossible to eat enough fruits and vegetables to supply all the vitamins and minerals needed for good health today. The more you are stressed, the more polluted your environment, the older you are, and the more ill health you have experienced, the more likely you are to benefit from supplementation.

There are lots of articles telling of the benefits of the vitamins found in fruits and vegetables. The truth of the matter is that food alone won't get the job done. You can get enough vitamin C in orange juice to prevent scurvy, but there is a whole quantum level of protection that vitamin C can provide that is only available through supplementation. There is enough nutrition in our food to prevent deficiency states, but to open the doors to a much higher level of benefit requires supplementation with vitamins and minerals. This higher level of benefit goes way beyond the prevention of deficiency states. The supplements are high-powered medicine. They may actually be more powerful than many prescription drugs.

In this section, we will look at the effects of antioxidants, aspirin, vitamins, minerals, and nutrients for a healthy heart and a longer life.

7 *Antioxidants*

When I started doing the research for this book over five years ago, I thought it would be almost entirely about drugs and their ability to reverse established blockages in the coronary arteries. As I methodically researched each of the drugs used to treat coronary heart disease, I came to the drug probucol. I discovered that probucol had been used in many experiments and had been clearly shown to prevent and reverse cholesterol deposits. This got my attention and I began to delve further.

Probucol does not lower blood levels of cholesterol like all the other drugs that have been shown to reverse the obstructions in the coronary arteries. I was intrigued. How could probucol do its magic without lowering cholesterol? I delved further and learned that probucol is an antioxidant. Could this antioxidant action be responsible for probucol's wizardry? The answer is yes.

As we learned in Part I, in order for LDL-cholesterol to become incorporated into the arterial blockage, it must first be oxidized. If you can stop the oxidation of LDL, you can stop the build-up of cholesterol in the arteries. **In my opinion, this is the most important breakthrough in cardiovascular research in the past decade and perhaps for all time!**

Antioxidants are substances that neutralize free radicals. Free radicals can oxidize or rust the tissues or cells they come in contact with. If free radicals are left alone and to their own devices, they will be very destructive in the body. Antioxidants are the only salvation from the demonic free radicals.

About three years ago, articles started appearing in the medical literature showing that the vitamins E, C, and beta-carotene had powerful antioxidant properties. The next step was to see if these vitamins could actually prevent cholesterol from being oxidized. You better believe they can! They are much more effective in halting this oxidation than I would have ever imagined. What's astonishing is that they work together in a synergistic fashion to accomplish this end.

There were two more questions for me to try to answer before I could be certain that these magic bullets would actually hit the target. The first was: do individuals with higher blood levels of these natural antioxidants have less coronary heart disease? Again, the answer was a resounding yes! And, finally, are people who supplement their diet with antioxidant vitamins protected? Absolutely!

In recent studies involving the use of antioxidants to prevent coronary heart disease, researchers showed that we could reduce cardiac events for men and women by about 40 percent. Let's assume this number is too high. Let's be very conservative and cut it in half to 20 percent. In 1994, we are expecting over 1,500,000 heart attacks, over 500,000 cardiac deaths, about 400,000 bypass surgeries, and at least 350,000 angioplasties. With the use of just vitamin E supplementation alone, and using the conservative 20 percent reduction figure, we could lower the 1,500,000 heart attacks by 300,000, the 500,000 deaths by 100,000, the 400,000 bypass surgeries by 80,000, and the 350,000 angioplasties by 70,000!!!!! If we just calculate the dollar savings on bypass surgeries alone, we get $3.2 billion this year ($40,000 x 80,000=$3,200,000,000)! Conservatively saving 100,000 deaths a year works out to 274 lives saved each day!

Each additional supplement could potentially add to the reduction in the heart attacks, deaths, and bypass surgeries calculated above. Could the sum of these supplements cut the incidence of coronary heart disease by more than half? It's a good bet they can.

VITAMIN E

In all my years of practicing medicine, there has not been a medicine, a drug, or a substance that has impressed me more than vitamin E. When I tell this to my fellow physicians they usually reply: "Yes, but it's all anecdotal. There is no data." They are wrong. Even I was surprised when I used my computer to check on the number of articles published on vitamin E in the National Library of Medicine during 1992. In that year alone, there were over 400 indexed articles. Pretty impressive for a vitamin with "no data."

When I told my friend, Karl Robinson, M.D., about my excitement over vitamin E and the antioxidants, he told me that his uncle, Junius Matt Rawlings, M.D., a professor and teacher at Wayne State University School of Medicine, had devoted his life to researching vitamin E and the antioxidants. Dr. Rawlings had amassed a tremendous amount of data, and after his death in 1976, his work was privately published by his colleagues. Because it was published privately, it was never seen by anyone. I asked my friend if he could get me a copy of his uncle's work and much to my delight, he was able find a copy of Dr. Rawlings' book, *Oxygen and Antioxidant Vitamins.*

Dr. Rawlings listed about 700 scientific references in his bibliography over twenty-five years ago. I don't know exactly how many of these articles dealt specifically with vitamin E and how many with the other antioxidants because the bibliography was organized by author rather than by subject. Clearly, the data, even in the 1970's, was substantially more than anecdotal. Dr. Rawlings was way ahead of his time. He was a real pioneer.

Two other vitamin E pioneers were Drs. Evan and Wilfrid Shute. They directed the Shute Clinic in London, Ontario, Canada, and they used vitamin E almost exclusively in their practice. In fact, in the 1970's the name Shute was synonymous with vitamin E. The Shute brothers treated over 35,000 patients with vitamin E. Dr. Wilfrid Shute's first book was called *Vitamin E for Ailing and Healthy Hearts* and his second, *Dr. Wilfrid E. Shute's Complete....Updated Vitamin E Book*. However, Dr. Shute was attacked and derided, and his findings ignored for over twenty years. Why was he attacked and derided? Because he wasn't scientific. He didn't have a clinical trial. His experience with over 35,000 patients was "anecdotal." Just think of all the lives that might have been saved if the "scientific community" had been more responsible and had scientifically and objectively tested the Shute brothers' experience.

Cardiovascular Benefits of Vitamin E

Vitamin E deficiency—a risk factor for coronary heart disease

I had been following the research in antioxidants for several years when I saw a research publication in 1991 that knocked me off my feet. The article appeared in *The American Journal of Clinical Nutrition* and showed that a low blood level of vitamin E was a better predictor of coronary heart disease than either elevated cholesterol levels or high blood pressure. In fact, low levels of vitamin E were more predictive than both high blood pressure and high cholesterol values combined! If vitamin E was low and cholesterol and/or blood pressure were elevated, the risk was even greater. In other words, elevated cholesterol and high blood pressure are higher risks for coronary heart disease when vitamin E blood levels are low.

This was classy research, too. It was sponsored by the World Health Organization and it looked at twelve populations across Europe. The statistics were impeccable and no one to date has challenged the validity of this study. This article was the turning point in the way that I now view coronary heart disease. For the first time, I began to have some insight into why some people with higher cholesterol levels might not have heart attacks. It also began to dawn on me that there was more to prevention than the standard AHA risk factors. That's not to say that these risk factors aren't important, it just means that they are not the whole story.

Vitamin E blocks LDL oxidation

Remember that the LDL-cholesterol cannot become incorporated into the arterial blockages unless it is oxidized. If antioxidants like vitamin E can block this oxidation, does it matter how high the cholesterol is? Can a high-risk LDL of 160 or 180 be reduced to a highly desirable functional level of 80 or 90 simply by protecting 50 percent of it from oxidation? Can this be the reason that higher levels of vitamin E are associated with lower risk of coronary heart disease? I think so and so did the researchers at the Center for Human Nutrition at the University of Texas Southwestern Medical School in Dallas.

There, in the early 1990's, Dr. Scott Grundy and his co-worker, Dr. Ishwarlal Jialal, first studied the effect of vitamin E on LDL-cholesterol in the test tube. They showed that if vitamin E and LDL are incubated together, the LDL becomes resistant to oxidation. The next step was to actually study the LDL of people who took vitamin E supplements. These researchers conducted a small clinical trial. If they could have done it on 6,000 people instead of just twenty-four people, we would have had an "official" clinical trial and there would be no more controversy about antioxidant supplements.

In this research project, Grundy and Jialal gave either a placebo or 800 international units (IU) of vitamin E daily to the participants. After twelve weeks, the vitamin E levels in the bloodstream had increased on the average of 4.4-fold in those who took the vitamin E. There was about a 50 percent decrease in LDL oxidation. The higher the vitamin E blood levels, the greater the resistance of LDL to oxidation.

For their encore, these same researchers repeated the experiment, only this time they gave vitamin E, vitamin C, and beta-carotene all together. These antioxidants complemented each other and an even greater degree of LDL protection was achieved. Good work! Thank you, Dr. Grundy.

Vitamin E and clotting

Vitamin E blocks platelet stickiness. In fact, the more vitamin E that is taken, the less the platelet stickiness. If the platelets don't adhere, the clotting can't start. This clotting connection is very hot in cardiovascular research these days. Big clinical trials are ongoing and others are being started to see if the use of anticoagulant blood thinners in combination with aspirin will prevent heart attacks. Personally, I'd much rather halt this dangerous clotting process with a safe, nontoxic vitamin than with the anticoagulant blood thinners.

More exciting news is that vitamin E inhibits vitamin K. Vitamin K is necessary for blood clotting. In fact, the anticoagulant blood thinners that are being used in the big clinical trials are drugs that inhibit vitamin K. Vitamin E, in a very large measure, will do exactly the same thing as these anticoagulant blood thinners. Vitamin E has the advantage that it not only blocks vitamin K, it also inhibits platelet stickiness and it is extremely nontoxic.

Vitamin E, angina pectoris, and angioplasty

When vitamin E levels are measured in patients with angina, they are found to be lower than those in angina-free patients. Preliminary studies suggest that vitamin E supplementation will prevent restenosis (reoccurrence of the narrowing of the artery) after angioplasty. The reason that I say that this is a preliminary report is that the number of patients in the study was not large enough to draw strong statistical conclusions. Vitamin E, however, did reduce restenosis by about 15 percent.

Vitamin E and HDL-cholesterol

Vitamin E supplementation has been shown to raise HDL-cholesterol. Other research, conducted on animals, has demonstrated that inclusion of vitamin E, even in a high-fat, high-cholesterol diet, will result in less arterial blockages.

Animals who were treated with vitamin E before the onset of heart attacks showed less damage to the heart, a smaller area of myocardial infarction, and a greater likelihood of survival.

When vitamin E raises HDL-cholesterol levels, it gives even more protection against coronary heart disease.

Noncardiovascular Benefits of Vitamin E

The most important noncardiovascular benefit of vitamin E that I found has to do with aging. Many researchers now believe that aging is an oxidative process. Vitamin E, one of the most powerful antioxidants, helps retard the aging process. It is even more powerful when combined with the other antioxidants.

It is also believed that oxidation plays a major role in the development of senile cataracts. Vitamin E has been shown to prevent cataract formation, although it does not reverse cataracts that have already formed. Preliminary studies have also shown significant slowing of the development of Parkinson's disease when vitamin E and vitamin C are supplemented together.

Reports are beginning to appear in the medical literature strongly suggesting that vitamin E may play an important role in the prevention of certain cancers.

Antioxidants, including vitamin E, will help protect the lungs from air pollution and smoking. Vitamin E supplementation has also been shown to boost the immune system in the elderly.

Should You Take Vitamin E?

That is the question that the *Johns Hopkins Medical Letter, Health After 50*, asked in their March, 1992 issue. Much to my surprise and delight, their answer was YES! No other medical institution has so publicly advocated any vitamin supplementation. I truly respect the editors of this health letter for evaluating the data and, in my opinion, coming to the only conclusion possible.

Is Vitamin E Safe?

I have reviewed the medical literature on vitamin E safety and I have gone through Dr. Shute's writings. My conclusion is that vitamin E is extremely safe. In animal studies, vitamin E has been shown not to cause cancer or birth defects. The only published precautions about vitamin E are related to its inhibition of vitamin K, the vitamin that is necessary for blood clotting. For this reason, vitamin E should only be used under a physician's supervision in patients who are taking anticoagulants or who are vitamin K deficient. The combination of anticoagulants and vitamin E could cause hemorrhage. **If you take an anticoagulant, do not take vitamin E unless you are guided by your physician.** Vitamin E may be used safely in combination with aspirin to retard platelet stickiness, which I believe is a good idea.

Cholestyramine (Questran, Cholybar) and colestipol (Colestid) are drugs that bind cholesterol in the intestinal tract and remove it from the body. However, these drugs will also bind the fat-soluble vitamins, including vitamins K and E. If cholestyramine or colestipol are being used to lower cholesterol, increased dosages of vitamin E may be needed. Also, since vitamin K is also likely to be removed by these drugs and become deficient, taking vitamin E supplements without vitamin K supplementation could lead to problems.

The bottom line here is that if you take cholestyramine or colestipol, you will need to work very closely with your physician in managing your supplements.

In order to find out what other potential precautions might be necessary in the use of vitamin E, I went back to Dr. Shute's book. Since he had treated over 35,000 patients with vitamin E at the time he wrote it, who could possibly know more? Here are some of his pearls of wisdom:

Iron

Inorganic iron will destroy vitamin E. Iron supplements should be separated from vitamin E supplements by eight to twelve hours. (Iron is an oxidant and may contribute to heart disease. Iron should not be taken unless there is a well-documented iron-deficiency anemia.)

Digitalis

Dr. Shute found that vitamin E enhanced the action of digitalis preparations (e.g. Digoxin) and that toxicity could occur if vitamin E was added to a regimen where digitalis was being used. If you take a digitalis preparation, do not take vitamin E unless you consult with your physician.

Rheumatic and congenital heart disease

Dr. Shute felt that vitamin E was a heart stimulant. He therefore cautioned about overstimulating a weakened heart or a heart that had mechanical obstructions to blood flow, such as mitral stenosis. In rheumatic heart disease, Dr. Shute would start with 75 IU of vitamin E a day and increase by 25 IU each month, with a maximum dose of 300 IU a day in chronic rheumatic heart disease patients.

Hypertension

Dr. Shute says that because of the heart-stimulating properties of vitamin E, it will further raise the already too high blood pressure in about one-third of all uncontrolled hypertensives. If the blood pressure is already controlled with medication, there is no problem. If the blood pressure is elevated, it should be controlled first and then the patient can start with low doses of vitamin E and build up slowly. I usually start with 200 IU per day in this situation.

Types of Vitamin E

Natural vitamin E is concentrated from vegetable oil, usually soybean oil. Synthetic vitamin E is usually made from petroleum or turpentine. Natural vitamin E is comprised of eight different substances, all of which have vitamin E activity. These natural vitamin E substances are all of the "d" or dextro form. The *d-alpha tocopherol* has the highest biological activity. The natural d-beta, d-gamma, and d-delta tocopherols and tocotrienols found in nature also have some biologic activity.

Synthetic vitamin E will be in the "dl" form. The "l" part of these tocopherols are not biologically active and may actually inhibit the activity of d-alpha tocopherol.

Mixed natural tocopherols means that the preparation contains d-alpha, d-beta, d-gamma, and d-delta forms. Since these occur naturally, some feel that they may have useful medicinal value. There is nothing wrong with taking pure *d-alpha tocopherol,* however, since it is the form of natural vitamin E that has been **proven** to be of value.

If the label says "dl," it's synthetic and not my first choice. I buy only natural d-alpha tocopherol plus or minus mixed tocopherols. The natural d-alpha tocopherol can be in a succinate, acetate, or nicotinate form. There is no hard data supporting one form over another. One investigator has found the succinate to have greater cancer-preventing properties in the test tube.

In all fairness, though, some of the successful research studies I reviewed used dl-alpha tocopherol and one study found dl-alpha tocopherol to be just as effective as d-alpha tocopherol in preventing LDL oxidation. So, it works, too. There is also some suggestion that the d-alpha tocopherol may be twice as potent as the dl-alpha tocopherol, but this has not been fully proven.

The bottom line is that, while all the answers aren't in yet on which type of vitamin E is the most effective, in the interim, I'm still choosing the d-alpha tocopherol.

How Much Vitamin E Should You Take?

In the studies I reviewed, the beneficial dosage of vitamin E ranged from 100 IU per day to 1,600 IU per day. The average therapeutic dose was 800 IU per day. Studies that examined the toxicity and safety of vitamin E have demonstrated that dosages up to 3,200 IU per day led to no consistent adverse effects. Because vitamin E is fat soluble, it is much better absorbed when taken with a meal that contains a little fat.

In the near future, blood testing to measure vitamin E blood levels and antioxidant activity will be more widely available. Until the time when dosage can be more precisely determined, a good average dose of vitamin E is 800 IU of d-alpha tocopherol daily.

If I were forced to choose only one supplement to take out of the dozens discussed in this book, it would be vitamin E. If I could then add a second supplement to the vitamin E, it would be vitamin C.

VITAMIN C

Over twenty years ago, Dr. Linus Pauling began his research on vitamin C and first received public attention in 1970 for his work when he published *Vitamin C and the Common Cold*. As of this writing, Dr. Pauling is ninety-three years young. I had the pleasure of hearing him speak on the subject of vitamin C and cardiovascular disease on May 16, 1992. He walked to the stage and up the four or five steps to the podium without help. He spoke clearly, logically, and brilliantly on his subject for one hour with no notes. I have the utmost respect and highest esteem for Dr. Linus Pauling. He is one of my heroes. Let's examine his ideas about vitamin C and atherosclerosis.

Dr. Pauling believes that coronary artery disease is a vitamin C deficiency state. He points out that premature coronary artery disease is essentially unknown in all the mammalian species that produce large amounts of vitamin C. About forty million years ago, when our prehistoric ancestors were eating huge amounts of vitamin C containing vegetation, a mutation occurred. The gene for the enzyme L-gulono-gamma-lactone oxidase mutated, and our ability to manufacture our own vitamin C was lost. At that time, it didn't make too much difference because enormous quantities of vitamin C were consumed daily in the vegetable-based diet. Today, it makes a difference.

Most animals can make their own vitamin C. The exceptions are: primates (including man), guinea pigs, and fruit-eating bats. If you examine the animals that make their own vitamin C, you find that they manufacture from 1,000 to 20,000 milligrams (1 to 20 grams) of vitamin C each day when compared to, and converted to, the weight of a human being. Dr. Pauling has long contended that the 60 milligram recommended daily allowance for humans is grossly inadequate.

Scurvy is a fatal disease caused by vitamin C deficiency. Sixty milligrams of vitamin C per day will prevent fatal scurvy, but it will not provide enough vitamin C to achieve optimum health.

If you examine the blood vessels of someone who dies of scurvy, you will see that the connective tissue of their blood vessels is weakened, and destabilized. The blood vessel walls have microscopic holes in them and there is bleeding through these holes into the tissues around the blood vessels. When this bleeding occurs near the skin, you see bruises.

Dr. Pauling's theory is that without vitamin C supplementation to at least the level of the animals that make their own vitamin C—1,000 to 20,000 milligrams per day—we will have weakened, unstable blood vessel walls. He calls this condition *subclinical scurvy*. Dr. Pauling speculates that atherosclerosis is the body's attempt to patch these weak spots and strengthen the blood vessel walls. In this scenario, the patching will thwart a major blowout of the artery and prevent a fatal hemorrhage.

Dr. Pauling postulates that the primary substance our body uses to try to repair the defective blood vessel walls is Lp(a). Lp(a) is similar in structure to LDL, but it has an extra appendage that resembles plasminogen, a substance involved in the clotting mechanism. As we discussed in Part I, Lp(a) contributes to atherosclerosis and coronary artery disease in two ways. One way has to do with its LDL-cholesterol component and the other is by facilitating clotting. Dr. Pauling, working with his associate, Dr. Matthias Rath, showed that vitamin C supplementation in guinea pigs (they, like humans, cannot make their own vitamin C) prevented both the deposition of Lp(a) in the arterial wall and the development of atherosclerosis.

Lp(a) levels vary considerably among individuals. Recent work has clearly shown that elevated Lp(a) levels is a strong predictor of coronary heart disease. Vitamin C may prevent the deposition of Lp(a) in the arteries, but this has not yet been proven in human beings. At the present time, there is no really good treatment to reduce elevated levels of Lp(a), although niacin, niacin plus neomycin, NAC, vitamin E, fish oil, anabolic steroids, and estrogen replacement in post-menopausal women have all shown some benefit in lowering Lp(a) levels.

Cardiovascular Benefits of Vitamin C

Vitamin C is water-soluble and has the ability to "bathe" the outside of the LDL molecule with antioxidant protection. Vitamin E and beta-carotene are both fat-soluble, so they can penetrate the fatty LDL molecule and protect it from the inside. These three antioxidants will work synergistically to protect the LDL from the treachery of oxidation.

There is some discussion in the literature as to which antioxidant is the most powerful. If vitamins C, E, and beta-carotene are all put in a test tube with oxidizers, the vitamin C will be totally used up before the other two are even touched. If a portion of the vitamin C remains, the other two won't even be called into play. This has led some researchers to the conclusion that vitamin C is the most important antioxidant. Vitamin C will also regenerate and reactivate the vitamin E that is used up in the process of blocking oxidation. This allows the vitamin E to be recycled and reused.

Vitamin C has been shown to be the only antioxidant that completely protects LDL from oxidant damage. In light of the absence of any significant adverse health effects of vitamin C, and because of its potential antioxidant activity, vitamin C tissue saturation in humans appears to be desirable.

Dr. Jialal, the man who has done the important antioxidant vitamin E work with Dr. Grundy, has also studied the antioxidant properties of vitamin C. He has shown that vitamin C is a very powerful inhibitor of LDL oxidation.

Dr. James Enstrom, from the UCLA School of Public Health, recently reported the results of a study he conducted, in which 11,348 adults, whose vitamin C intake totaled as little as 500 mg a day, decreased their overall mortality and cardiovascular mortality.

RESEARCH

In Dr. Enstrom's ten-year prospective epidemiologic study, those people who got 140 to 150 mg of vitamin C from their diet each day, and who took at least another 150 mg of supplemental vitamin C, were considered to be in the high-intake category. People in the low-intake group got less than 50 mg of vitamin C per day in their diet. The middle group got more than 50 mg in their diet, but did not take a vitamin C supplement. The men in the highest intake group had a 42 percent lower mortality rate when compared with the men in the lowest intake group. The women only had a 10 percent reduction in overall mortality. Cardiovascular mortality for men and women in the highest intake group were reduced 45 and 25 percent, respectively.

Vitamin C may also be helpful in raising HDL. The higher the vitamin C levels in the bloodstream, the higher the HDL.

Vitamin C has been shown to help lower LDL-cholesterol by getting the LDL into the bile so it can be excreted from the body in the bowel movement. In addition it has also been shown to decrease platelet stickiness and reduce clotting. Furthermore, there is a strong association of vitamin C supplementation and higher HDL, lower LDL, and lower blood pressures.

When blood samples are taken at the time of a heart attack, vitamin C and vitamin E levels are both low. No one knows for sure which comes first—the low levels or the heart attack. It may take researchers another five or ten years to solve this riddle. For my part, I want to make sure that my vitamin C and E levels are high enough so that there is plenty to go around if they're going to be used up.

Vitamin C and blood pressure

I was able to find six studies published in 1991 and early 1992 showing a statistically significant benefit of vitamin C on blood pressure. These studies found that vitamin C effects were mild, but definite, and that the lowering of the systolic blood pressure was greater than that of the diastolic pressure. All these studies were carried out on mild or borderline hypertension, so don't throw away your blood pressure medication. Vitamin C is just one of the many supplement weapons in our arsenal to be used in the war against hypertension and coronary heart disease.

Noncardiovascular Benefits of Vitamin C

Vitamin C and cancer

On September 10-12, 1990, the National Cancer Institute, in conjunction with the National Institute of Health, sponsored a symposium on vitamin C. This symposium was largely the result of Dr. Linus Pauling's efforts. There were many reviews on vitamin C presented. One review showed that in people with higher dietary intake of vitamin C, there was evidence of a statistically significant reduced risk of cancer.

Vitamin C has also been found to be protective against stomach and intestinal cancer and may reduce the risk of cancer of the larynx, mouth, esophagus, pancreas, lung, breast, and uterine cervix.

Cataracts

Like vitamin E, vitamin C may help prevent cataracts.

Is Vitamin C Safe?

If you take too much vitamin C, you will get diarrhea and/or flatulence. This is quite rare at dosages under 2,000 mg a day and may not occur at dosages in excess of 10,000 per day.

Because vitamin C is cleared from the body by the kidney, I recommend that you consult your physician and reduce dosage of vitamin C if you have kidney disease. Vitamin C has also been associated with oxalate kidney stones, so anyone with a history of kidney stones should consult their physician before taking vitamin C. Lastly, a rare type of hemolytic anemia, G6PD deficiency, can be aggravated by vitamin C.

Most vitamin C is made from corn. People who are allergic to corn can get vitamin C made from sago palm in the health food store.

If you are taking large doses of vitamin C (over 3,000 mg per day), and you abruptly stop taking it, you may develop an acute deficiency of vitamin C. This is a rare reaction but deserves mention. If, for some reason, you must decrease vitamin C intake, do so in increments over a week to diminish the likelihood of this rebound phenomenon.

How Much Vitamin C Should You Take?

Many of the clinical studies show benefits of vitamin C at dosages as low as 200 mg per day. The RDI for vitamin C is 60 mg a day. Dr. Linus Pauling takes 18,000 mg per day. I take 10,500 mg per day. As you can see, there is a wide range of effective dosages. If you are not currently taking vitamin C, you might start with 500 mg three times daily and build up to 1,000 mg three times a day with meals. Based on the current literature, that dosage should be more than adequate for prevention purposes. If you have coronary heart disease and you want more protection, you could go up in 500 mg increments. I have not personally prescribed over 12,000 mg per day on a long-term basis.

I buy the best vitamin C I can get. In the past I have used less expensive vitamin C and gotten upset stomach. The least expensive, most effective way to take vitamin C is in powder or crystalline form. A quarter of a teaspoon of the crystals usually has about 1,000 mg of vitamin C. Read the label to know exactly how much your product has. Five hundred milligram tablets or capsules will be more convenient for many people.

BETA-CAROTENE

Like vitamin E, beta-carotene is a fat-soluble, antioxidant carried on or within the LDL particle, where it protects LDL from oxidation. Beta-carotene is converted to vitamin A in the body. For this reason, it is also called pro-vitamin A. Unlike vitamin A, however, large doses of beta-carotene do not cause toxicity. The body will not convert the beta-carotene to vitamin A if making the conversion will result in toxic amounts of vitamin A.

Beta-carotene has many functions in the body that have nothing to do with vitamin A. Beta-carotene is a member of the carotenoid family and has more pro-vitamin A activity than any of the other family members. Over forty different carotenoids are found in fruits and vegetables, including carrots, squash, tomatoes, salad, leafy vegetables, dried fruits, fresh strawberries, fresh melon, broccoli, and brussel sprouts.

Several epidemiologic studies have shown that people who eat the most beta-carotene containing fruits and vegetables have the lowest rates of certain cancers, coronary artery disease, and death from coronary heart disease.

> **RESEARCH**
>
> **Dr. J. Michael Gaziano of the Harvard Medical School reported on the results of his beta-carotene research at the April, 1992, meeting of the American College of Cardiology. He followed 1,299 men and women over age 65 (average age 72) for almost five years. He kept track of their intake of foods high in beta-carotene. During the study period, there were 270 deaths, 161 of which were due to coronary heart disease. According to Dr. Gaziano, the study found an "inverse relationship of consumption of fruits and vegetables high in beta-carotene and subsequent death from cardiovascular disease. The association persisted after controlling for all available cardiac risk factors. Those food items highest in beta-carotene content were associated with the greatest reduction in cardiovascular disease deaths."**

Even modest supplementation with beta-carotene has been shown to raise HDL-cholesterol levels. This could contribute to the reduction in deaths due to cardiovascular disease among patients with higher dietary beta-carotene intake.

Cardiovascular Benefits of Beta-carotene

Beta-carotene as an antioxidant

Dr. Ishwarlal Jialal of the Center for Human Nutrition at the University of Texas Southwestern Medical Center, Dallas, has worked with beta-carotene as well as vitamins C and E. He has shown in the test tube that beta-carotene will block LDL oxidation and LDL uptake by macrophages. In fact, beta-carotene is over twenty times more powerful in blocking LDL oxidation in the test tube than is vitamin E. However, when LDL oxidation is measured in people who take antioxidants, vitamins E and C are much more powerful than beta-carotene in preventing LDL oxidation. This has led some researchers to suggest that the beneficial effects of beta-carotene are due to something other than its antioxidant action.

Like vitamins C and E, beta-carotene has actually been shown to reduce the number of major coronary events. Beta-carotene has also been shown to increase HDL-cholesterol levels.

RESEARCH

A study is currently being directed by Dr. Charles H. Hennekens, professor of medicine and preventive medicine at Harvard Medical School. The Physicians' Health Study, the only one of its kind so far to report its results, is an on-going study of more than 22,000 U.S. male physicians. The doctors are taking aspirin and/or beta-carotene and/or a placebo. In this study, 333 men had a history of coronary heart disease. One-hundred-six of these men took beta-carotene, 50 mg every other day, and the rest took placebos. Those who took the beta-carotene had a 51 percent reduction in major vascular events (heart attack, stroke, bypass surgery, or cardiac death) when compared to the placebo controls. Interestingly, there were *zero* vascular events in those who took an aspirin tablet every other day in addition to the 50 mg of beta-carotene every other day. Because the numbers were too small and because the study was not designed to answer the question about prevention of coronary heart disease, Dr. Hennekens believes it is premature to recommend beta-carotene supplementation for the general public.

Beta-carotene and coronary disease in smokers

An unexpected and very exciting finding from the Physicians' Health Study was that beta-carotene protected male smokers from coronary heart disease. The group with the highest intake (greater than 14,000 IU per day) of beta-carotene had a 70 percent lower risk of heart attack, death from heart attack, or the need for angioplasty and bypass surgery when compared to the group with the lowest beta-carotene intake! Even very modest amounts of beta-carotene consumption (the equivalent of half a carrot a day) provided some protection from coronary disease in smokers.

Noncardiovascular Benefits of Beta-carotene

Beta-carotene and cancer

Preliminary studies have shown that beta-carotene can reverse leukoplakia, a premalignant condition of the mouth. While no definite link has been proven for other cancers in human beings, there is unequivocal evidence that individuals who eat more fruits and vegetables and those with higher blood levels of beta-carotene have less cancer. Some animal studies have shown that beta-carotene supplementation will prevent certain cancers from developing. Beta-carotene supplementation has been shown to help protect smokers from some of the precancerous effects of tobacco smoke.

Beta-carotene and the immune system

Recent studies have shown that massive beta-carotene supplementation in AIDS patients will improve T-cell ratios and benefit the immune system.

In one study, where progressively larger doses (up to 300 mg a day) of beta-carotene were given to try to find changes in the immune system, no immune changes were detected. However, increases in HDL-cholesterol were noted at all levels of beta-carotene administration.

Beta-carotene and stroke

As I mentioned above, beta-carotene is converted to vitamin A in the body. The higher the beta-carotene intake, the higher the blood levels of vitamin A. Very recent studies have shown that the higher the vitamin A blood level, the lower the death rate from a stroke and the greater the likelihood of a complete recovery from a stroke.

Is Beta-carotene Safe?

Beta-carotene is extremely safe. I could only find two side effects documented in the medical literature. The first is that too much beta-carotene can, on rare occasion, cause the skin to turn yellow.

The second, and potentially more serious, side effect has to do with combining beta-carotene and heavy alcohol intake. Baboons were studied at Mount Sinai School of Medicine in New York. When heavy alcohol intake was combined with large doses of beta-carotene (30 to 45 mg of beta-carotene/1,000 calories) there was evidence of toxic liver changes. However, in this study the baboons were given 50 percent of their total caloric intake as alcohol. They made the baboons chronic alcoholics. If your alcohol intake is greater than two drinks per day, periodic blood tests to make sure there is no liver damage wouldn't hurt. If your alcohol intake is 50 percent of your total calories, like the baboons, you should forget about the beta-carotene and check yourself into an alcohol rehabilitation program.

How Much Beta-carotene Should You Take?

In the Physicians' Health Study, where beta-carotene supplementation was associated with decreased coronary heart disease, the dose was 50 mg every other day. That is 83,333 IU every other day. For me, it is too difficult to keep track of every-other-day dosage, so I recommend 30 mg or 50,000 IU every day in conjunction with vitamin E and vitamin C supplements.

SELENIUM

I have followed the medical literature on selenium, an essential trace mineral, for several years. I knew that selenium would have to play an important role as an antioxidant, because it is necessary for the production of the essential antioxidant enzyme, glutathione peroxidase. Dr. Rawlings had collected research studies from the 1960's showing a key antioxidant role for selenium.

Selenium and vitamin E work synergistically as antioxidants. Excess selenium intake can be toxic. Vitamin E protects against selenium toxicity. For this reason, I only recommend selenium supplementation when vitamin E is also being taken.

Cardiovascular Benefits of Selenium

Nothing that I would call definitive has yet been published to show that selenium supplementation will prevent coronary heart disease. Several epidemiologic studies have shown a relationship between low selenium intake and/or low blood selenium levels and coronary heart disease. The best study to date was published in late 1992 by Dutch investigators. They showed that middle-aged Dutch men with the lowest blood levels of selenium had the highest risk of coronary heart disease.

Noncardiovascular Benefits of Selenium

There are numerous reports in the medical literature strongly suggesting a beneficial role of selenium in the prevention of cancer. Paradoxically, excesses of selenium have also been shown to cause cancer.

How Much Selenium Should You Take?

In 1980, the National Research Council established a "Safe and Adequate Daily Dietary Intake" of 50 to 200 mcg of selenium per day for adults. In 1989, the recommended dosage was reduced to 70 mcg per day for men and 55 mcg per day for women. The average intake of selenium in the U.S. is about 110 mcg per day. Excessive selenium intake can be toxic. Toxicity has not been reported with doses less than 900 mcg per day.

I do not recommend selenium supplementation of more than 200 mcg per day. When selenium is supplemented, vitamin E supplementation should always accompany it to help guard against any possible side effects. However, vitamin E can be supplemented without selenium.

Notice that the amount of selenium is extremely small. The dose is in micrograms (mcg). A microgram is 1/1,000 of a milligram (mg).

CO-ENZYME Q 10 (CoQ10)

This powerful antioxidant is known as co-enzyme Q 10, CoQ10, ubiquinol, or ubiquinone. Data is accumulating very rapidly showing a wide variety of beneficial actions on the heart for this potent substance that is ubiquitous (hence its name) in the body. We both manufacture it and get it in our diet.

CoQ10 may be the most important antioxidant of all. When CoQ10, vitamins E and C, and beta-carotene are all added to a test tube containing lots of free radicals, the CoQ10 will be used up first. If there is enough CoQ10 in the test tube, the vitamins won't even be called into play. If there is not enough CoQ10 to neutralize all the free radicals, vitamin E will come into play once the CoQ10 is used up. Vitamin C will recharge the vitamin E, and only when all the C and E are spent will the beta-carotene start to be used. CoQ10 is the first line of defense.

PAINLESS Rx

Having all the antioxidants present in sufficient quantity is the way to get the maximum protection from coronary disease.

Cardiovascular Benefits of CoQ10

CoQ10 has been shown to improve cardiac function in heart failure due to cardiomyopathy (a weakening of the heart muscle) and to reduce episodes of angina pectoris and nitroglycerine use in coronary artery disease.

When I treat a patient with coronary heart disease who is still having angina pain, despite full doses of the traditional antianginal drugs (nitroglycerine, long-acting nitrates, beta-blockers, calcium channel blockers, etc.), I always include CoQ10 in my supplementation regimen.

It has been found that in patients with coronary heart disease, ubiquinone levels are low. It has also been shown that CoQ10 may be even more effective as an antioxidant than either vitamin E or beta-carotene. When CoQ10 is supplemented, blood ubiquinone levels go up and LDL is protected from oxidation. Like vitamin E, CoQ10 is fat-soluble, so it is able to penetrate the LDL molecule and protect it from oxidation from the inside. Like vitamin E, it is also better absorbed when taken with a little fat in the diet.

There are a couple of recent studies in the medical literature showing that CoQ10 can significantly lower elevated blood pressures. In one of these studies, there was also a significant fall in LDL-cholesterol and a small, but statistically significant rise in HDL.

One of the most important discoveries about CoQ10 is that the HMG-CoA reductase-inhibiting class of cholesterol-lowering drugs (lovastatin, simvastatin, and pravastatin) also block the body's ability to produce CoQ10. This results in: 1) a decreased blood level of CoQ10, which could lead to a decrease in cardiac function; 2) LDL that is vulnerable to oxidation; 3) higher blood pressure; 4) higher LDL; 5) lower HDL; and 6) more angina. I prescribe CoQ10 for everyone taking one of these cholesterol-lowering drugs.

How Much CoQ10 Should You Take?

The average dose of CoQ10 used in the beneficial studies was 100 mg per day. Higher dosages have also been used without reports of toxic side effects. CoQ10 is well tolerated and the only downside to its use is that it is quite expensive. It is available in the health food store.

BIOFLAVONOIDS

Bioflavonoids have potent antioxidant properties. They are discussed in detail in the section on herbs (see Chapter 9), and with red wine (see Chapter 11), and green tea (see chapter 15).

ANTIOXIDANTS AND NUTRIENTS WORK TOGETHER

When I see a patient in my office with angina, I use a whole spectrum of vitamin and mineral supplements, including vitamin E. CoQ10 and L-carnitine, magnesium, vitamin C, and N-acetyl-cysteine also have beneficial effects on angina, and they all seem to work synergistically. You will see how each nutrient helps in a slightly different way as we go along.

As we discussed, vitamin C recharges vitamin E so that it can be reused. You get a lot more mileage from the vitamin E when vitamin C is also on board. In several studies, the more antioxidants on board, the lower the risk.

In my opinion, combining antioxidants—the more the better—will result in the most efficacious state of affairs. The antioxidants work together so that the whole is greater than the sum of the parts.

Most researchers agree that the antioxidants work in concert with each other. Each antioxidant has its own special field of action, and when all the antioxidants are present together, the net effect is enhanced. The optimum dosage of each is still in the process of being worked out.

THE FUTURE OF ANTIOXIDANTS IN MAINSTREAM MEDICINE

With all this information suggesting that antioxidants will protect against coronary heart disease, why have they not yet become mainstream medicine? In medicine today, nothing is accepted as dogma and mainstream until it undergoes a clinical trial. That means that you have to prospectively study a large group of people who received the treatment and compare their results to a similar group who received a placebo. The whole process is double-blinded so the researchers and the participants won't know who is getting what. There has not been a clinical trial on the antioxidants as yet, and for that reason the medical establishment is unwilling to go out on a scientific limb, unwilling to break the clinical trial rule, unwilling to risk prescribing a safe, nontoxic therapy that conservatively has the potential to save at least 274 lives a day from vitamin E alone! Are they right or are they being too rigid? Let's look more closely at the available data.

The National Heart, Lung and Blood Institute (NHLBI) held a workshop on September 5 and 6, 1991, in Bethesda, Maryland, on "Antioxidants in the Prevention of Atherosclerosis." The conclusion of this conference was that clinical trials using natural antioxidants were justified. I quote from the proceedings of the workshop: ". . . clinical studies will allow us to 'fine-tune' our understanding of these natural antioxidants—beta-carotene, vitamin E, and vitamin C . . . trials using high, but safe, doses could be undertaken in the near future. **Close surveillance and repeated physician visits would be unnec-**

essary because there are few concerns about safety." The scientists further stated: "Because these micro nutrients, used at reasonable doses, have **no known toxic side effects**, the trial could be done on a large scale with minimum surveillance and therefore at a reasonable cost." I placed the highlight for emphasis.

It's now 1994, and the first clinical trial has just been started. It takes several years after a clinical trial begins before the results are forthcoming and recommendations are made. The clock has been ticking since 1991, when the experts in the field overwhelmingly decided that the antioxidants were safe. How many lives have been needlessly lost while we are waiting for the results of the clinical trials? Let's see if we can get an estimate.

On May 20, 1993, two extremely important papers appeared in the same issue of the *New England Journal of Medicine*. I had been waiting with baited breath for these two articles since November, 1992. It was then that I heard the preliminary data presented at the annual meeting of the American Heart Association in New Orleans. The earlier data had shown a 30 percent average coronary risk reduction in men and women who took vitamin E supplements. So, when the final report was published and showed an even greater average reduction of 40 percent, I was ecstatic. Let's take a closer look at each of these truly exciting studies.

The first publication dealt with women. Researchers from Harvard Medical School and Harvard School of Public Health followed over 85,000 female nurses for over eight years. There was a 41 percent reduction in the number of heart attacks and deaths due to coronary heart disease in the nurses who took vitamin E supplements. There was no benefit from eating foods rich in vitamin E. Only those women who took the vitamin E supplements and took them for two years or longer benefitted. Dosages of less than 100 IU of vitamin E per day were associated with little or no apparent benefit. Also, there was no suggestion of a greater decrease in risk with higher daily doses.

The second paper reported on male health care professionals—dentists, veterinarians, pharmacists, optometrists, osteopathic physicians, and podiatrists. In this study, also from Harvard, there was a 37 percent reduction in the number of fatal and nonfatal heart attacks, angioplasties, and bypass surgeries. This benefit only came to those men that had taken vitamin E supplements for two years or longer and in a dose of at least 100 IU daily. For the men, there was an additional advantage in taking higher dosages of vitamin E. Those men who took the most vitamin E—an average daily dose of 419 IU—had an average risk reduction of 41 percent. Like the nurses, the men who ate vitamin E-rich foods did not benefit. Only supplementation with vitamin E was able to reduce the risk of coronary heart disease. In this study, a high intake of vitamin C was not associated with a lower risk of coronary artery disease.

The official conclusion from both of these studies? You guessed it. "Don't take vitamin E until we have the results of a clinical trial!"

Why This Apparent Vitamin/Antioxidant Paradox?

Almost all the researchers involved in vitamin and antioxidant research (Dr. Pauling is one of the exceptions) say it is too early to recommend antioxidant vitamin supplementation. I disagree.

The antioxidants are extremely safe. So safe, in fact, that the researchers at the NHLBI workshop in September, 1991, gave a green light to begin large-scale studies with only minimal surveillance because of there being so "few concerns about safety." These are the same researchers that are being publicly quoted now as saying that people should not start taking vitamin supplements!

I think I know the answer to this apparent paradox. If everyone began taking the antioxidant supplements, it would be impossible to conduct the studies necessary to prove the benefits or lack of benefits of the antioxidants. The researchers are trying to insure that they will be able to definitely answer these important questions. That's their job. That is what they do for a living.

Being a clinician, my job and my approach are different. The antioxidants may save lives. They are safe. I use them. If the researchers show they don't help, we can all stop taking them. No harm will have been done. Because of the safety of these agents, there is little to lose and much to gain. For many people, slowing or halting the atherosclerotic process now will be lifesaving.

PAINLESS Rx

A low-cholesterol, very low-saturated fat, moderate monounsaturated-fat diet, plus antioxidants, may make a huge difference in the prevention and control of coronary heart disease. That is what I recommend for my loved ones, for my patients, and it is what I do for myself.

In my opinion, there is no need to wait five or ten years until the dedicated scientists prove the value of the antioxidants. Five or ten years could be too late for too many.

8 *Aspirin*

Aspirin is neither a food nor a nutritional supplement. It is a drug that is available over the counter without a prescription. I believe that supplementation with aspirin can play an important role in the prevention of heart attacks.

In the late 1980's, I began following the literature and collecting the important research on the role of aspirin in the treatment and prevention of coronary heart disease. In the first six months of 1993 alone, the size of my file on aspirin almost doubled. In February, 1993, the American Heart Association published recommendations for the use of aspirin in the prevention and treatment of heart disease and stroke. They cautioned that the decision to use aspirin in the prevention of coronary disease should be made on an individual basis in conjunction with a physician or other health care provider. **I agree with this admonition. Aspirin is a powerful drug and any decision about long-term aspirin use is best made in consultation with your physician.** They further cautioned that aspirin should always be an adjunct, not an alternative, to risk factor management. They meant that if you continue to a eat a lot of saturated fat, not exercise, and not take care of your blood pressure, then don't expect aspirin to protect you. I agree with this admonition as well.

The important questions about aspirin are: (1) How might aspirin be helpful? (2) Who will benefit from aspirin? (3) What are the side effects and dangers? And, (4) what dose will be most effective and give the lowest incidence of adverse reactions?

WHAT DOES ASPIRIN DO?

Aspirin blocks cyclooxygenase, an enzyme formed inside the blood platelets. Without this enzyme, the platelets cannot produce a substance called thromboxane A_2. Without thromboxane A_2, the platelets can't stick to each other. The inhibition of this enzyme lasts for the lifetime of the platelet, about ten days.

As we have discussed, the obstructions in the arteries grow when LDL is oxidized and added to the plaque. They also grow when small platelet clots form on their surface. When a blood clot forms at the site of a fissure or tear in the plaque, a heart attack occurs. The first thing to happen when this heart attack-producing blood clot forms is for the platelets to stick together.

Aspirin may help slow plaque growth, and it will definitely help prevent a heart attack. The current evidence is much more supportive of aspirin preventing heart attacks than it is for aspirin slowing plaque growth.

PAINLESS Rx

My own personal theory is that if vitamin E is added to aspirin, then the combination will enhance the blockage of plaque formation and also add additional benefit in preventing a heart attack. They will work synergistically. At the present time, there is no clinical trial to test this hypothesis.

Since aspirin prevents the formation of blood clots in the arteries, any condition caused by clots, plaque, blockages or obstructions in the arteries could potentially benefit. This includes stroke and peripheral vascular disease (cholesterol build-up in the arteries leading to the legs) with claudication (pain in the legs during exertion).

Peripheral Vascular Disease

In the Physicians' Health Study, there was a 54 percent decrease in the need for surgery for peripheral vascular disease in those doctors who had no symptoms of claudication at the beginning of the study and who were given aspirin. In those doctors who were known to have peripheral vascular disease at the beginning of the study, there was an 85 percent reduction in the need for surgery in those who were given aspirin.

Bottom line on peripheral vascular disease and claudication:

Aspirin can be very helpful.

Stroke

There are three kinds of strokes: thrombotic, hemorrhagic, and embolic. A thrombotic stroke occurs in the same way as a heart attack, except that the end organ is the brain instead of the heart. A blood clot forms at the site of an atherosclerotic plaque and there is a brain infarction. As you might guess, if aspirin is protective against heart attacks, it would stand to reason that it would protect against a thrombotic stroke, and it does.

An embolic stroke occurs when a clot that is formed outside of the brain travels to the brain and blocks or plugs up the artery in which it is traveling. You might guess that since aspirin can prevent clots, it would also prevent embolic stroke. You would be partially right. All the data is not in yet, but it appears that aspirin is helpful in this situation, albeit not as protective as in thrombotic stroke.

A hemorrhagic stroke takes place when there is bleeding into the brain. You might guess that aspirin would contribute to bleeding because of its ability to block platelet function. You might further guess that for this reason, aspirin would increase the number of hemorrhagic strokes. You would be right once again.

Nonetheless, aspirin is useful in the primary prevention of strokes because the number of embolic and thrombotic strokes are so much greater than the number of hemorrhagic strokes. When aspirin is used to try to prevent strokes in patients who are at a high risk, the benefit is in the range of a 15 to 20 percent reduction in the total number of strokes.

When aspirin therapy was compared to surgery for the prevention of stroke, the study had to be stopped early because the aspirin patients were doing so much better than the surgery patients.

Aspirin and Colon Cancer

When I first saw a headline in the newspaper saying that aspirin would cut colon cancer deaths by 40 percent, I thought it was phony. I checked it out and sure enough, there was the article in the number-one authoritarian medical publication, the *New England Journal of Medicine.* American Cancer Society researchers studying more than 660,000 men and women found that those who took aspirin sixteen or more times a month for at least a year were 40 percent less likely to die from colon cancer than those who took no aspirin at all. Those who took aspirin less than sixteen times a month also lowered their risk in proportion to the amount of aspirin they took.

Other maneuvers discussed in this book that help lower the risk of colon cancer are: calcium and selenium supplementation and increased amounts of insoluble fiber in the diet (see Chapters 7, 9, and 14).

WHO WILL BENEFIT?

This question will have to be answered in regard to prevention as well as for the actual treatment of established coronary heart disease. Primary prevention means preventing disease in someone who is not known to have any disease. Secondary prevention means preventing more disease in someone who already has the disease.

Primary Prevention

There are two major studies that have looked at this question, one from the U.S. and one from England. Unfortunately, both studies only involved men, so we will have to extrapolate to women. I think we can safely do that based on some additional research that included women.

Let's look at the U.S. study in detail. The British results are comparable.

The Physicians' Health Study was a real clinical trial for aspirin, so the results are considered dogma and mainstream medicine. Over 22,000 male U.S. physicians, aged forty to eighty years, were given either an aspirin (325 mg) or a placebo every other day. Half of the doctors also got 50 mg of beta-carotene every other day. The study was stopped after five years in 1988. The reason was that there had been such a striking reduction in the number of heart attacks in the men taking the aspirin that the question that the study had been set up to address was answered—a 44 percent reduction in the number of heart attacks, to be precise. There was, additionally, an 18 percent reduction when nonfatal heart attack, nonfatal stroke, and death from a cardiovascular cause were lumped together.

There were subgroups that derived more benefit than others. Diabetics and those with high blood pressure benefitted more than nondiabetics and those with lower blood pressures. **There was no benefit for men under 50 years of age and the benefits increased with advancing age**. Men with all levels of cholesterol were helped, but those with lower cholesterol may have been helped more.

The information on women comes from a similar study on nurses. This study was not a clinical trial, because the nurses were not given aspirin versus placebo in a prospective, double-blind fashion. The aspirin use by the nurses was carefully documented, but these results are not considered dogma or mainstream. The nurses who were previously free of coronary disease symptoms and who took from one to six aspirins per week had 25 percent fewer heart attacks. **Only women over fifty years of age benefitted from regular aspirin use.**

The American College of Chest Physicians has recommended aspirin for all individuals with risk factors for coronary artery disease. These include obesity, diabetes, elevated LDL-cholesterol, strong family history of coronary disease, and smoking.

Smokers are clearly at an increased risk of coronary heart disease. The risk decreases when smoking is stopped. Many physicians are reluctant to give smokers information about the protection from smoking that they can get by using aspirin, antioxidants, and the B-vitamins for fear it will be interpreted as covert permission to continue smoking. There is good preliminary data showing that all smokers may benefit from aspirin.

PAINLESS Rx

My belief, for which there is not yet conclusive data, is that in smokers, aspirin in combination with vitamin E will prove to be even more protective than either aspirin or vitamin E alone. I also believe that this will hold true for nonsmokers as well.

Bottom line for the use of aspirin in the primary prevention of coronary disease in men and women :

(1) over age 50
(2) diabetes
(3) high blood pressure
(4) elevated LDL
(5) strong family history of coronary disease
(6) smokers over age 30

Secondary Prevention of Coronary Disease

The information about secondary prevention comes from several sources, including the Physicians' Health Study. In a subset of 333 physicians who had angina, there was a 30 percent reduction in subsequent heart attacks in those who took aspirin. One of the unexpected and striking findings was that in the sub-subset of physicians who took both aspirin and beta-carotene, there were no heart attacks. The investigators are unwilling to make too much of this finding because they say the study was only designed to find out about aspirin and heart attack. The purpose of the beta-carotene arm of the study was to look at cancer prevention.

Numerous studies have demonstrated an improved survival and a reduction of new heart attacks in heart attack survivors who take aspirin. In addition, patients with stable angina, unstable angina, and silent ischemia have all had fewer heart attacks and increased survival with aspirin therapy. There has also been a decreased need for bypass surgery and angioplasty with aspirin use. In one study, the death rate in aspirin takers was one-third that of nonaspirin users.

A study from the University of Minnesota has shown that aspirin will reduce total mortality and coronary heart disease mortality in smokers who have had a previous heart attack.

Aspirin has been shown to help keep the arteries open after angioplasty and increase survival up to 42 percent after bypass surgery.

Current information strongly suggests that if you chew and swallow one adult-strength aspirin at the very first sign of an acute heart attack, your chances of surviving that heart attack are improved. This applies even if you are taking aspirin every day anyway.

Dr. Charles Hennekens, professor of medicine at Harvard Medical School and a man I very much admire, was quoted in the December, 1992, *Medical World News*: "Aspirin is still not being utilized optimally in the treatment of acute heart attacks. It should be the drug of choice, the first drug you give when they have a heart attack, but it's not. When it becomes so, I think we'll have saved 5,000 to 10,000 more lives in the U.S. each year."

Bottom line for the use of aspirin in the secondary prevention of coronary disease in men and women :

(1) documented coronary disease
(2) previous heart attack
(3) angina
(4) unstable angina
(5) silent ischemia
(6) angioplasty and/or coronary bypass

IS ASPIRIN SAFE?

There are only two types of problems with aspirin: bleeding and gastrointestinal (GI) irritation. Hemorrhagic stroke is a manifestation of the bleeding problem. GI irritation can cause pain and discomfort and could even lead to a bleeding ulcer. The solution to the GI problem is to use buffered or enteric-coated aspirin, to use the lowest possible effective dose of aspirin, and to take the aspirin with a meal. Lower dosages may also help reduce the incidence of hemorrhagic stroke.

Blood pressure that is out of control, alcoholism, bleeding disorders, active peptic ulcer disease, and advanced kidney or liver disease are situations where it is probably best not to use aspirin. ***Decisions about aspirin use are best made in consultation with your physician.***

HOW MUCH ASPIRIN SHOULD YOU TAKE?

As the research on aspirin has evolved, it has been learned that lower dosages will do the job and that the lower the dose, the fewer the side effects. Early studies used 1,000 mg or more of aspirin a day. The Physicians' Health Study used 325 mg every other day. Swedish investigators have used 75 mg a day effectively, and Dutch researchers have shown that a 30 mg-a-day dose is just as effective as a larger dose in preventing strokes. Studies are underway in this country to test 100 mg every other day and to test a timed-release, low-dose aspirin. Initial studies suggest that the timed release, low-dose aspirin may cause the least amount of bleeding.

It takes a few days for the lower dosages to get all of the platelet thromboxane A_2 inhibited, whereas the higher dose will do it quickly. That's why the dose at the time of a heart attack is 325 mg. Chewing it before swallowing will get it into the system even faster. If there is no emergency, you can just start with a daily low dose of aspirin.

Enteric-coated, or buffered, aspirin has fewer GI side effects. The only low-dose, enteric-coated aspirin tablet that I have found is Bayer's 81 mg "adult low strength" tablet. That's what I use. When a lower dose enteric-coated tablet or a low-dose, timed-release preparation becomes available, I will probably switch to one of them.

A final note before closing: acetaminophen (Tylenol) has no significant effect on platelets and cannot be substituted for aspirin to achieve the effects listed above.

9 *Other Vitamin and Nutrient Supplements*

For most of my professional career, vitamins have not been respected. In fact, those physicians who prescribed vitamins were more often than not considered quacks. Over the past three years, vitamin and mineral supplements have begun to get some of the respect that they so justly deserve.

The whole concept of vitamin supplementation recently got a big boost when *Time, Newsweek, The New York Times, U. S. News & World Report,* and *Medical World News* all ran favorable, highly visible stories on vitamins. Even the superconservative Center for Science in the Public Interest came out in favor of vitamin supplementation!

The medical literature is now replete with literally thousands of recent references documenting the utility and benefits of vitamin supplements. Vitamins can save lives, and there is an enormous scientific justification for taking them. The time for vitamin supplementation is now!

B-COMPLEX VITAMINS

The B-complex vitamins include: thiamine (B_1), riboflavin (B_2), niacin (B_3), pyridoxine (B_6), cobalamin (B_{12}), folic acid, biotin, and pantothenic acid.

The B-complex vitamins are the facilitators of almost every important biochemical reaction that takes place in the body. For years, the standard party line has been that we get all the vitamins we need from our diet and that vitamin supplements are not necessary. You may have also heard the one about all that vitamins do is give you expensive urine. Well, that's all part of a dying paradigm, an old theory that belongs in the file with the one about the world being flat. I believe that this is the dawn of a new era and a new paradigm, and I am glad to be a party to the new line of reasoning. The modern concept is that vitamin supplementation is a useful tool in the prevention of degenerative diseases and the preservation of optimum nutrition and better health.

The B-complex vitamins are the cornerstone in the foundation of this new concept because they are so intimately involved in so many biochemical processes in the body. From helping the immune system to lowering cholesterol and homocysteine, the B-complex vitamins are invaluable.

Like the antioxidants, the B-vitamins also complement each other and should always be taken together for maximum benefit. I will now go through some of the data on the B-vitamins that have the greatest impact on the heart and give you some of the specifics.

Vitamin B_6

Dr. Jules Constant of the State University of New York at Buffalo recently reviewed the role of vitamin B_6 in atherosclerosis. He cited over thirty-five references showing a relationship of pyridoxine levels (B_6) to coronary heart disease, elevated serum cholesterol, atherosclerosis, and degenerative changes in the arteries. Since most studies show a deficiency of B_6 in coronary heart disease, he suggests raising the recommended daily allowance of vitamin B_6.

Pyridoxine has been shown to be often deficient in the elderly. When vitamin B_6 is supplemented in elderly people who are deficient, their immune system functions better.

Excessive amounts of vitamin B_6 (over 1,000 mg per day) have been reported to cause nerve damage. There is one case in the literature where suspected toxicity occurred at a dosage of 200 mg per day. For this reason, I personally do not prescribe more than 100 mg of vitamin B_6 per day. I routinely prescribe 50 mg daily.

Niacin

Vitamin B_3, which is also called niacin, is one of the most important supplements when it comes to reducing LDL-cholesterol and raising HDL-cholesterol. Of all the agents used to accomplish this end, only niacin has been definitely shown to reduce mortality from all causes and to increase lifespan. Niacin can save lives!

Niacin by itself can lower LDL, Lp(a), and triglycerides. It consistently raises HDL, even when other means to do so have failed. When used with drugs, niacin has one of the best track records for reversing established obstructions in the arteries.

Niacin is the least expensive of all the agents used to treat cholesterol problems. It costs between $50 and $250 per year to use niacin, as compared with about $2,000 a year for cholesterol-lowering drugs like Mevacor.

With all these beneficial features, you would think that almost everyone would be taking niacin. When treatment beyond diet is required to lower LDL-cholesterol, triglycerides, and/or Lp(a), or to raise HDL-cholesterol, niacin is the agent of first choice. Niacin probably accomplishes these beneficial effects by inducing a low-grade toxicity in the liver. This mildly toxic, low-grade hepatitis slows the rate at which the liver produces LDL, triglycerides, and Lp(a). While no one wants to take anything that will create liver toxicity, the facts are that taking the niacin properly and for the right reasons does foster longer life.

Is niacin safe?

Many of the difficulties with niacin are due to this toxic action on the liver. Not everyone can take niacin. At least 15 percent of those who try to take niacin cannot tolerate it because of side effects or liver toxicity. I have used niacin successfully in very carefully selected patients for over fifteen years. It is my firm belief that niacin should only be used under the supervision of a physician. It can definitely be a double-edged sword, and it is too dangerous to be used without adequate supervision, even though you can buy it on your own in the health food store. I know of several deaths due to liver failure caused by unsupervised use of niacin.

How much niacin should you take?

Most people can safely take 50 to 150 mg of niacin a day, and I recommend this as part of an overall supplement program. However, this is not enough to derive the full therapeutic effects on LDL and HDL. There is some suggestion that this level of supplementation (50 to 150 mg) may work synergistically with chromium in raising HDL-cholesterol. Niacin should be taken with meals and a cool beverage to prevent flushing.

Precautions

Please, don't try to take therapeutic dosages of niacin on your own! If your LDL-cholesterol remains high and/or your HDL-cholesterol stays too low after employing the other strategies discussed in this book, then definitely ask your physician about the possibility of using niacin.

B-vitamins for Homocysteine

As we discussed in Part I, homocysteine is an amino acid that has been found to be elevated in the blood of patients with premature coronary artery disease. It is considered an independent risk factor for coronary heart disease in men. Homocysteine does its dirty work by injuring the blood vessel walls and causing intravascular clotting.

One of the problems with identifying individuals with high homocysteine is that most physicians do not routinely measure homocysteine levels when doing laboratory work. Although 25 to 35 percent of patients with premature coronary heart disease have no cholesterol abnormalities, some of these individuals will have elevated blood levels of homocysteine and will benefit from treatment with vitamins B_6, B_{12}, and folic acid.

Homocysteine elevations result from several different genetic disorders. Homocysteine could be the cause of premature coronary heart disease when there is a strong family history of coronary disease and most, or all, of the traditional risk factors (e.g., elevated LDL-cholesterol or low HDL-cholesterol) are absent. A recent (1992) study published in the *Journal of the American Medical Association* concluded that elevated homocysteine levels are an independent risk factor for coronary heart disease. An even more recent (1993) study documented that vitamin therapy is an efficient, cost-effective way to manage homocysteine.

I do not routinely test for homocysteine levels. I do routinely prescribe those nutrients that are known to lower homocysteine levels. Vitamin B_6, folic acid, and vitamin B_{12} are all intimately involved in the metabolism of homocysteine and all have been found to be low where homocysteine levels are high.

If homocysteine blood levels are known to be very high, then the dose of folic acid that has been shown to be effective is 5 mg per day. Other studies have shown vitamin B_6 and vitamin B_{12} to be more effective than folic acid in lowering homocysteine. Most experts in the field recommend taking all three B-vitamins for maximum protection from homocysteine.

Precautions

If pernicious anemia (an anemia due to vitamin B_{12} deficiency) is present, vitamin B_{12} must be given by injection because it can't be absorbed from the intestinal tract. If pernicious anemia is present but has not been diagnosed, folic acid supplements will correct the anemia, but the nerve degeneration that accompanies the pernicious anemia will continue unabated. That's the only potential danger of taking folic acid supplements. The best solution to this dilemma is to take a vitamin B_{12} shot each month and take 800 mg of folic acid by mouth each day.

There have been reports of vitamin B_6 toxicity at dosages of 2,000 mg per day. I have seen one case report of toxicity at 200 mg per day. Fifty to 100 mg per day is a safe dose without physician supervision. Higher dosages require a physician's supervision.

Documented elevations of homocysteine should be treated under the supervision of a physician.

Dr. Linus Pauling believes that vitamin C should be added to the list of supplements that may be helpful in protecting against homocysteine. I hope by now that you have already added vitamin C to your list of supplements and that this is just a moot point.

Bottom line on supplements to lower homocysteine:

Prevention

Vitamin B_{12}

Pernicious anemia present: 1,000 mcg intramuscular each month.

No pernicious anemia: 50-500 mcg by mouth daily.

Vitamin B_6

50-100 mg by mouth daily.

Folic Acid

400-800 mcg by mouth daily.

Who else will benefit from the B-vitamins?

Elderly people are more likely to be deficient in the B-vitamins and more likely to benefit from supplementation. A recent study showed that the number of days each year that older people suffered from infections was cut in half when modest vitamin supplementation was employed.

How much B-vitamin complex should you take each day?

I usually prescribe 50 to 100 mg of B_1, B_2, B_3, and B_6. The dose of B_{12} is 50 to 500 mcg and the dose of folic acid is 400 to 800 mcg.

AMINO ACIDS

Amino acids are the building blocks of protein. When taken in food, they have no particular medicinal effects. When given in large doses as a single amino acid, they can have profound therapeutic effects in the body.

N-acetyl-cysteine (NAC)

N-acetyl-cysteine (NAC) is a sulfur-containing amino acid that has at least three possible beneficial roles in the treatment of coronary heart disease. First, it is a major constituent of glutathione peroxidase, the powerful antioxidant enzyme that also requires selenium for its production. Glutathione peroxidase is one of the most important antioxidants in the body.

NAC has not been widely studied. Italian researchers showed that patients undergoing coronary artery bypass surgery had improved heart function and reduced oxidative stress when NAC was given during surgery. Another study has shown no antioxidant benefit from NAC.

The second and perhaps most important potential use for NAC is in angina pectoris. Several studies have shown that NAC can re-establish sensitivity to nitroglycerine after patients have become tolerant to it. After taking nitroglycerine for a while, some people will no longer respond to it. This is called tolerance. NAC may sometimes help make the nitroglycerine work again. The amino acid arginine can sometimes also do the same thing.

The third possible role for NAC is in reducing levels of Lp(a). Lowering Lp(a) with NAC may not be a good thing to do, however. It may lower it by using it up in the clotting reaction. Other natural therapies that are better for lowering Lp(a) include exercise, niacin, fish oil, and vitamins E and C. If Lp(a) is known to be elevated, and especially if coronary heart disease is known to be present, all of these measures could be used simultaneously.

Precautions

Diabetics should not use NAC without the supervision of their physician, as NAC could aggravate diabetes. If Lp(a) is significantly elevated, or if you are trying to reverse tolerance to nitroglycerine, treatment should definitely be under the supervision of your physician.

How much NAC should you take?

NAC is available in the health food store in 500 and 600 mg capsules. The oral dosage is not well established because most of the research has been done using intravenous NAC. I have used NAC in conjunction with other nutrients to successfully re-establish sensitivity to nitroglycerine. I have not gone above 1,200 mg per day. In the intravenous studies, much higher dosages were used.

NAC is **not** a supplement that I use routinely for all heart patients or for prevention. I have only used it to help re-establish sensitivity to nitroglycerine.

L-carnitine

Although L-carnitine is relatively unknown in traditional cardiology, it has powerful and beneficial effects on the cardiovascular system. Technically, L-carnitine is not an amino acid because it is not used for protein synthesis. However, it is produced in the body from two amino acids (lysine and methionine) and three vitamins (C, B_3, and B_6).

L-carnitine initially got my attention when I read a case report of severe congestive heart failure that responded dramatically to supplementation with L-carnitine and CoQ10. When I started researching L-carnitine, I was amazed to find literally hundreds of articles describing its powerful effects on the body.

L-carnitine carries fatty acids into the cells so they can be burned. Without adequate amounts of L-carnitine, fat cannot be utilized as fuel. Normal heart muscle gets about 60 percent of its total energy from the burning of fatty acids. Several studies have shown that L-carnitine will help fuel a failing heart.

In addition, L-carnitine has antioxidant properties and can protect and limit the damage to an injured heart muscle at the time of a heart attack. It has also been shown to increase the amount of work the heart can do before angina pain occurs.

If all this weren't enough, L-carnitine also has been shown to lower LDL-cholesterol and triglycerides and to raise HDL-cholesterol levels. In patients who develop elevated cholesterol and triglycerides after hemodialysis for kidney failure, those with the lowest HDLs have the best response to L-carnitine. I have seen significant falls in triglyceride levels with L-carnitine.

There are other forms of carnitine that are not naturally found in the body. They can be toxic. D-carnitine, DL-carnitine, and "racemic" carnitine should never be used. Only L-carnitine should be used.

Is L-carnitine safe?

In a few studies, triglyceride levels went up after L-carnitine administration. When L-carnitine is used, blood levels of cholesterol, HDL, and triglyceride should be followed closely. Rarely, slight gastrointestinal disturbances have been reported and even more rarely, a body odor has been noted after L-carnitine administration.

How much L-carnitine should you take?

The exact dosage for L-carnitine is unknown. A recent study showed improved exercise tolerance in patients with angina using 300 mg of L-carnitine three times daily. Other studies have used 2,000 mg daily with benefit and without toxicity. I usually start with 500 mg per day and, if necessary, build up to 2,000 mg daily in divided dosages. I have not seen any adverse side effects from this regimen. Like CoQ10, L-carnitine suffers from being quite expensive and like CoQ10, the expense is usually justified by the good results achieved. L-carnitine is available in the health food store.

L-lysine and L-arginine

There is some preliminary data on the use of these amino acids in cardiovascular disease, and they are included here more for the sake of completeness than because they have proven efficacy or safety. There has been a flood of new research on arginine in the medical literature lately and my guess is that in the near future arginine will have an established role in the fight against heart disease.

Arginine has been shown to be deficient in patients with elevated cholesterol levels and angina, and when supplemented, to reduce angina and dilate the coronary arteries. In addition, recent studies have even shown that arginine will prevent the build-up of arterial obstructions in animals fed a high-cholesterol diet. Arginine is needed for the inner lining of the arteries to make a relaxing factor that will expand the arteries. This relaxing factor will not only open the coronary arteries and relieve angina, it will also relax the arteries and lessen hypertension.

I was pretty excited about these findings until I came across another article showing that cancer patients given huge supplements of arginine (30 grams per day) had an increase in a tumor growth factor. On the other hand, I found an article showing that the same 30-gram megadose of arginine would stimulate the production of the immune system's beneficial killer cells. Nevertheless, I am reluctant to recommend vigorous arginine supplementation except under the close supervision of a physician. I believe that it may be useful and safe at doses of 1 to 3 grams per day in patients with refractory angina, high blood pressure, or elevated LDL-cholesterol levels, but this remains to be proven.

Dr. Linus Pauling has reported the use of large doses of lysine in conjunction with vitamin C supplementation in three patients with angina. There was definite improvement in these cases. Whether the lysine acted by stimulating L-carnitine production or by some other mechanism is unknown.

As mentioned above, this information on lysine and arginine is included only for completeness. I am not recommending their use unless under the supervision of a physician.

DHEA—A PRELIMINARY REPORT

DHEA is the acronym for dehydroepiandrosterone, a steroid hormone produced by the adrenal gland. Blood levels of DHEA fall with age. DHEA levels have also been found to be lower in men with documented obstructions in their coronary arteries and men who die of heart attack. This is not due to age alone, because even younger men with more blockages have less DHEA. Surprisingly, there was no relationship between DHEA levels and the extent of the blockages at autopsy in men.

In rabbits with high cholesterol levels, DHEA prevented the build-up of arterial obstructions.

The DHEA levels do not appear to correlate with heart disease in women. Perhaps this is, in part, due to the extra protection already afforded to women by estrogen hormones.

Other studies have purported to show beneficial effects of DHEA on arthritis, cancer, the immune system, diabetes, memory, osteoporosis, and obesity. It sounds almost like a panacea. It may turn out to be just that, but I believe it is still premature to recommend supplementation with DHEA. Other adrenal hormones, such as cortisone, have definite therapeutic benefits. However, when they are given on a daily or even an every-other-day basis, they often cause enormous side effects and problems. In addition, DHEA is a prescription drug and is currently only imported from Europe.

I am prepared to wait another year or two for more data before I personally take or recommend the use of DHEA.

HERBS AND THE HEART

Herbs are plants that have medicinal properties. Until just recently, on the grand scale of time, virtually all medicines were herbal. Today there is no profit in herbs because they can't be patented. The pharmaceutical companies would not do the research needed to get FDA approval for a substance that they could not patent. I recently saw studies on an old herbal preparation for the prostate gland. The herb, saw palmetto, actually did a better job on enlarged prostate glands than the new high-priced drug Proscar. However, your doctor won't be seeing any four-page, four-color advertisements for saw palmetto in his favorite medical journal. There is just no profit in it.

Gum Guggul

I'm always looking for natural or herbal substances that can be used for the heart. So, when one of my patients asked me about gum guggul (also called guggulipid and guggulsterone) I was surprised that I hadn't heard of it. It's not a name I would quickly forget. So, I headed off to the medical library to see what I could find. To make a long story short, there were about twenty articles on guggulipid, all in medical journals from India. No work had been done on this herb in any other part of the world. I figured this was OK, because the plant only grows in India. I was able to get a hold of a few of the articles, and I was delighted to learn that this plant substance could lower LDL-cholesterol levels and raise HDL-cholesterol. In the research that showed lowering of LDL and raising HDL, 1,500 mg or more per day of an *unstandardized* herbal preparation were used. The dosage recommended on the bottles of the guggulipid that I was able to obtain was 25 mg three times daily of a *standardized* herb. I wasn't really sure about the correct dosage, but I decided to see if the guggul at the recommended dose was as effective as the Indian reports said it was.

I tried the standardized guggulipid on a few patients at 25 mg three times daily and then at 50 mg three times daily. I did not see any change whatsoever in their cholesterol or triglyceride values at either dosage level. Going even higher with the dosage would have made the cost of this herbal therapy as high as that of some of the more expensive American cholesterol-lowering drugs that have been proven to be effective. And, guess what? An Indian company holds the patent on guggulipid. I learned that natural or herbal doesn't always mean better or cheaper.

Beta-sitosterol

Cholesterol belongs to a family of compounds called sterols. The adrenal hormones, estrogen, and testosterone all contain this sterol nucleus. There is no cholesterol in the plant kingdom, but there are plant sterols. Human beings cannot readily absorb plant sterols. We have sterol receptors in our intestine that will grab cholesterol as it passes through the gut. Once a sterol receptor grabs a cholesterol molecule, it will be absorbed into the body. When we eat plant sterols, such as beta-sitosterol, they too are grabbed by the sterol receptors in our intestinal tract. This fills up the receptor and the receptor will try to pull the plant sterol into the body, but it is not very successful. Only a tiny fraction of the plant sterol is normally absorbed. For some reason, long distance runners seem to absorb more plant sterols than other people.

Apparently, the receptors will let go of the plant sterol after a while and it will pass out of the body in the bowel movement. If a cholesterol molecule happens to be passing by a sterol receptor when this receptor is busy trying to absorb a plant sterol, guess what happens? You guessed it. The cholesterol molecule will just keep on going and eventually pass out of the body in the bowel movement.

This brilliant hypothesis was tested and proven by Dr. Scott Grundy of the Center for Human Nutrition at the University of Texas Southwestern Medical School in Dallas. You remember Dr. Grundy. He's the man who showed that supplementing with vitamin E will make the LDL-cholesterol resistant to oxidation.

Dr. Grundy showed that mixing beta-sitosterol with eggs would prevent the absorption of the egg-cholesterol into the body. The cholesterol in the eggs passes out of the intestine in the bowel movement.

Dr. Grundy is currently completing another study with beta-sitosterol. In this study, he is showing that taking beta-sitosterol as a nutritional supplement will actually lower LDL levels.

Let me tell you how I use beta-sitosterol. I love eggs. They are one of my favorite foods. After I learned about antioxidants, I began to eat a few whole eggs instead of just the egg whites (which contain no cholesterol), because I figured that even if my cholesterol went up a little, if the LDL didn't get oxidized, it wouldn't get incorporated into blockages anyway. I fried my eggs in olive oil, knowing that the monounsaturated fatty acids would also afford me some protection (see Chapter 11). But I still felt guilty. Twenty-five years of thinking that egg yolks were poison was not easy to overcome. Dr. Grundy changed all that for me. Now I take three 200 mg capsules of beta-sitosterol about five to ten minutes before I sit down to my eggs—another example of what to do when you can't do what you should do! And no more guilt! Just pure joy. Thank you, Dr. Grundy.

One more helpful point on the subject of eggs. The new eggs on the market have not gotten the good press that they deserve. These Good News eggs have about 50 percent less saturated fat than regular eggs. Since it's the saturated fat that drives up the LDL (see Chapter 11), these new eggs are, in my opinion, a definite improvement. When cooked in olive oil and preceded by beta-sitosterol, the Good News eggs are just that—good news and good eating.

Beta-sitosterol can be taken before any cholesterol meal. If you eat a lot of saturated fat, it won't make any difference how much beta-sitosterol you consume—your LDL will still go up. High-cholesterol, lowfat situations where beta-sitosterol is useful are: seafood such as shrimp, hamburgers made from flank steak, a larger than average portion of chicken or turkey breast, etc.

Beta-sitosterol is found throughout the plant kingdom. Soybeans are an excellent source and this may explain in part the cholesterol-lowering action of soybeans. A diet enriched with beta-sitosterol could also help block the reabsorption of the cholesterol that enters the intestine from the liver via the bile. This may well be the mechanism of the cholesterol-lowering effect that Dr. Grundy is seeing in his current research. Beta-sitosterol has been used in one study with children who have hereditary cholesterol elevations. Beta-sitosterol was chosen because of its lack of toxicity and side effects in these children who will have to take it over a long period of time. The dosage of beta-sitosterol in this study was 1,000 mg three times daily.

Pure beta-sitosterol is available in the health food store in 200 mg capsules as Blockaid 200 from a company named Solaray. Other companies have packaged beta-sitosterol along with other nutrients of less proven value. I prefer to use the Blockaid 200, which contains only beta-sitosterol.

Bioflavonoids

Bioflavonoids are compounds found in fruits, berries, vegetables, tea, and wine. Although first discovered in 1936, their usefulness as medicinal substances is only now beginning to be appreciated. Green tea contains substantial amounts of the bioflavonoid catechin. This bioflavonoid is probably responsible for the ability of green tea to prevent cancer (see Chapter 15), which has been widely reported in the lay press recently. You have also seen a lot of articles about red wine and the "French Paradox" (see Chapter 11). The French believe that one of the things that keeps their incidence of coronary heart disease so low is their intake of red wine. Red wine is loaded with catechin and other bioflavonoids.

These bioflavonoids have been widely tested in animals and they have beneficial effects on several important causative factors in heart disease. They have been shown to lower LDL levels, block LDL oxidation, and inhibit platelet stickiness. As I review the literature, I see more and more articles each month on the beneficial effects of the bioflavonoids.

Not enough human research has been conducted to make specific dosage recommendations for the bioflavonoids. Bioflavonoid capsules are available in the health food store and several companies combine vitamin C and bioflavonoids in one capsule. Twinlab actually makes a product called Wine & Tea Polyphenols (bioflavonoids are polyphenols) made from red wine and green tea. The only side effect that I have seen from any of these products is allergic reactions.

If you decide to try and include the bioflavonoids in your supplementation regimen, start with a low dose and build up slowly. I take about half of my total vitamin C supplement as vitamin C combined with bioflavonoids.

d-limonene

d-limonene is a major ingredient in the essential oil of orange and other citrus fruits. Like the bioflavonoids, studies have been done mainly in animals thus far. The thing about d-limonene that caught my eye was a study showing that it acts just like the cholesterol-lowering drugs Mevacor, Zocor, and Pravachol in the test tube. It blocks the enzyme HMG-CoA reductase, which is necessary for cholesterol production in the body.

The Japanese have injected d-limonene directly into the gallbladder to dissolve gallstones in human beings. There are also over ten recent studies in the medical literature showing anticancer activity of d-limonene in animals. In addition, there are over ten recent articles describing the highly allergic nature of d-limonene.

The only source of d-limonene that I have been able to find is a product called Citrus-Power made by Nature's Herbs and available in health food stores. Anyone allergic to citrus will be allergic to this product, because d-limonene is truly the essence of the citrus fruit. This product could be used as an adjunct in a regimen to lower LDL levels. If you choose to use it, start with the smallest dose and build up slowly. If you find you are allergic to d-limonene, stop it right away.

Garlic

Because garlic is a food first and a supplement second, I have described the benefits of garlic in Part III: Food to Nourish Your Heart. Deodorized garlic pills and capsules are a good alternative for those who want to insure a consistent daily intake of garlic and/or are concerned about the potential for garlic body odor. The usual dose is two to four capsules or pills per day.

Lecithin

For most of the past twenty-five years, I've been hearing that lecithin will lower cholesterol and protect the arteries. I made several previous attempts to verify this claim with no success. I decided for this book that I would spend as much time as it took in the library to answer the question once and for all. I headed off to the library fully prepared to spend the entire day researching this matter.

Much to my delight, I quickly found a recent article that had already reviewed the subject thoroughly. The author had gone back to the first published article on lecithin in 1943 and found twenty-two subsequent articles where the effect of lecithin on serum cholesterol had been studied.

I was hoping to find documentation of lecithin's benefits so I would have still another effective natural therapy to recommend to you. Unfortunately, there is no convincing evidence that lecithin does anything useful. Save your money. It will be much better spent on antioxidants such as vitamins E and C and beta-carotene.

FISH OIL

When I first started reviewing the literature on fish oils, I was very enthusiastic about their possibilities. I was able to find research showing over twenty benefits for the cardiovascular system from fish oils. As I delved further into the medical literature, I was able to find a negative study for just about every proposed benefit—that is, a study showing that the benefit did not occur. My conclusion after reviewing over a hundred studies is that fish oil supplements should **not** be part of the standard routine for the prevention and reversal of coronary heart disease.

There are a couple of problems with the fish oils. They are polyunsaturated fatty acids and as such are prone to oxidation. When they oxidize they can in turn oxidize LDL-cholesterol. They should never be taken unless accompanied by substantial antioxidant supplementation. The second problem with fish oils is that they often raise LDL levels. I have used them on several occasions to try to lower elevated triglycerides and even though the triglycerides came down, the LDL went up. So, I'm not sure I actually accomplished anything.

Eating fish two to three times per week, however, may be an acceptable alternative. Once coronary disease is established, being a vegetarian is probably the most powerful dietary maneuver a person can do to reverse the coronary disease. Eating vegetarian, plus fish two or three times a week, would be a very close second.

One possible role for fish oil supplementation is in preventing restenosis after coronary angioplasty. Several studies have been done to evaluate fish oil supplements in blocking restenosis, which occurs as often as 45 percent in the first six months after angioplasty. Most studies have shown no benefit from the fish oils. However, a recent study using 15,000 mg a day of Max EPA (a proprietary fish oil) did show less restenosis in those patients taking the Max EPA. Of special note is that those who also ate the most fatty fish had an additional benefit on top of the fish oil supplements. This is quite remarkable, because the amount of omega-3 fatty acid from the supplements was 100 times greater than the intake from the dietary fish. The control subjects who ate more fish also did better than control subjects who did not eat fish.

If fish oil supplements are used, I do not recommend cod liver oil because of its high vitamin A and vitamin D content. Therapeutic doses of cod liver oil will result in intake of too much vitamins A and D. Fish oil supplements, when indicated, are best used under a physician's supervision.

10 *Minerals*

Several minerals deserve attention in regards to preventing and reversing coronary heart disease. The minerals generally have a rather narrow therapeutic range in which they are beneficial. Above this therapeutic range, they can cause side effects, which can be toxic or even cause death. Below the therapeutic range, mineral deficiency can be a major contributor to coronary heart disease, hypertension, sudden death, diabetes, elevated levels of LDL-cholesterol, increased oxidized LDL, lowered HDL-cholesterol, platelet stickiness, and increased clotting. Let's look at each mineral individually.

MAGNESIUM

From a cardiovascular point of view, magnesium is the most important mineral. Magnesium facilitates energy production in virtually every cell in our body and is the activator for over 300 biochemical enzymes necessary for optimum metabolic well-being. Without adequate amounts of magnesium, our cells lose their vigor. Magnesium plays an important role in balancing calcium and potassium—two other extremely important minerals.

Cardiovascular Benefits of Magnesium

Magnesium may lower your chances of dying if you have a heart attack. The documentation of this mighty mineral's ability to save lives is growing at a brisk pace. As always, animal experiments pave the way for human trials. In magnesium-deficient dogs with experimentally induced heart attacks, the amount of heart muscle death is greater when compared to dogs who are not deficient in magnesium.

Over ten years ago, the first randomized trial to test for benefits of magnesium in the treatment of acute heart attack in humans was reported. Over the next ten years, six more studies were completed. In 1991, investigators at the National Heart, Lung and Blood Institute in Bethesda, Maryland, and Oxford University in England published the results of a meta-analysis. This sophisticated statistical technique enables researchers to combine the results of these seven studies. In those who received magnesium in addition to conventional therapy, the death rate was reduced by 55 percent!! All seven studies included only 1,301 patients, so some researchers believe the numbers are too small to advocate magnesium therapy routinely in acute myocardial infarction (heart attack).

The life-saving benefits of magnesium in these studies probably occurred due to magnesium's ability to calm and stabilize the heart rhythm and prevent arrhythmias like ventricular tachycardia and ventricular fibrillation. In February, 1992, Israeli researchers reported on another 169 patients: 2 percent of those treated with intravenous magnesium died in the hospital compared to 15 percent of those who received a placebo!

If you need more proof, there is another study involving 2,316 patients. Half of these heart attack patients received intravenous magnesium when they were brought to the hospital and half received no magnesium. The death rate twenty-eight days later was 7.8 percent in the magnesium group and 10.3 percent in those who did not get the magnesium—about a 24-percent increase in survival!

All the answers are not in yet on magnesium's ability to save lives when given in the hospital at the time of a heart attack. The latest study (November, 1993) was just reported at the AHA meeting in Atlanta, Georgia. In this study magnesium did not offer protection when given at the time of the heart attack.

Well, I think it's time to take action on the information that we have available. Almost everyone can benefit from magnesium supplementation. You don't have to wait until you get a heart attack. And you don't have to risk not getting magnesium, if you need it, when you arrive at the hospital. You can supplement with a little magnesium every day to be sure that you do not have a magnesium deficiency.

Besides preventing death at the time of the heart attack, magnesium may also play an important role in preventing coronary heart disease. Studies have shown that people who ingest increased amounts of magnesium from hard water or in their diets are less likely to develop coronary disease and sudden death than are those who have lower magnesium intake. The mechanism by which magnesium prevents sudden death is primarily through calming and stabilization of the heart rhythm. However, there are several other beneficial effects of magnesium on the cardiovascular system.

Magnesium and cholesterol

I was only able to find one recent study in human beings suggesting that a diet high in magnesium lowered LDL-cholesterol and triglycerides and caused a slight increase in HDL-cholesterol. This study was from India and the magnesium-rich foods were fruits, vegetables, beans, peas, and nuts. It's hard to know for sure if it was the high magnesium content of these foods or the fact that they were free of cholesterol and saturated fats that made them so beneficial.

Very recent preliminary but extremely important studies in animals are showing that having enough magnesium on board gives added antioxidant protection.

Magnesium and blood pressure

Numerous studies have attempted to look at the relationship between dietary magnesium and blood pressure. In studies where people's diets are analyzed to determine how much magnesium they are eating, there is a strong association between increased magnesium intake and decreased blood pressure. These findings have led other investigators to give magnesium to people with high blood pressure to see if supplemental magnesium will lower blood pressure. These studies do not show a clear-cut benefit from magnesium supplementation and have been a disappointment to me.

This is not particularly surprising. I would not expect a single panacea to reverse hypertension. The two proven natural ways to lower blood pressure are with weight loss (if you are overweight) and exercise. In salt-sensitive people, salt restriction will also lower blood pressure. In these salt-sensitive individuals, magnesium as well as potassium and calcium supplementation may augment the beneficial blood pressure response to salt restriction.

Magnesium and diuretics

Besides diet, the most common cause of magnesium deficiency is diuretic therapy. Diuretics are used in the treatment of high blood pressure and congestive heart failure. The diuretics cause the kidney to lose magnesium and potassium. Several studies have shown that potassium cannot be fully replaced unless magnesium is also given. Both magnesium and potassium stabilize the heart's rhythm, and are protective against sudden death due to ventricular fibrillation and ventricular tachycardia.

Magnesium, the vasodilator

Magnesium relaxes blood vessels. It was this finding, in conjunction with the epidemiological studies regarding magnesium and blood pressure, that led to the trials of magnesium as an antihypertensive agent. Some believe that this relaxing or opening up of the blood vessels is an additional benefit in acute myocardial infarction. The vasodilatation decreases the work of the already stressed heart. This same advantageous mechanism also applies to congestive heart failure.

Some cases of angina pectoris due to coronary artery spasm are due to magnesium deficiency. And don't forget the dog study where the size of the heart attack was reduced by magnesium. This may well be in part due to the dilatation of the coronary and the peripheral arteries by magnesium.

Is magnesium a calcium channel blocker?

A powerful class of drugs that has proven benefits in coronary heart disease and hypertension are the calcium channel blockers. Because of the intimate counter-balancing interactions of calcium and magnesium, it is believed that magnesium acts as a calcium channel blocker. The calcium channel blocking drugs are used to treat hypertension, angina, and congestive heart failure. Sounds like a pretty good overlap with magnesium to me. In addition, recent studies have shown that calcium channel blocking drugs will block or slow the build-up of the atherosclerotic plaque.

A few studies have shown that magnesium will inhibit platelet stickiness and block the clotting reaction. Magnesium may also prolong or intensify oral anticoagulants.

Magnesium and diabetes

As many as 25 percent of patients with diabetes have magnesium deficiency. It has been proposed that magnesium is lost from the kidney due to the increased urination in diabetes. A few investigators believe magnesium deficiency contributes to the complications of diabetes. Other studies suggest that magnesium deficiency actually makes the diabetes worse, creating a vicious cycle.

Noncardiovascular Benefits of Magnesium

The intimate dance that magnesium does with calcium has lead some physicians to the conclusion that magnesium is just as important as calcium in the prevention and treatment of osteoporosis.

Magnesium alone or in conjunction with calcium and vitamin E will stop leg cramps.

Magnesium deficiency alone or in conjunction with a low-fiber diet is a major cause of constipation.

Is Magnesium Safe?

There are three specific situations of importance in which magnesium supplementation can be dangerous. When kidney function is impaired, the body will not be able to rid itself of excess magnesium, and toxic amounts can build up rapidly. **Do not take magnesium supplements if kidney function is impaired**. Another potentially hazardous condition is that of heart block—a condition in which the electrical impulses generated in the top of the heart (the atrium) cannot travel to the bottom of the heart (the ventricle). Magnesium has the ability to calm an excitable heart rhythm and prevent fatal rhythm disturbances. If the rhythm is already too calm or too slow and a heart block is present, magnesium supplementation can further aggravate this state. If a pacemaker is in place to treat the heart block, magnesium can be used, but only under a physician's supervision.

The third contraindication to magnesium supplementation is the use of anticoagulants. Since magnesium may intensify or prolong the anticoagulant action, serious or fatal hemorrhage could occur. Magnesium should only be supplemented under the supervision of a physician if anticoagulants are being taken. Magnesium will, however, compliment aspirin and vitamin E in providing protection from clotting in those not taking anticoagulants.

I have reviewed the drug interactions of magnesium and I find two additional interactions of lesser importance. The first is that magnesium can block the absorption of tetracycline, an antibiotic, from the intestinal tract. So if you are taking magnesium and your physician prescribes an antibiotic, be sure and tell your physician. The other interaction is with the group of oral antidiabetic medications called sulfonylurea drugs. These include Glucotrol and Micronase. Only magnesium hydroxide, which is the form of magnesium found mainly in antacids, is listed as a possible cause of the blood sugar getting too low when used in conjunction with the sulfonylurea drugs. I could not find any other major interactions or contraindications. The more medicine you take, the more likely you are to have a drug interaction. **If you are on prescription medication, check with your physician before taking magnesium or any other supplement.**

The major side effect of magnesium supplementation is diarrhea. Magnesium is the active ingredient in Milk of Magnesia. It will act as a laxative if you take too much. A recent study found magnesium to be the cause of about 5 percent of all "unexplained" diarrhea. I have used this side effect therapeutically in some people with chronic constipation.

One last precaution. Several years ago, a well-known health authority was appearing on a national television program. He was nervous. He took lots of magnesium to calm and stabilize his nervous system. It did. He died on national television of a magnesium overdose.

Types of Magnesium

Magnesium is available in many forms. Some authorities feel that magnesium chloride is the best, but it is more likely to irritate your stomach. Magnesium oxide is the least expensive form of magnesium, but is more likely to cause diarrhea at lower dosage levels.

I have tried essentially all the different forms of magnesium on my patients and on myself, and I have come to the conclusion that magnesium chelated with amino acids, such as aspartate, alpha-ketoglutarate, citrate, and taurinate are best. You can always try the less expensive magnesium gluconate and magnesium oxide—and if this works for you, you will save money.

How Much Magnesium Should You Take?

Before supplementing with magnesium, be sure you have normal kidney function as measured by a blood test (BUN and Creatinine). **Do not take magnesium if you have a heart block or are taking anticoagulants**. If there are any questions, be sure and check with your doctor.

The recommended daily dietary allowance for magnesium is 280 mg for adult women and 350 mg for adult men. Pregnant and lactating women need more. Most Americans get about half this amount in their diet. I take 500 mg of magnesium in supplements daily. Always take calcium in conjunction with magnesium. They balance each other and work together. The dosage of magnesium should be 50 to 80 percent of the calcium. So, if you take 1,000 mg of calcium, the magnesium dosage is 500 to 800 mg per day. For 1,200 mg of calcium, it is 600 to 960 mg of magnesium.

Because magnesium is involved in so many biochemical reactions involving the B-complex vitamins, you get more mileage from your magnesium when you also take a balanced formulation (50 to 100 mg) of the B-complex vitamins.

CALCIUM

Calcium, along with magnesium and potassium, plays a major role in cardiovascular health. Each mineral plays a beneficial role when present in the proper amount. Too little as well as too much can be injurious. And, they must be present in the proper balance with each other and sodium for optimum results.

Calcium intake, like magnesium intake, has been associated with a lower risk of developing hypertension. There have been many studies where calcium has been given to individuals and their blood pressure response has been followed. Over half of these studies showed significant blood pressure lowering.

RESEARCH

In these studies, the magnitude of the average fall in blood pressure is not great—5 to 7 points (mm Hg) of systolic blood pressure (the top number) and 3 to 4 points of diastolic blood pressure (the bottom number). According to David A. McCarron, M.D., the researcher who has studied hypertension and calcium perhaps more than any other investigator, "about 30 to 45 percent of hypertensive individuals fall into this 'calcium-sensitive' category."

Just about the same percentage of people who will decrease their blood pressure with salt restriction will also decrease their blood pressure with calcium supplementation. There is some cross over and overlap between calcium- and sodium-sensitive individuals. Those mineral-sensitive people who restrict salt while adding calcium, magnesium, and potassium may have a substantial reduction in blood pressure and may not need to take high blood pressure drugs. If the mineral modifications alone were not enough, CoQ10 and vitamin C may also be supplemented in conjunction with them.

With high blood pressure, the bottom line is the control of the blood pressure. If natural nondrug methods work, great. If they don't work, you must take whatever medication is necessary to lower the blood pressure into as near a normal range as possible. Only by controlling the blood pressure can you reduce your risk of coronary heart disease.

The above-mentioned average blood pressure reductions due to calcium supplementation are modest. However, they are averages. Some people in the studies with calcium supplementation had falls in systolic blood pressure of over twenty points (mm Hg).

The amount of calcium is also crucial. Some people who had an initial fall in blood pressure with moderate calcium supplementation got an increase in blood pressure when the calcium dosage was pushed higher.

The same thing also happens in some people who restrict salt. Moderate salt restriction will cause a fall in blood pressure, and severe salt restriction will cause the blood pressure to go back up in some people.

Calcium, Colon Cancer, and Cholesterol

Several studies have shown a reduction in the incidence of colon cancer when calcium intake is increased. In these studies, calcium intake of over 1,200 mg per day was associated with a 75 percent decrease in colon cancer. It is thought that calcium binds the bile salts, some of which may cause or promote colon cancer.

This same mechanism probably explains how calcium supplementation lowers blood cholesterol levels. One recent study has shown about a 4 percent fall in LDL-cholesterol and a 4 percent rise in HDL-cholesterol when men and women were supplemented with calcium carbonate. The cholesterol enters the intestinal tract with the bile salts. When the cholesterol and bile salts are bound by the calcium, they cannot be reabsorbed. This is the same mechanism as the cholesterol-binding resins and the soluble fiber. Dietary fiber will work hand-in-hand with the calcium to reduce the risk of colon cancer and to lower blood cholesterol levels.

One word of caution is in order. A very recent study from England (1993) has shown an increase in the rate of growth of colon cells when calcium is supplemented. The exact significance of this finding is as yet unclear. The big question is: could this increased growth rate promote cancer of the colon? I don't know the answer to this question, and I am still using moderate calcium supplementation while I keep my eyes and ears open for more data. I advise you to do the same.

Calcium and Osteoporosis

Adequate calcium intake is necessary to maintain the structural integrity of the bony skeleton. Weight-bearing exercise such as walking is also required. If you are a woman, estrogen is also necessary. I have been impressed with the difficulty in maintaining healthy bones after menopause when estrogen replacement is lacking. Exercise and calcium alone seem to be enough for men.

Types of Calcium

Bone-meal calcium is often contaminated with lead. Calcium citrate may raise blood aluminum levels and aluminum deposits are often seen in the brains of many Alzheimer patients. Calcium chloride may cause intestinal irritation.

Calcium carbonate is the most widely used calcium supplement, and it is also the least expensive. In order for calcium carbonate to be absorbed into the body, it must first dissolve in the stomach. This requires stomach acid. As we get older, the stomach makes less hydrochloric acid and consequently it might be harder to utilize calcium carbonate. In this situation, calcium lactate or calcium gluconate might be the best choice.

As with magnesium, calcium chelated with amino acids often works well. One way to tell if your calcium supplement will dissolve in your intestinal tract or not is to put it in vinegar. This acidic solution will mimic your stomach acid. If the calcium pill does not dissolve in thirty to forty minutes (stirring every five to ten minutes) in the vinegar, it won't dissolve in your body and you need to try another calcium supplement.

How Much Calcium Should You Take?

I suggest 1,000 to 1,200 mg of calcium per day for adults. If you have a history of high blood calcium levels or kidney stones, or are taking vitamin D, consult your physician before taking calcium supplements. If you consume a lot of dairy products in your diet (only nonfat dairy products are recommended), you can reduce your calcium supplementation proportionately.

Precautions

As blood vessels get older and more atherosclerotic, they tend to calcify. Ingesting too much calcium could enhance this calcification process. Also, vitamin D will facilitate the calcification process. In my opinion, adults who get even a minimal amount of exposure to the sunlight do not need vitamin D supplementation. The sunlight will activate our own natural vitamin D. Too much vitamin D and too much calcium may accelerate the calcification and aging of our arteries.

POTASSIUM

Potassium, like magnesium and calcium, is important in blood pressure regulation and maintenance of a normal, healthy, heart rhythm. These three minerals interact and balance each other. If potassium and magnesium are both low in the body and you replace only the potassium, it will not correct the potassium level in the bloodstream. You must also replace the magnesium. In fact, just replacing the magnesium will actually raise the blood level of potassium. Magnesium replacement will block the potassium loss by the kidney. That's how intimate their relationship is.

The most common cause of potassium (and magnesium) deficiency is diuretics used to treat hypertension and congestive heart failure. A low level of potassium caused by diuretics has been associated with unstable heart rhythms, high blood sugar levels (diabetes), and elevated triglycerides.

Potassium and Blood Pressure

The degree to which potassium can lower blood pressure is by no means established. In one study, 81 percent of those who increased their dietary potassium intake reduced their blood pressure medication by 50 percent. Nearly 40 percent of those eating the potassium-rich foods were able to discontinue drug therapy altogether.

Once again, the bottom line on blood pressure is that it is lowered and controlled. Do not stop your blood pressure medication. Employ the techniques and recommendations in this book. Monitor your blood pressure with your doctor. If the blood pressure comes down into the normal range, your doctor will, if possible, lower the amount of blood pressure medication. Remember, the two proven means of lowering blood pressure are to lose weight if you are overweight and to exercise.

English researchers conducted a meta-analysis of thirteen studies that used potassium to try to lower blood pressure. They found that potassium definitely lowered blood pressure.

Potassium is just one of the several tools you have at your disposal. My own experience is that when multiple nutritional therapies are used together, the results are improved. The supplements tend to be synergistic in their action.

Potassium and Stroke

Potassium has been shown to markedly decrease the number of deaths related to stroke in both men and women.

RESEARCH

Dr. Louis Tobian, a professor of medicine at the University of Minnesota Medical School in Minneapolis and a well-respected hypertension researcher, recently spoke to the American Society of Hypertension at their annual meeting. Dr. Tobian reported on the results of a 12-year study in a Southern California retirement community.

Women over age 50 who ate more than 67 mEq of potassium a day (one mEq of potassium is equal to 40 mg of potassium) were virtually free of stroke death. Those women eating less than 49 mEq of potassium a day had a stroke death rate of 5.3 per 100 individuals.

(continued on next page)

RESEARCH (continued)

When men consumed more than 76 mEq of potassium a day there were no stroke deaths. An intake of less than 59 mEq a day for men resulted in 3.4 stroke deaths per 100 individuals. The protection afforded by potassium is independent of other risk factors for stroke.

The average healthy American diet contains from 2,000 to 3,000 mg of potassium per day (50 to 75 mEq). The good news is that you don't have to increase your dietary potassium very much to be in the protective range if you are already getting several servings a day of fruits and vegetables. You just have to be sure to continue to eat your fruits and vegetables.

Potassium Supplementation

If you take diuretics, you may well need potassium supplementation. Your doctor will have to take a blood sample and measure the serum potassium level. In my opinion, the potassium level should be above 4.2 mEq/L. This was the level that showed protection against malignant rhythm disturbances in patients with a heart attack.

The amount of supplemental potassium you take will depend on the serum level. Usually about 40 mEq (1,600 mg) of potassium a day will maintain potassium balance and keep the serum level at 4.2 mEq or greater for people on diuretics. The most potent potassium supplements are by prescription only. The reason for this is that if the potassium gets too high in the bloodstream, this too can cause potentially lethal heart rhythm disturbances.

If the kidneys are working properly, they will excrete any excess potassium. So the amount of potassium supplemented is dependent on the amount of potassium lost and how healthy the kidneys are. The best way to do this is by monitoring the blood levels of potassium and with kidney tests (BUN and Creatinine). Your doctor should monitor these tests and prescribe the potassium supplements.

Food Sources of Potassium

Fruits, vegetables, potatoes, peas, beans, fish, and skim milk are the best sources of potassium. A medium banana supplies 450 to 650 mg of potassium. Half a cantaloupe gives 650 to 850 mg. A medium potato, baked, with skin provides 650 to 850 mg. Spinach, lentils, split peas, and all types of beans are excellent sources of potassium. A large glass of orange juice (8 oz.) provides about 400 to 500 mg of potassium.

PAINLESS Rx

The more fruits and vegetables you eat, the more potassium you will get. Add beans and peas to your diet to get an additional 600 to 1,000 mg of potassium per cup. And all these foods are zero cholesterol and zero saturated fat—absolutely essential in your heart-healthy diet.

Health Food Store Potassium

Potassium preparations in the health food store usually contain 99 mg of potassium per tablet or capsule. If you are taking diuretics, you need serious potassium supplementation. Prescription potassium plus blood monitoring is the correct way to go. For maintenance and preventive medicine, you will get more mileage out of increasing the fruits and vegetables in your diet than by taking the health food store potassium. Daily intake of a banana, a big glass of orange juice, a baked potato, a cup of spinach, and a cup of beans will provide enough potassium to put almost everyone in the stroke-protection zone.

Is Potassium Safe?

Since potassium is excreted from the body by the kidneys, impaired kidney function could result in excess potassium in the body. Fatal heart rhythm disturbances have occurred from excessive potassium in the bloodstream. People with defective kidney function should not even eat foods rich in potassium. **If there is any question about your kidney function and potassium supplementation, check with your doctor first and let him or her monitor your blood levels.**

I have never heard of a serious complication from too much dietary potassium in a person with normal kidney function.

SELENIUM

This important antioxidant mineral is discussed in the antioxidant section (see Chapter 7).

CHROMIUM

Chromium has several important functions in the prevention and reversal of coronary heart disease.

Chromium and Glucose Tolerance Factor (GTF)

The story on GTF chromium has been unfolding since the 1950's, when researchers initially found that a component of yeast would prevent diabetes in animals. This factor was named GTF. Subsequent work found *tri*valent chromium to be an integral part of GTF. (*Hexa*valent chromium, used to tan leather and plate chrome bumpers, is highly toxic.)

This *tri*valent chromium is bound to niacin and amino acids in the GTF. GTF chromium vigorously enhances the action of insulin. Without GTF, the potency of the available insulin is markedly decreased. This weakened insulin action will greatly restrict the body's ability to use glucose. The body will then respond by making more insulin. But, the insulin is still ineffective and the blood sugar will rise. This is precisely the state of affairs seen in maturity onset (Type II) diabetes.

I don't mean to suggest that all maturity onset diabetes is due to chromium deficiency. However, when chromium is deficient and it is supplemented, elevated glucose (blood sugar) and insulin levels fall towards normal within a few weeks. If there is no chromium deficiency, chromium supplementation will not help. Since chromium deficiency is not uncommon, I believe that every maturity-onset diabetic deserves a trial of chromium supplementation to see if this will improve diabetic control.

Diabetics lose more chromium than nondiabetics. Chromium is washed out of the body along with the glucose in the diabetic urine. Athletes who perspire heavily also have higher chromium losses.

Syndrome X, Chromium, and Insulin Resistance

One of the important risk factors for coronary heart disease to emerge over the past few years is that of insulin resistance. It has been known for many years that diabetes that comes on later in life is strongly associated with an increased risk of coronary heart disease. These individuals have elevated or higher than normal insulin levels in their bloodstream and there is a resistance in the body to the action of insulin. So, the body makes even more insulin to try to overcome this resistance. This insulin resistance and elevated levels of insulin are very often associated with high levels of triglycerides, low levels of HDL-cholesterol, and high blood pressure.

This constellation of abnormal risk factors was named "Syndrome X" by Gerald Reaven, M.D., a professor of medicine and chief of endocrinology at Stanford University School of Medicine in Palo Alto, California. Dr. Reaven's research has dealt with trying to find the cause of this so-called "Deadly Quartet," another name for the syndrome coined by Norman Kaplan, M.D., of the University of Texas Southwestern Medical School in Dallas.

Interestingly, the blood sugar levels in the early stages are not elevated. The increased insulin production is able to keep the blood sugar levels in check, but the cost of this compensation is substantial. The elevated insulin drives the triglycerides up and the HDL-cholesterol down. Insulin will also stimulate the growth of plaque and blockage in the arterial wall and worsen high blood pressure.

In my opinion, this syndrome cries out for a trial of chromium. Chromium will not only increase insulin sensitivity, it will also raise HDL-cholesterol and sometimes lower total cholesterol, triglycerides, and LDL-cholesterol.

Chromium, Cholesterol, and Arterial Plaque

One of the major types of drugs used to treat high blood pressure is the beta-blockers. One of the major side effects of beta-blockers is that they lower HDL-cholesterol. Because of reports that chromium might raise HDL-cholesterol levels, investigators at the University of North Carolina at Chapel Hill (the institution at which I did my internal medicine training) studied HDL-cholesterol levels in patients with high blood pressure who were being treated with beta-blockers. During the two months of chromium supplementation (they used 600 mcg of chromium picolinate per day) the HDL-cholesterol went up a whopping 16 percent. This is even more impressive because of the known HDL-lowering action of the beta-blockers. Total cholesterol and triglycerides did not change in this study.

Other studies have also shown chromium to raise HDL-cholesterol and to lower LDL-cholesterol, total cholesterol, and triglycerides. If chromium could, in fact, cause these beneficial changes in the blood lipid (fat) pattern, you would expect that it might be able to reverse blockages in the arteries. In a study done on rabbits, it was found to do just that. Interestingly, the amount of reversal in the rabbits was not dependent on the blood lipid levels. I'm not sure what to make of this finding, but before leaving the research on chromium, I want to point out one more study.

Chromium and Lifespan

Gary Evans, Ph.D., of Bemidji State University in Minnesota, made an amazing announcement at the 1992 annual meeting of the American Aging Association. He supplemented laboratory rats with three different formulations of chromium. At the end of forty-one months, the only rats still surviving were those supplemented with chromium picolinate. And 80 percent of that group were still alive, while all the others had died. Dr. Evans did get my attention. Just one more tiny piece of evidence supporting chromium supplementation. In this case, specifically chromium picolinate.

Do We Get Enough Chromium in Our Diet?

There is growing evidence that marginal chromium deficiency is widespread in the United States. The National Research Council RDA for chromium is 50 to 200 mcg for adults. Numerous studies have shown that dietary chromium is commonly deficient. Very recent studies have shown that the elderly have increased chromium losses and often consume less than 30 mcg of chromium per day.

In my opinion, there is more than enough evidence to support supplementing with chromium. I base this conclusion on chromium's potential to increase insulin sensitivity and balance blood sugar, raise HDL-cholesterol, and lower LDL-cholesterol and triglycerides. These results have all been accomplished in human beings. The animal studies showing reversal of blockages and improved longevity all need further study.

Is Chromium Safe?

In reviewing the literature, the only potential side effect of *tri*valent chromium that I could find was that it might interfere with iron metabolism and lower the blood count and ferritin levels in rats (see iron below). This might actually be a beneficial effect.

What Type of Chromium Is Best?

There are several sources of *tri*valent chromium GTF. Until recently, the main sources were chromium chloride, which may be poorly absorbed, and brewers yeast, which is not always standardized for chromium content. Also, many people are allergic to brewers yeast.

The other two major sources of chromium are chromium picolinate and chromium polynicotinate. These two forms of chromium are proprietary and the manufacturers are intensely competitive, each claiming to have an advantage over the other. I spent much more time than I had anticipated in researching to decide if there was, in fact, an advantage of one form of chromium over the other.

More of the studies have been done with chromium picolinate and chromium chloride. However, it appears that all forms of *tri*valent chromium are effective.

How Much Chromium Should You Take?

Studies reported in the medical literature with human beings have safely used 600 to 800 micrograms (mcg) of chromium daily over a period of a few weeks to up to two months. As a longterm supplement, I would suggest 200 mcg per day. It may take several weeks or even a few months to totally replenish deficient body stores of chromium, but 200 mcg is a safe dosage over the long haul.

IRON

For years, it has been known that pre-menopausal women have fewer heart attacks than men of the same age. It was always assumed that this benefit was due to a protective effect of the female hormone estrogen. In 1981, Jerome L. Sullivan, M.D., Ph.D., was the first to postulate that iron loss through menstruation might account for this benefit enjoyed by women. He was led to that hypothesis after seeing some data showing that women who had a simple hysterectomy (the ovaries are not removed and estrogen secretion is left intact) also had an increased risk of coronary disease. Dr. Sullivan continues to champion the concept that depletion of iron stores through menstruation is what really protects pre-menopausal women.

More recently, researchers from Finland have reported that men with high stored iron levels have an increased risk of having a heart attack. This work, which was published in October, 1992, stimulated American investigators to examine blood samples that had been collected over a number of years and frozen as well as dietary data that was already in the computers ready for analysis.

Abstracts of this American research were published in early 1993 and the research presented to the American Heart Association Cardiovascular Epidemiology meeting in March, 1993. The official medical journal publication of this research, which sometimes takes up to a year after the material is presented at a medical meeting, is not yet available.

This American research from Harvard Medical School in Boston and Loyola University Stritch School of Medicine in Maywood, Illinois, does not confirm the Finnish research and shows a weak, if any, connection between dietary iron intake, body iron stores, and risk of heart attack. So, all the hoopla may have been for naught.

The reason that the correlation of iron with coronary heart disease seems to make sense is that iron is a known oxidizer of LDL-cholesterol. It was thought that higher body stores of iron would result in more oxidized LDL-cholesterol and hence more uptake of LDL into the arterial blockages. This fit with the Finnish research because in that study, the higher the LDL levels, the greater the risk from the high iron stores.

While the researchers work out the details, just keep taking your antioxidants (vitamins C and E, beta-carotene, CoQ10, and selenium). This will protect you from all known causes of LDL oxidation, including iron. Definitely don't supplement with iron unless there is unequivocal iron deficiency. This will give you the best protection that I can recommend at this time.

If you want to do more to try to protect yourself from any potential negative effects of excess iron stores, consider donating a pint of blood every four to six months. I have not completely discarded the iron hypothesis. It is logically appealing and it may well turn out to have real merit. I recently donated my first unit of blood since being in medical school.

You have to watch your vitamin supplements carefully because many multivitamin preparations contain iron. However, more and more vitamin companies are now giving the public a choice of iron-free supplements.

ZINC AND COPPER

Just as calcium and magnesium are codependent minerals, so are zinc and copper. They balance each other, and each plays an important role in the body's ability to deal with cholesterol and oxidation.

One of the problems with trying to assess the roles of copper and zinc is that blood levels of these minerals don't always reflect body stores or dietary intake. So, it's very difficult to draw meaningful conclusions based on blood levels. Long-term dietary studies have not been done.

Copper

The same Finnish researcher who reported on iron as a risk factor for coronary heart disease, Dr. Jukka T. Salonen, has also published data showing a similar role for copper. In Dr. Salonen's study, the plaque-promoting effect of elevated LDL-cholesterol is present only, or at least much stronger, in men with high blood copper levels. Remarkably, he also found that a low blood level of selenium will greatly increase the body's ability to grow artery-blocking cholesterol plaque. In still another study, Dr. Salonen showed that men with the highest levels of blood copper had a four-fold higher risk of heart attack.

In the research laboratory, copper is often used to induce oxidation of LDL-cholesterol. Another study, this one by someone other than Dr. Salonen, showed that the higher the blood levels of copper, the lower the blood levels of HDL-cholesterol. Copper not only stimulates LDL oxidation, it also diminishes the levels of protective HDL.

Diabetics have higher blood copper levels than nondiabetics. Diabetics with vascular complications of diabetes have higher blood copper levels than diabetics without these complications.

Would it be a good idea to induce copper deficiency?

NO! Copper is essential in the body. Copper deficiency causes anemia and in some studies low levels of copper will raise LDL and lower HDL-cholesterol. Copper deficiency has also been associated with aneurysms or weakness of the aorta. We don't need to deplete our body's essential copper stores. We need to insure a *normal* level of copper and to do everything possible to prevent the copper from being oxidized.

How do you protect the body from the adverse effects of copper?

PAINLESS Rx

ANTIOXIDANTS! ANTIOXIDANTS! ANTIOXIDANTS! Vitamins C and E, beta-carotene, selenium, and CoQ10, and perhaps a little zinc.

Zinc

Both zinc deficiency and zinc supplementation have been reported to cause HDL-cholesterol to fall. Since zinc and copper balance each other, it's not too surprising to find the same up-and-down relationship to HDL with zinc that is seen with copper. Looking at one without the other is only half the picture. Zinc may retard the absorption of copper and, in fact, they compete for binding sites and absorption in the intestinal tract.

As we get older, our vision often gets worse. One cause of this is cataracts, which may, in part, be prevented or retarded by antioxidants. Another cause of age-related failing vision is macular degeneration—a degenerative process in the eye that leads to blindness. It is the leading cause of blindness in older people. Zinc may slow the progression of macular degeneration.

So, it looks like zinc supplementation may be beneficial. There are actually at least another ten good reasons to supplement with zinc—from boosting the immune system to improving wound healing. Diabetics are also prone to zinc deficiency.

Zinc and Copper Recommendations

Supplement with 30 to not more than 50 milligrams (mg) of zinc per day. Balance the zinc with 2 mg of copper per day, and take a full measure of daily antioxidants to protect against oxidized copper.

Part III

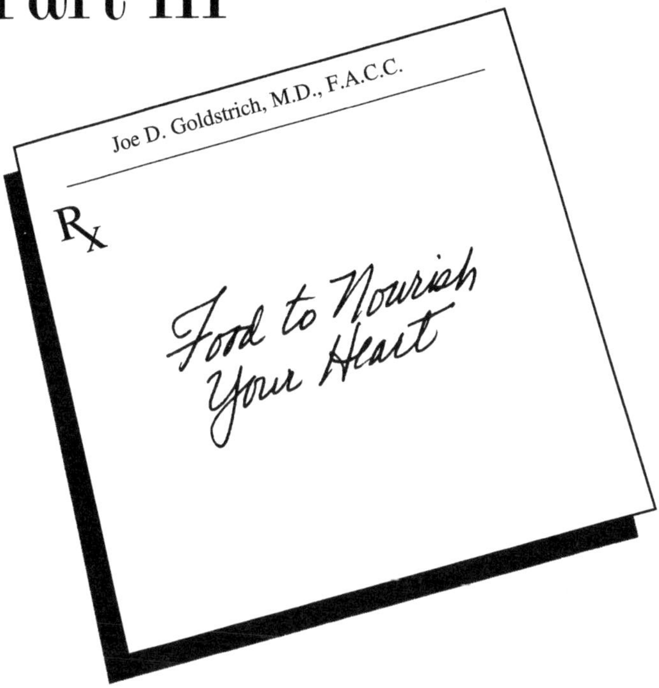

As I get older, I hope that I get wiser. I want to enjoy my life to the fullest, and I also want to be as healthy as possible. In my younger days, I thought that being healthy required a high level of deprivation. My new wisdom has taught me that deprivation does not always mean good health. The people who live around the Mediterranean Sea don't deprive themselves. They eat some of the most exciting and delicious cuisine in the world. They season with herbs, garlic, and onions. They use olive oil liberally. They enjoy a glass of wine with their meal. They relish their fruits and vegetables. They are not deprived. They find great pleasure in their diet, and they have the lowest rates of cardiovascular disease in the world!

One of the main lessons in this section on food is simply to learn how to eat as people in the Mediterranean basin do. This will be a truly painless prescription! I personally enjoy this Mediterranean-style food more than any other cuisine. Not to eat it would be real deprivation for me. If you learn the lessons here, you will find great pleasure in eating a heart-healthy diet.

If I had to pick the one element of the Mediterranean diet that is the most important, it would clearly be olive oil. There are three reasons why this monounsaturated oil is so important. We have already looked at the first reason. The people who use olive oil as their exclusive dietary oil have the lowest rates of heart disease in the world.

The second reason is that olive oil is resistant to oxidation. So, it won't contribute to LDL oxidation like the polyunsaturated oils. The olive oil will actually help protect the LDL-cholesterol from oxidation.

The third and final reason is that olive oil will raise the good HDL-cholesterol and lower the bad LDL-cholesterol. This will lower the risk of coronary heart disease. There is no other dietary regimen, including a 10 percent fat diet, that will result in this optimum situation of a higher HDL and a lower LDL. Other monounsaturated fats, such as those found in nuts and avocados, will do the same thing.

In this section, we will see what roles the Mediterranean diet, cholesterol, protein, carbohydrates, sugar, fiber, coffee, tea, and salt play in a heart-healthy lifestyle.

11 *The Mediterranean Way*

THE FRENCH PARADOX

For many years, it has been known that the amount of coronary heart disease in the Mediterranean countries of Europe is quite low. The Greeks eat more red meat than any other country in Europe, yet their coronary disease rate is one of the lowest in the world. French women are heavy smokers and they have one of the lowest heart attack rates. What could be the cause of this protection from coronary heart disease in the Mediterranean countries?

The November 17, 1991, edition of "60 Minutes" addressed this question and raised several other issues. I got a transcript of the program from Journal Graphics so I could study "The French Paradox" in detail. There were several important points made to try to explain why the French have considerably less coronary disease than Americans, despite a diet that contains more fat. The three important features of the program are:

(1) The French scientists believe that their substantial wine (red) consumption is very protective. I'll tell you the whole alcohol and wine story shortly. They believe this is the most important factor.

(2) The French believe that their relaxed attitude and slow eating helps the digestion (along with the wine) and that this de-stressed eating is protective.

(3) Lastly, they believe that whole milk increases coronary heart disease (and I agree—it is full of fat and cholesterol) but that cheese is different. Dr. S. Renaud, a French

> scientist, has done research showing that in rats, the fat in the cheese comes out in the bowel movement whereas the fat from whole milk gets absorbed into the body and participates in raising LDL-cholesterol levels. I'm not ready to buy this cheese argument totally, and I haven't added unlimited cheese back to my diet just yet. In fact, despite the apparent French Paradox, the overwhelming majority of evidence is against the fat and cholesterol found in cheese and dairy products. Throughout the world, diets low in dairy fat—from the Japanese to the Eskimos—are associated with the lowest coronary heart disease rates.

Nonfat dairy products have not been around long enough to stand the test of time. But it appears that they are healthy and acceptable. Nonfat milk, fat-free cheese, nonfat yogurt, and nonfat cottage cheese all fall into this category. If you use 2 percent milk instead of nonfat milk, you increase the saturated fat content from zero to about 32 percent of the calories. Nonfat milk is much better than lowfat or 2 percent fat or whole milk.

As we get older, many of us lose our ability to digest milk. The major nutrient in dairy products is calcium. Because of the gas and bloating that occurs if you can't properly digest milk, it may be reasonable to pass on the milk and dairy products and take a calcium supplement instead.

Interestingly, in France, the farther one lives from the Mediterranean Sea, the higher the coronary heart disease rate. They use less olive oil in the north of France. Even so, the coronary heart disease rate in northern France is about half of ours in the United States.

OLIVE OIL

Olives are plentiful in the countries around the Mediterranean and the "table spread," so to speak, is olive oil. They actually put it on their bread the way we use butter and margarine in this country. Some of the lowest coronary rates in the world are in the Mediterranean countries. As I said earlier, the Greeks eat more red meat than any other country in Europe.

When I visited Greece in 1989, I was impressed with several things. The meat was lean. The feta cheese was delicious. The olives were succulent. Many smoked tobacco. They mopped up the olive oil from their plates with some of the best-tasting bread I have ever put in my mouth. The feta cheese intake of the Greeks may support the French speculation about cheese not being harmful.

Cardiovascular Benefits of Olive Oil

The effect of olive oil in the diet has been studied. Researchers from Italy and the State University of New York at Buffalo evaluated 4,903 Italian men and women who were twenty to fifty-nine years of age. They found that increased consumption of butter was associated with significantly higher blood pressure, higher serum cholesterol, and higher blood sugar levels in men. In women, only the blood sugar level was higher. In both sexes, consumption of olive oil, and to a lesser degree other vegetable oils, was associated with lower cholesterol, lower blood sugar and lower systolic blood pressure. They concluded that eating butter may adversely affect coronary heart disease risk and that using vegetable oils is associated with a lower risk. The main vegetable oil used was olive oil.

Substituting olive oil for other fats (e.g. butter) will lower LDL-cholesterol, raise HDL-cholesterol, reduce oxidized LDL, and hopefully bring our coronary risk down to the level of the Greeks and the Italians.

I have recently noticed that quite a few restaurants in this country, especially Italian, are now pouring out a saucer of olive oil—sometimes with herbs such as basil—to put on the table instead of butter. I applaud this action. I have found that if they don't do this as part of their normal routine, they will in most instances do so on request.

What Is the Best Olive Oil?

Olives are pressed several times to extract all the oil from them. The olive oil that comes from the very first pressing is called extra virgin. That's the best. Heat is generated by the pressing and to get more oil, you have to press harder and harder, generating more and more heat. It's almost like the oil has already been fried. Also, the oil from the subsequent pressings becomes acidic, and chemicals are used to reduce the acidity. Other chemicals are also used to try to increase the yield of oil from the subsequent pressings. Extra virgin oil contains the least acid, less than 1 percent, and has the most distinctive taste. The second pressing is called virgin olive oil and it has from 1 to 3 percent acid. Blended olive oil has an even higher acid content.

The above terminology is for imported olive oil. A slightly different terminology is used in this country. Domestic olive oil from the first pressing is called virgin. There is no domestic extra virgin olive oil. Refined domestic olive oil has had more than one pressing and the lowest U.S. grade is called residue oil.

Olive oil smokes at 390 degrees. The better the olive oil, the lower the smoke point. Smoking oil is oxidized oil. Never eat food cooked in oil that has been heated to the smoke point. That oil is rancid/oxidized/spoiled. You have to be careful when you cook with olive oil not to get it too hot.

The Orientals know a trick that is very useful. They use it in wok cooking, but it can also be used in the fry pan. If you add water and oil (olive) to the **cold** fry pan and then heat it slowly, the water will boil at 212 degrees and turn to steam. This helps keep the oil cooler and prevents its smoking and oxidizing while the steam helps do the cooking. **Caution: never add water to hot oil because it will splatter and burn you.**

I like to use the best grades of olive oil available on my bread and for salad dressings and sauces. I enjoy the unique flavors of the different virgin and extra-virgin olive oils.

Olive Oil Is Rich in MUFA

Olive oil is rich in MUFA (monounsaturated fat). MUFA is only one of the many different kinds of fats and oils. Others include saturated fat, polyunsaturated fat, trans-fat, tropical oils, cocoa fat, coconut oil, fish oil, rice bran oil, lecithin, partially hydrogenated fat, hydrogenated fat, omega-3, omega-6, stearic acid, oleic acid, and more and more and more.

Fat is a necessary nutrient for health. Our bodies require the essential fatty acids in order to maintain a number of important and vital body functions. The problem in modern-day society is that we eat too much fat and too many nonessential fatty acids. The result is that we gain weight and plug up our arteries.

There are so many different kinds of fat that it is very easy to get overwhelmed, lost, and confused in the jungle of fat terminology. In order to make intelligent decisions about what to eat, you have to have a working knowledge of these fats.

Oxidation of fats

When a fatty acid oxidizes it does so at the site of a double bond. The double bond is broken and oxygen is picked up at this fracture site. This oxygen-carrying fractured fatty acid will then have the ability to attack LDL-cholesterol and other molecules and oxidize them. Polyunsaturated fatty acids have the most double bonds, so they are the most susceptible to oxidation.

Explaining the terms

Hydrogenated and saturated fats (SFA) are the same things. Unsaturated fatty acids have double bonds. When double bonds take up hydrogen, they become single bonds and the fat is said to be hydrogenated or saturated (with hydrogen). If some of the double bonds are converted to single bonds and some remain double, the fat is said to be partially hydrogenated. If the hydrogens line up on the same side of the fat, it is a cis-fatty acid. If the hydrogens line up across the fatty acid, it is a trans-fatty acid. In nature, fatty acids are always cis, never trans. Partial hydrogenation results in trans-fatty acid formation. If a fat has more than one double bond it is a polyunsaturated fatty acid (PUFA). If it has only one double bond, it is a monounsaturated fatty acid (MUFA).

Now that the terms are defined, we can take a closer look at each of the individual fats:

PUFA: lowers LDL **and** HDL.

PUFA: are readily oxidized and will oxidize LDL, facilitating its conversion into plaque. There is some evidence to suggest that diets high in PUFAs are associated with an increased risk of cancer.

SFA: raises LDL and lowers HDL. The more SFA in the diet, the higher the death rate from coronary disease. SFA facilitates clotting.

MUFA: lowers LDL and may raise HDL. This is the healthiest kind of fat to eat. Olive oil and canola oil fall into this category.

Trans-Fatty Acids will raise LDL and lower HDL just like SFA.

Oleic Acid: the major MUFA in olive oil. It is resistant to oxidation.

Stick margarine is loaded with trans-fatty acids. Tub margarine has less.

Butter is pure SFA.

Skim/nonfat dairy products have had all the fat and cholesterol removed.

Tropical oils (coconut, palm) are SFA.

OTHER OILS RICH IN MUFA

Only three recommended cooking oils have over 50 percent of their fatty acids as MUFA: olive, canola, and high oleic sunflower oil.

High Oleic Sunflower Oil

High oleic sunflower oil is a result of special breeding or genetic engineering. It has about 80 to 82 percent MUFA compared to about 70 to 77 percent for olive oil and 58 to 62 percent for canola. The high oleic sunflower oil has a higher smoke point than olive oil (450 vs 390 degrees) or canola oil (440), so it has more resistance to oxidation (good) than olive or canola oil. Since it is also very low in saturated fats (10 percent vs 14 percent for olive oil and 6 percent for canola oil), it is low in trans-fatty acids, too.

The only drawback to high oleic sunflower oil that I can see is that people have not been using it for centuries as they have olive oil. Olive oil has stood the test of time, while the high oleic sunflower oil still has to prove itself. Because of its resistance to oxidation, higher smoke point, and the fact that it is relatively tasteless, high oleic sunflower oil will probably start appearing more and more in commercial products. I'm willing to give it a try. At the present time, high oleic sunflower oil is only available commercially.

Regular sunflower oil is not the same thing as high oleic sunflower oil. Regular sunflower oil is 69 to 77 percent PUFA, 13 to 20 percent MUFA, and about 11 percent SFA. The PUFAs are readily oxidized and can therefore oxidize LDL. They should be avoided.

Canola Oil Is Special

Canola oil contains 58 to 62 percent MUFA, 32 to 36 percent PUFA and about 6 percent SFA. It has less SFA than any other oil. There are two major PUFAs in vegetable oil—linoleic and linolenic. Canola is rich in linolenic, an essential, beneficial fatty acid. The problem is that the double bonds of linolenic acid (there are three of them—linoleic only has two) can break and become oxidized. Canola has a higher smoke point than olive oil, but if it does smoke, there will be more oxidation because there is more PUFA. I keep canola oil on hand but don't use it as much as olive oil.

Another benefit of canola oil is its ability to decrease platelet stickiness and lower the clotting tendency, further protecting against coronary artery disease. It is better than olive oil in this regard. The best canola oil (cold pressed) is obtained in the health food store.

FLAX SEED OIL (LINSEED OIL)

The use of medicinal flax seed oil dates to the fifth century B.C., when Hippocrates recommended its use. The long history of flax seed oil use is detailed by Udo Erasmus in his excellent book, *Fats and Oils*. He is a strong advocate of flax seed oil and goes into great detail about its purported benefits in his book.

Flax seed oil, like canola oil, is a rich source of the polyunsaturated essential fatty acid, linolenic acid. Flax seed oil is the richest source known for linolenic acid. Because the three double bonds are easily broken and oxidized, flax seed oil must be kept in the refrigerator in a bottle that excludes light.

Twenty years ago, Scandinavian researchers touted the cardiac benefits of flax seed oil for cardiac patients, but not much has been written lately. I found one recent article saying that when vitamin E and flax seed oil were given together, there was a fall in LDL-cholesterol, an increase in HDL-cholesterol, platelet clotting factors were reduced, and the expected antioxidant effect of vitamin E was evident.

Linolenic acid is an omega-3 fatty acid. It is the only major source of omega-3 fatty acids for vegetarians. The linolenic acid must be converted to Eicosapentaenoic Acid (EPA) before it is beneficial (see Chapter 13). Only a small amount of linolenic acid is actually converted into EPA. The most efficient and healthy way to get the EPA is to eat fish.

I don't take flax seed oil as a supplement. It can be used as a supplement or as an ingredient in salad dressing. Many people enjoy its nutty flavor. Trans-fatty acids in the diet will reduce the effectiveness of the conversion of linolenic acid to EPA. Vitamins C, B3, B6, zinc and magnesium are also required to fully utilize the flax seed oil. Increased antioxidants, especially vitamin E, are necessary when the diet is supplemented with extra flax seed oil.

RICE BRAN OIL

Recently, several favorable articles on the effects of rice bran oil have appeared in the medical literature. Rice bran oil comes from the brown bran, high-fiber outer shell of rice. This bran layer is removed when brown rice is processed to make white rice. The oil from this bran coat will lower LDL-cholesterol and triglycerides and not lower HDL-cholesterol. These beneficial changes could not be predicted from the fatty acid composition of the rice bran oil. There appears to be something else in the oil that affords the beneficial results.

Rice bran oil is now available in health food stores. At the present time, I do not recommend that you make it your primary oil. More research needs to be done. I do recommend that you incorporate more brown rice into your diet—it's a much better food than white rice. The brown rice not only has this cholesterol-lowering oil, it's a great source of fiber.

WHEAT GERM

A recent study showed that raw wheat germ will lower LDL cholesterol and triglycerides. Partially defatted wheat germ was not as good as whole, raw wheat germ. So, like the rice bran oil, something in the oil faction of this whole grain (wheat) has a beneficial effect on serum cholesterol.

Eat the whole grain brown rice and whole grain wheat for a healthy, natural, nutritious diet. When you eat the whole grains, you not only get the helpful oils, you also get the beneficial fiber (see Chapter 14) and all the additional nutrition of the whole grain. And, you get these healthful nutrients in perfect balance—just the way the good Lord put them there. There is no need to supplement your diet with rice bran oil, wheat germ oil, or wheat germ.

HOW TO STORE OIL

Oil is oxidized by air (oxygen) and heat. Once you open the bottle, the air factor comes into play. Oxidation is minimized if oils are stored in the refrigerator. Saturated fat (like butter and margarine) is solid in the cold refrigerator. Canola oil has the lowest SFA content and will remain liquid in the refrigerator. Olive oil turns semisolid. This is a drawback, but I still keep my bottle of olive oil after it has been opened in the refrigerator to deter/prevent oxidation. You can let the bottle of olive oil sit outside of the refrigerator until it returns to room temperature and a more fluid state. I am too impatient for this, so I just shake the bottle to homogenize it and then pour it while it is still cold. That seems to work for me.

Always buy small bottles of oil. The bigger bottles will have more air exposure by virtue of being opened more and will have more opportunity to oxidize than a small bottle.

FINDING THE FAT IN THE SUPERMARKET

If you want to learn more about choosing foods with low saturated fat content off the supermarket shelves, there is a book that will be very helpful. *The Living Heart Brand Name Shoppers Guide*, by DeBakey, Gotto, Scott, and Foreyt, is excellent. They break down thousands of brand name products as to their calories, fat, saturated fat, and cholesterol content. There is information here that is not readily available from other sources.

Bottom line on choosing fats:

Why Not PUFA and SFA (instead of MUFA)?

SFA raises LDL cholesterol.
PUFAs are more likely to oxidize.

Butter vs Margarine

For Butter:
No trans-fatty acids.

Against Butter:
Loaded with SFA and cholesterol.

For Margarine: (Squeeze or soft tub is better than stick.)
Less SFA, no cholesterol.

Against Margarine:

Contains trans-fatty acids which raises LDL and lowers HDL.

The winner? Neither! It is best not to use either butter or margarine. If you need to put some fat on your bread or vegetables, try a little olive oil like the Italians and Greeks who have the lowest coronary heart disease risk. If you must use margarine, use the diet tub margarine or the liquid squeeze bottles—they have less trans-fatty acid and less SFA.

AVOCADOS AND NUTS

Four very important research papers published in 1992 and 1993 have shed new light on the role of dietary fat in the treatment of coronary heart disease. The same health-food enthusiasts who knew that fertile eggs from well-fed chickens had something good to offer were all the while snacking on nuts and eating avocado and alfalfa sprout sandwiches for lunch. In the early 1980's, shortly after I left the Pritikin Longevity Center, I tried to convince some of these devotees to see the error in their ways, but they were steadfast in their belief that what they were doing was healthy. Their conviction was so convincing, I began to crack a few nuts in the fall and mix up an occasional guacamole, my ambivalence overshadowed by the sheer joy of my taste buds. I tolerated this low level of guilt and irresolution until four recent articles set me free.

Three of the articles are on nuts and one is on avocados. All demonstrate the cardiovascular benefits of lowering LDL-cholesterol and/or improving the ratio between LDL-cholesterol and HDL-cholesterol.

RESEARCH

In the avocado study from New Zealand, fifteen women aged thirty-seven to fifty-eight were given either the most rigorous American Heart Association (AHA) diet (Phase III) or a high complex carbohydrate diet enriched with avocado. Both diets lowered total cholesterol, but the AHA diet lowered HDL more than LDL, while the avocado diet lowered only LDL. The avocado diet was more effective than the AHA diet!

The first nut article was an evaluation of 31,000 California Seventh-Day Adventists, who already live seven years longer than the average American because of their healthy diet. Those who ate any kind of nuts more often than once a week had significantly fewer heart attacks. Those who ate the nuts more than five times a week had the lowest heart attack rates. The most frequently consumed nuts were peanuts, almonds, and walnuts. Technically speaking, peanuts aren't even nuts, they are legumes. These "nuts" all have a high MUFA content and a low SFA content.

Four additional important pieces of information came out of this study: (1) Eating more cheese resulted in a higher heart attack rate. (2) Whole wheat bread provided protection from heart attacks when compared to white bread. (3) Men who ate beef more than three times a week had a higher risk of a fatal heart attack. This was not true for women who ate beef. And (4) the heart attack rate was independent of egg consumption. Whether you ate eggs or not made no difference.

The second nut study involved supplementing the diet with almonds. Almonds, like avocado, are rich in MUFA. Men and women supplemented their diet with about three and one-half ounces of raw almonds a day for nine weeks. The results showed about a 10 percent fall in total cholesterol and LDL with no change in HDL. As would be expected, these results are similar to the avocado study. Both studies supplemented the diet with MUFA and found that the LDL falls and the HDL stays the same. This improved ratio of HDL to LDL is protective against coronary heart disease.

(continued on next page)

RESEARCH (continued)

The third and last nut study involved walnuts. Walnuts have more PUFA than MUFA. In this study, total cholesterol, LDL, and HDL all fell. LDL fell 9 times more than the HDL, so the ratio of HDL to LDL was improved.

If you increase your PUFA intake, you must also be sure that you have adequate antioxidant protection. But, that's always true. And wouldn't we be better off choosing nuts with a high MUFA content instead of walnuts? The high MUFA "nuts" are: hazelnuts, almonds, pistachios, and peanuts.

GARLIC

One of the biggest and most pleasant surprises to me in doing the research for this book was discovering the potential benefit of garlic and, to a lesser extent, onions. I guess if I had to pick the unique dietary factors that make up the Mediterranean diet, they would include olive oil, red wine, and garlic. The surprise was that so much research had been done on the medicinal effects of garlic, although the research may not be as pure as I would like. This is because often the companies that manufacture the deodorized garlic preparations used in the studies were sponsors of the studies. Nevertheless, there is a substantial body of research showing therapeutic benefits of garlic. There is some controversy over whether cooking the garlic inactivates its beneficial effects or not. Benefits have been shown, however, for both cooked and raw garlic as well as aged garlic extract, garlic oil, and dried garlic powder.

Over the past twenty years, I have met about a dozen people who claimed to eat raw garlic every day. The amount ranged from a regular clove to an elephant ear clove to a whole head of garlic each day. All these people claimed extraordinary benefits from the garlic. One elderly Italian man was vigorous and active into his eighties. The most common claim was that they never got a cold. Most ate their garlic with the evening meal or at bedtime. They claimed that the garlic odor of their body was less strong during the day with night-time consumption. One divorced man in his fifties claimed his wife left him because she couldn't stand his smell and he wouldn't give up his raw garlic.

Another drawback to the raw garlic is that its allicin content, the active ingredient in garlic, varies considerably from garlic batch to garlic batch—as much as tenfold. But don't be discouraged. Dried garlic pills that are deodorized and standardized for consistent allicin content are now available. In Germany, deodorized garlic pills are one of the most popular over-the-counter medicinal preparations sold.

Cardiovascular Benefits of Garlic

Studies showing reductions in LDL-cholesterol and triglycerides have been done using a German deodorized garlic powder (Kwai) and a Japanese deodorized aged garlic extract (Kyolic). The LDL-cholesterol fell 10 to 12 percent and the triglycerides about 17 percent. In the Japanese study (done at Loma Linda University in California), the HDL-cholesterol had a slight but significant increase.

The exact mechanism by which garlic achieves the beneficial cholesterol changes is not completely worked out. It appears that the active ingredients in the garlic inhibit cholesterol production in the liver, very similar to the HMG-CoA reductase inhibiting drugs like Mevacor (lovastatin), Zocor (simvastatin), and Pravachol (pravastatin).

In both the Japanese and German studies, four pills or capsules were taken each day. The magnitude of the benefits on LDL, HDL, and triglycerides are about equal to those beneficial changes seen with rigorous dietary restrictions or with some cholesterol-lowering drugs. About 20 percent of the participants in the German study got a garlic odor to their body.

Garlic also appears to beneficially retard clotting by reducing platelet stickiness and activating clot breakdown (fibrinolysis). The blood is also thinned, fibrinogen is reduced, and blood flow through small blood vessels is improved. The action on the platelets is very similar to that of aspirin, which has been well studied and shown to reduce the risk of heart attack.

Garlic may cause a very mild reduction in blood pressure and in a few studies, it has been shown to lower blood sugar levels.

Noncardiovascular Benefits of Garlic

There are numerous studies showing that garlic can prevent cancer in animals. It has been shown to enhance the immune system, and some of the compounds in garlic have antibiotic properties.

Precautions

Eating large amounts of garlic may cause gastrointestinal irritation. People with ulcer disease, hiatus hernia, and sensitive stomachs may be particularly susceptible. So, if you are going to add raw garlic to your diet, start slow with very small amounts to be sure you can tolerate it and build up slowly. Body odor will probably be the limiting factor if you build up slowly. Also, some people are allergic to the deodorized garlic pills and capsules.

A few years ago, I got excited about the beneficial effects of garlic and I ate several raw cloves at one meal. I got one heck of a case of esophageal irritation and heartburn.

ONIONS

Garlic and onions come from the same family. The botanical name for garlic is *allium sativum* and that of onion is *allium cepa*. They are both bulbs that belong to the lily family. They are both rich in sulfur-containing compounds. It is thought that these sulfur-containing compounds are responsible for their medicinal effects. With one exception, no one is marketing onion pills and consequently not much research has been done on onions lately. Twinlab does combine onions in their garlic preparation. However, looking back in the literature over the past twenty years, I have found several articles on onions showing that they, too, can lower cholesterol and retard clotting.

ALCOHOL

There are five questions about alcohol consumption that must be addressed and answered.

1. Will you live longer if you drink alcoholic beverages?

The answer to this question depends on how much you drink and who you are. **Heavy** alcohol consumption is associated with an increased mortality. Not only are fatal and nonfatal auto accidents increased, but alcohol consumption is associated with about 41 percent of deaths from unintentional falls; 47 percent of drownings in those younger than 15 years; 69 percent of deaths in boating accidents; 49 percent of episodes of interpersonal violence, such as murder or attempted murder; 39 percent of partner battering; 50 percent of reported rapes; and 39 to 50 percent of deaths in fires, according to Marilyn Aguirre-Molina, Ed.D., of the Robert Wood Johnson Medical School, University of Medicine and Dentistry of New Jersey.

In addition, heavy alcohol consumption is associated with cirrhosis of the liver, bleeding esophageal varices, sudden death, stroke, cardiomyopathy (a weakening of the heart muscle), heart rhythm disturbances, hypertension, and cigarette smoking—all of which can shorten your life. Alcoholism takes a heavy financial, emotional, and social toll not only on alcoholics but also on their families, their coworkers, and the whole community.

The key word here is **heavy**. **Heavy** drinking will shorten your life and make it miserable. Moderate drinking (about two drinks per day) may lengthen your life and hopefully make it happier. The mortality curve associated with alcohol consumption is U-shaped. The highest mortality comes at both ends. Those that don't drink at all and the heavy drinkers have the highest mortality. The moderate drinkers—those in the middle—have the lowest overall mortality.

RESEARCH

At a conference sponsored by the Alcoholic Beverage Medical Research Foundation, Arthur Klatsky, M.D., of the Kaiser Permanente Medical Center in Oakland, California, reported a 20 percent decrease in premature death in those people who have three to five drinks a day. One-or-two-a-day drinkers were 10 percent less likely to die prematurely. Those who had six or more drinks a day had a 30 percent increased risk of premature death. Dr. Klatsky is the originator of the U-shaped mortality curve.

There is a fine line between decreased risk of premature death and increased risk of premature death. The difference between five and six drinks a day is too fine a line for me. Many people who drink even three or four drinks per day are alcoholic or pre-alcoholic. Other studies on cardiovascular mortality show definite benefit from two to three drinks per day.

As I was doing the final editing on this book (December, 1993) the current issue of the *New England Journal of Medicine* came across my desk. The title of the lead article read: "Moderate Alcohol Intake, Increased Levels of HDL, . . . and Decreased Risk of Myocardial Infarction."

I felt really good knowing that the information that I am presenting to you is truly state of the art.

2. Will alcohol lower your risk of cardiovascular disease?

The answer, again, depends on how much you drink. Alcohol can actually cause heart disease. There are many studies that show that alcohol will worsen hypertension, raise triglycerides, and cause heart rhythm disturbances—all of which can increase cardiac risk. Long-term, heavy alcohol consumption can actually cause cardiomyopathy.

A recent article in *Circulation*, the cardiologists' main medical journal, reviewed the effects of alcohol on the heart and concluded that light to moderate alcohol intake is protective against heart disease in men. We'll talk about women in a minute.

The Harvard School of Public Health's study—a subset of the Physicians' Health Study—showed that an **increased** amount of alcohol intake correlated with a **decrease** in coronary heart disease among men.

RESEARCH

In this health professionals' follow-up study, the participants were 44,000 male dentists, veterinarians, pharmacists, osteopathic physicians, optometrists, and podiatrists. They filled out a health questionnaire in 1986 at the beginning of the study. Those who had coronary disease were excluded. Two years later, 96 percent of the living participants answered questions about newly diagnosed coronary disease in the past two years. Causes of death were determined from autopsy reports and hospital records. There were a total of 350 confirmed fatal and nonfatal coronary events during the 72,290 person-years follow-up. After adjusting for the important coronary heart disease risk factors, including dietary cholesterol, dietary fat, and fiber intake, there was a striking *inverse* relationship between increasing alcoholic intake and coronary heart disease. The relative risk of coronary disease was almost half in those men who consumed the equivalent of two drinks per day compared to nondrinkers.

A similar study from California did not show as strong a result in men, but did find a significantly higher risk of coronary disease in women who gave up drinking between 1964 and 1974 than in those who continued to drink.

Another study showed that men who died of coronary heart disease were more likely to have never been drinkers. In this study, up to fifty-six drinks per week had a 40 percent reduction in fatal and nonfatal coronary disease compared to nondrinkers. The reduction was greater in women than in men in all drinking categories.

Dr. David Blankenhorn, who pioneered research on the regression of coronary artery disease in humans, reported that subjects who did not develop new obstructions in their coronary arteries drank more alcohol than those subjects who did develop new obstructions.

In my opinion, there is enough evidence to support the concept that mild to moderate alcohol intake will lower overall mortality in men and cardiovascular mortality in both sexes. Heavy alcohol consumption is detrimental to good health, no matter who you are.

3. How does alcohol reduce cardiovascular mortality?

And

4. Does red wine have special properties that other forms of alcohol don't have?

There are several possible mechanisms whereby alcohol may favorably affect coronary risk. One mechanism is through HDL-cholesterol, but this is controversial. Most studies show that alcohol will raise HDL. A few studies show no increase in the ratio of HDL to total cholesterol. There is even controversy about the fraction of HDL that alcohol increases. Some studies have shown that the type of HDL that increases after alcohol is not the type of HDL that is active in protecting the arteries. Other studies do show an increase in useful HDL after alcohol intake.

Another premise is that alcohol interferes with clotting and platelet stickiness. This was the conclusion of a French study from their equivalent of our National Institutes of Health (INSERM). Another French study showed beneficial effects on inhibiting platelet stickiness from *red* wine, but not from white wine or other alcohol. These same researchers also found that red wine had a stronger enhancing effect on HDL-cholesterol than either white wine or other alcohol.

As discussed earlier, the French have a much lower rate of coronary disease than would be expected from their saturated fat intake and smoking habits. They do drink a lot of red wine, especially with meals. Some would argue that the red wine with a relaxed meal is an antistress strategy that helps lower their risk.

Another possibility is that the red wine contains something special that is protective. The search for these special ingredients has now centered on compounds found in the skin of the grapes used to make the red wine. The substance or substances are most likely bioflavonoids. These bioflavonoids have been shown to act on the liver to block cholesterol production, similar to the drugs like lovastatin, pravastatin, and simvastatin. They also exhibit a powerful antiplatelet stickiness action that protects from clotting. These same bioflavonoids are also found in nonalcoholic grape juice, so there is an alternative for abstainers.

White wine also contains these bioflavonoids, but at about 10 percent of the level found in red wine. A recent study from northern California showed that white wine drinkers enjoyed a slightly greater protection from coronary disease than red wine drinkers or other alcohol imbibers. This is somewhat opposite to what the French have found and needs to be confirmed.

Still another potential benefit of the bioflavonoids is that they have been shown to have antioxidant capabilities. This has only been demonstrated in the test tube thus far.

In summary, then, wine, probably by virtue of its bioflavonoids and alcohol content, has a beneficial effect on coronary disease. Red wine may be better than white, but there is some evidence that white wine is also helpful.

And, lastly,

5. What to do with all this information?

I'm reminded of a case that one of my colleagues told me about last year. One of his patients, an elderly widower in his seventies, was complaining of not being able to sleep. My colleague, not wanting to prescribe sleeping pills, suggested a brandy or a cocktail at bedtime to relax the gentleman and help him sleep. He had been a teetotaler all his life. He tried it and it worked. In fact, it made him feel so good he began to drink to relax during the day. Within six months, he was a full-blown alcoholic and needed to be hospitalized to withdraw from alcohol. I'll never forget this story, and I do not want to be responsible for anyone becoming addicted to alcohol.

If you don't drink, don't start. There are plenty of other beneficial things you can do to reduce your risk of coronary disease and heart attack. If alcohol does not agree with you or you are an alcoholic who no longer drinks or you choose not to drink for religious or moral reasons, or for any other reason for that matter, that's OK—**do not start to drink alcohol**. If you enjoy a little alcohol and it is no problem for you, **don't feel guilty about averaging one or two drinks per day**. Drinking more than that will not improve your overall survival and it may contribute to your early demise. I believe the French may have something to teach us about enjoying life. I enjoy a little wine with my dinner. I am not prejudiced against either red or white wine—I enjoy both.

Remember that alcohol consumption can aggravate high blood pressure and high triglycerides. **If you have either of these problems and you are now consuming alcohol, I would advise you to stop drinking alcohol** and see what happens to the triglycerides and the blood pressure. If they improve off alcohol, don't drink—drinking alcohol will increase your risk of coronary disease and heart attack by raising the blood pressure and/or triglycerides. If you have a cardiac rhythm disturbance, alcohol can make it worse (so can caffeine and nicotine). Stop the alcohol and see what happens. Remember, moderation is the secret.

One last word about women and alcohol. There has been some suggestion that women who drink moderately have an increased risk of breast cancer. Recent studies have shown that alcohol increases estrogen blood levels in pre-menopausal women and that this may be the mechanism by which alcohol increases the risk of breast cancer. In the pre-menopausal years when estrogen is already present, women are at a lower risk of coronary heart disease anyway. Pre-menopausal women probably won't derive as much overall benefit from alcohol as will men. They will need to take this information into consideration as they formulate their own overall preventive health plan.

12 *Cholesterol*

Cholesterol is a waxy substance manufactured only by animals. There is no cholesterol in the vegetable kingdom. It makes me mad to see labels on greasy, fatty, unhealthy products that say "no cholesterol," as if the product were healthy and good for you. Not everything that is cholesterol-free is healthy, and not everything that contains cholesterol is unhealthy. Fish, which are members of the animal kingdom, have cholesterol and fish is healthy to eat.

As we saw in Part I, the correlation between high cholesterol levels and heart disease is well-documented. The less cholesterol in our diet, the less cholesterol our bodies must get rid of. The less cholesterol we eat, the farther our antioxidants will go to keep the LDL-cholesterol from oxidizing and depositing in our arteries.

CHOLESTEROL AND SATURATED FAT

When cholesterol is packaged with saturated fat, its negative effects are multiplied several fold. Since almost all animal fats are saturated, whenever animal flesh is eaten, all visible fat should be trimmed away. This includes chicken and turkey skin and the "hidden" fowl fat, the little globs of greasy yellow and white fat that are concealed in the crevices of the meat. For chicken and turkey, the best choice is the breast, with all visible fat and skin removed. For beef, it is flank steak with all visible fat removed.

The more saturated fat we eat, the higher we will drive our serum cholesterol and LDL-cholesterol. The saturated fat will block production of the receptors that remove cholesterol from the bloodstream. Because it is the combination of saturated fat and cholesterol that is so toxic, you can't look at one without the other.

William E. Connor, M.D., and his wife, Sonja L. Connor, M.S., R.D., have written two very important books that make this concept very easy to understand—*The New American Diet* and *The New American Diet System* (Simon and Schuster). They developed the CSI or Cholesterol Saturated Fat Index to take into consideration both of these factors. Their books will help you choose the foods with the lowest cholesterol and saturated fat content. Plus, there are some terrific, healthy recipes in both books.

HOW MUCH CHOLESTEROL SHOULD YOU EAT IN A DAY?

The answer to this question depends on who you are and what you want to accomplish. Many cardiologists will tell you that if they had coronary disease, they would become vegetarians. Since cholesterol is found only in animal products, a true vegetarian diet would contain no cholesterol. Many people call themselves vegetarians, but what they really mean is that they eat no animal flesh. People who eat dairy products and eggs are called lacto-ovalo vegetarians.

The diet that will have the most power in reducing LDL-cholesterol is a cholesterol-free diet. This could include egg whites and nonfat dairy products. Reversal of coronary artery disease is most likely with the lowest intake of cholesterol and fat. This will cause the greatest reduction in LDL-cholesterol. The lower the LDL, the more likely reversal.

What you take in with your cholesterol is just as important as how much cholesterol you take in. As I mentioned above, the combination of saturated fat and cholesterol is unhealthy, whereas fish oils plus cholesterol appear to be a healthy combination. This is true even though fish contains the same amount of cholesterol per pound as does beef, chicken, turkey, veal, or pork. However, beef, chicken, turkey, veal, and pork contain saturated fat, while fish contains omega-3 fatty acids. Omega-3 fatty acids are polyunsaturated and can be healthy if accompanied by enough protective antioxidants (polyunsaturated fatty acids are very susceptible to oxidation).

Whole milk, whole milk yogurt, butter, cheese, cream, sour cream, whipping cream, and cream cheese all contain cholesterol and saturated fat and should be highly limited or totally eliminated from the diet. Nonfat dairy products have most of the fat and cholesterol removed and are acceptable in your heart-healthy diet.

It is interesting to note that milk consumption is lower in the Mediterranean countries and they have the lowest incidence of coronary disease. France and England have similar fat consumption, but the English drink more milk and have more heart disease. In Japan, where milk consumption is extremely low, Japanese males have a low incidence of coronary disease, despite heavy cigarette smoking and much high blood pressure. The Greenland Eskimos eat lots of fish and drink essentially no milk and have almost no coronary heart disease. And, just to show you that it's not an easy matter to figure out, the United Kingdom has the second lowest meat consumption in the European community and the second highest coronary heart disease rate, while Greece has the highest red meat consumption and one of the lowest rates of coronary heart disease. Perhaps it's the olive oil, garlic intake, and the exclusion of milk products in the Greek diet that gives them their protection. In addition, the meat that I saw when I visited Greece was extremely lean.

Even if you do everything else right, the amount of cholesterol you eat will influence your blood LDL-cholesterol level. A recent study showed that healthy men who exercised, limited their saturated fat intake, and limited their total fat intake, still raised their LDL-cholesterol when dietary cholesterol increased from 200 to 600 mg per day. In some cases, the LDL was raised by more than 25 percent.

RESEARCH

Another study from Germany showed that individuals who ate meat or sausage daily had average cholesterol levels of 242 for men and 255 for women. Those who ate meat and sausage less than once per week had average cholesterol values of 218 for men and 205 for women. The HDL-cholesterol levels were not different.

To control serum cholesterol, you need to limit meat and saturated animal fats. Vegetarianism takes this to the extreme and is a viable alternative if you have significant coronary disease and you want to maximize your chances of reversing or halting the build-up of plaque in your arteries.

Additional studies demonstrate that when exercise and saturated fat intake are held constant, and cholesterol intake is raised from 200 to 600 mg per day, the LDL-cholesterol will rise on the average about 10 percent. The response will vary from individual to individual, ranging from a high of about 25 percent increase in LDL to even a slight fall in LDL in an occasional person. The point is that some people are more sensitive to dietary cholesterol than others. The only way to know for sure how you will respond is to have a blood test after you make a significant dietary change. If you can't or won't do that, the safe thing to do is to eat less cholesterol.

PAINLESS Rx

If you have coronary disease, consider eating a lowfat vegetarian diet like the one Dr. Dean Ornish recommends in his book, Dr. Dean Ornish's Program for Reversing Heart Disease (Random House). The supplements that I told you about in Part II will also be extremely helpful. If you don't have heart disease, but you want to do all that you can to prevent it, you could use a basic lowfat, vegetarian diet and add some fish, nonfat dairy products, and a little olive oil to the program.

This painless prescription is quite palatable and very healthy. I do this, and maybe 4 or 5 times a month I will eat a portion of chicken or turkey breast. Sometimes I will add minced clams to my pasta sauce and when I feel like I need more protein, I eat as many hard boiled egg whites as I want.

DIETARY CHOLESTEROL GUIDELINES

The American Heart Association (AHA) Step 1 diet allows 300 mg of cholesterol a day. I believe that is too much. That translates to about a pound of beef, fish, pork, veal, chicken, or turkey each day. Healthy people do not need that much cholesterol or protein. The Step 2 diet allows 200 mg of cholesterol a day, which I believe is a healthier choice for everyone. Again, if you have heart disease, strongly consider a lowfat, vegetarian diet with maybe six ounces of fish three or four times a week. Any of the Pritikin books or the McDougall books or the Ornish books will tell you the specifics of a very lowfat, extremely low-cholesterol diet.

EGGS

An egg contains between 200 and 250 mg of cholesterol and roughly 6 grams of fat. About half the fat is saturated and half is oleic acid—the same fat that is in olive oil. **All** of the fat and cholesterol are in the yolk. The egg white is pure protein. If you fry the egg in butter, margarine, or bacon grease, you will be adding trans or saturated fat, and this will drive the LDL-cholesterol even higher. Poached, soft- and hard-boiled eggs are healthier. It's the saturated fat that you take in with your egg cholesterol that makes it even less healthy.

Version 1

The good news about eggs is that you can get 98 percent of the good egg taste and be 100 percent cholesterol-free if you just use the egg whites. I make delicious egg-white omelets with mushrooms, onions, green and red pepper, other vegetables, and picante sauce. A little touch of olive oil in the nonstick fry pan and I don't feel the least bit deprived. Try it, you'll like it!

Within the overall limits of cholesterol intake, you can eat eggs (poached, soft-, and hard-boiled). That would mean a maximum of one egg per day with no other animal protein on those days. You would be a lot better off if you only did this one or two days a week and made fish the main source of your animal protein. You can also eat unlimited amounts of hard-boiled egg whites.

Version 2

I love eggs. They are one of my favorite foods. However, for the past twenty-five years I have eschewed egg yolks, limiting myself to egg-white omelets and hard-boiled egg whites. Recently, I have made three important discoveries that have changed my whole perspective on eggs.

The first discovery is the supplement beta-sitosterol, which was described in detail in Part II. The beta-sitosterol prevents the absorption of cholesterol from the intestinal tract. If the cholesterol isn't absorbed, it can't raise the LDL level. Beta-sitosterol can neutralize much of the cholesterol in eggs and other cholesterol-containing foods. Nothing, however, will neutralize saturated fat. It must be drastically reduced and eliminated.

The second discovery is the new eggs that are on the market that have reduced cholesterol and reduced amounts of saturated fat. The egg people have discovered that if they feed the chickens a healthier diet, the chickens will lay healthier eggs. The health-food enthusiasts who only buy their eggs at the health food store have known this for years. These healthier eggs go by different names regionally. In my part of the world, they are called Good News eggs.

A new egg is due out on the market soon that will contain predominantly omega-3 fish oils without any fishy smell. I look forward to this additional healthy egg choice.

The currently available healthier eggs contain a total of about 4 grams of fat, as opposed to 6 grams in the regular eggs. One gram of the fat is saturated, one gram is polyunsaturated, and two grams are monounsaturated. Two grams of saturated fat in two eggs is less than the amount of saturated fat in a 4-ounce serving of canned red salmon. Not perfect, but quite acceptable to an egg lover a couple of times a week. If I fry my egg, I do it in a nonstick pan and use a little bit of olive oil. This further improves the ratio of saturated to monounsaturated fat. On days that I eat eggs for breakfast—I usually eat two eggs—I often do not eat any more animal protein or cholesterol for the rest of the day.

The third and final discovery was that eating these eggs as I have described above, along with the beta-sitosterol, has actually resulted in a fall in my blood cholesterol and LDL-cholesterol level. I feel particularly good about this because I also know that my LDL is well protected from oxidation by the generous amounts of antioxidants that I have in my system.

A recent study from South Africa showed that healthy young men who ate three, seven, or fourteen eggs per week and did not otherwise change their diet had no change or elevation of their blood cholesterol levels over the seven months of the study. In all probability, these subjects were less sensitive to the effects of dietary cholesterol in raising their serum cholesterol. In the study about nuts that we described in the last chapter, Seventh-Day Adventists who ate eggs had no increase in their rate of coronary heart disease.

PAINLESS Rx

I still don't have all the answers. I'm trying to learn as much as I can in order to make my own life healthier and happier. If you are trying to reverse coronary heart disease, you are still better off becoming a vegetarian. Egg yolks would not be part of a vegetarian diet. If you love eggs and you are on a prevention program as I am, you shouldn't feel guilty about eating eggs a couple of times a week in the manner that I have described above.

13 *Protein*

We need protein in our diet. The questions are how much and what kind? We derive a significant amount of protein from animals. However, all animal flesh contains cholesterol and saturated fat. If we reduce the amount of animal flesh, and therefore protein in our diet, we will lower our cholesterol intake, which will lower our serum LDL-cholesterol. Lowering saturated fat intake will also lower LDL.

A recent interesting study compared four groups: (1) pure vegetarians (vegans), (2) vegetarians who also ate dairy products and eggs (lacto-ovalo vegetarians), (3) vegetarians who ate fish but not red meat, and (4) meat eaters. Total and LDL-cholesterol was lowest in the vegans and increased progressively in the lacto-ovalo vegetarians, fish eaters, and meat eaters. Also, the more PUFA and the less SFA in the diet, the lower LDL-cholesterol. They also found that alcohol raised HDL-cholesterol.

The Tarahumara Indians of Mexico eat a diet based on corn and beans, fruits and vegetables, and small amounts of game, fish, and eggs. Coronary disease is extremely rare in the Tarahumara. Researchers from the University of Oregon recruited twelve Tarahumara Indians to look at the effect of the typical unhealthy American diet on their blood values. After just five weeks on the American-style diet, the Indians raised their total cholesterol from 121 to 159. Their LDL went up 39 percent. They also gained an average of more than eight pounds each.

Interestingly, their HDL also went up 31 percent. The LDL to HDL ratio was a little higher (not good) but the absolute level of HDL was higher (good). The increased fat in the diet raised the HDL. The opposite happens when we go on a lowfat, weight-reducing diet—the HDL falls (not good). This is yet another argument for the Mediterranean-type diet that allows olive oil, some animal protein, and restricts saturated fat and cholesterol. Maintaining the HDL levels has very strong protective value.

When cholesterol (not fat) is added to a lowfat diet, the LDL goes up and the HDL stays the same. All these studies combined teach us that: (1) total cholesterol needs to be restricted, (2) both the kind of fat, and (3) the amount of fat eaten is important. A low-cholesterol, lowfat diet where the major fat intake is MUFA or olive oil is best.

RED MEAT

All the answers on red meat are not in yet. For many years, I completely avoided red meat because it is such a rich source of SFA. Recent research, mainly by Dr. Scott Grundy at the Center of Human Nutrition at the University of Texas Southwestern Medical School in Dallas, has shown that beef contains a significant percentage of its fat in the form of stearic acid, a fatty acid that does not raise the LDL level because it does not shut off the production of LDL receptors.

RESEARCH

Dr. Grundy and his coworker, Dr. Margo Denke, conducted their study at the Dallas VA Medical Center. They fed ten men, fifty-one to seventy-two years old who already had high LDL-cholesterol, a diet with 40 percent of the calories from fat. There were four different test diets: butterfat, beef tallow, cocoa butter, and olive oil.

Butterfat raised the LDL-cholesterol the most—to an average of 164. Beef tallow was lower at 156, followed by cocoa butter at 148, and olive oil at 140. Cocoa butter did not raise the LDL as much as beef because cocoa has 35 percent stearic acid and beef tallow only has 22 percent stearic acid. As you can see, butter will drive the LDL up and olive oil will hold the LDL down.

Bottom line on beef:

Some *lean* beef can be incorporated into a healthy diet. The emphasis is on **lean**. Butter should be avoided.

Sources of Lean Red Meat

Remember, even if you find the leanest beef available, the beef is animal protein and contains cholesterol. You will do better if you eat red meat in moderation.

Flank steak that has been trimmed of visible fat is the leanest red meat. A 3-ounce portion contains five grams of fat and about 160 calories, making it about 28 percent fat. (Each gram of fat contains nine calories. Five grams of fat is 45 calories. Forty-five calories is 28 percent of 160 calories). Lean game such as venison, rabbit, elk, moose, and antelope are all in the same ballpark.

According to an article in *U.S. News and World Report* (May, 1992), lean buffalo has only 15 percent of its calories in fat and is becoming more widely available. However, I haven't seen it in the stores yet.

I'm a real fan of the Healthy Choice brand (ConAgra). In my opinion, they have done an outstanding job of producing and making available healthy lowfat, low-calorie, low-cholesterol meals. They have produced extra-lean hamburger meat that comes in a sausage-like roll. It is found next to the ground beef in the supermarket. The fat content is the same as flank steak—28 percent, and it tastes delicious.

If you buy ground hamburger meat in the grocery store, even the so called "lean," it is apt to have over 50 percent of its calories from fat. "Regular" chopped meat will have 50 to 70 percent of its calories from fat—way too much.

Weight Watchers has two lines of frozen meals that I like. One is called "Ultimate 200" and the other is "Smart Ones." All of the items have less than 200 calories per package and the "Smart Ones" have no more than one gram of fat per serving. For lunch today, I had the Ultimate 200 London Broil in mushroom sauce. One hundred ten calories, 25 mg of cholesterol, and one gram of saturated fat. A delicious, lean red-meat meal with about as few calories as you could find in a meal anywhere.

I keep a supply of these Weight Watcher products and Healthy Choice frozen meals in the freezer of the refrigerator in my office. My rule of thumb is that if the meal has fewer than 300 calories and less than five grams of fat (total fat content), then it is acceptable. There are dozens of choices including beef, chicken, shrimp, fish, and turkey. Meals can be ready in about five minutes or less in the office microwave.

CHOCOLATE

Like beef, chocolate contains stearic acid. Stearic acid is a saturated fatty acid that does not raise LDL-cholesterol because it does not shut off production of LDL receptors. Chocolate is high in calories and full of sugar. Don't get me wrong—I love chocolate. After my sojourn with Nathan Pritikin, I totally excluded chocolate from my diet. However, after reading Dr. Grundy's research, I have allowed myself occasional chocolate treats. Thank you, Dr. Grundy.

If you are trying to reverse coronary disease, it is best to forego the chocolate. If you are on a prevention program, an occasional sample of chocolate won't be harmful. If you eat it, don't feel guilty. Enjoy it, and thank Dr. Grundy.

FISH

In this section, I will focus entirely on the effects of eating fish. We have already discussed the use of fish oil supplements in Chapter 9. Obviously, there is a big overlap in that the fish oil supplements are made from edible fish. There are significant differences, however. Just about everyone can benefit from eating more fish. Hardly anyone will need to take fish oil supplements.

About twenty years ago, Scandinavian researchers first noticed that Greenland Eskimos had low death rates from coronary artery disease. Their diet was studied, and it was found that they eat about 14 ounces of fish or whale meat per day, 365 days per year.

The lowered coronary disease rate in the Greenland Eskimos was found **not** to be genetic. Danish Eskimos who eat the standard Danish diet have high coronary disease rates similar to the Danish.

In Japan, where coronary heart disease rates are among the lowest in the world, the average fish consumption is about three and one-half ounces per day, 365 days per year. The very lowest coronary rates in Japan are on the island of Okinawa, where fish consumption is about twice as high as on the Japanese mainland.

In 1985, a landmark study was published in the *New England Journal of Medicine* that showed lower death rates among men who ate an ounce of fish a day over a twenty-year period.

RESEARCH

Professor Kromhout and his colleagues at the University of Leiden in the Netherlands reported on the relationship between fish consumption and coronary heart disease in a group of men in the town of Zutphen, the Netherlands. The unique aspect of this study was that it spanned twenty years. Over this twenty-year period, the death rate from coronary heart disease was more than 50 percent lower in those men who consumed at least 30 grams (about one ounce) of fish per day, 365 days per year, than among those who did not eat fish. They concluded that eating as little as one or two fish dishes per week may be of value in the prevention of coronary disease.

A more recent study showed that in male survivors of heart attack a moderate intake (10 to 11 ounces) of fatty fish per week decreased total mortality by 29 percent. This effect occurred without any reduction in serum cholesterol levels and corroborates the results from Zutphen.

What is it about fish that affords this high-powered protection? Current research suggests that it's the fats and oils in the fish that produce the benefits. These fats are called omega-3 fatty acids and there are two of them: Eicosapentaenoic Acid (EPA), which has five double bonds, and Docosahexenoic Acid (DHA), which has six double bonds. These double bonds make the fish oils polyunsaturated (PUFA), so that when fish and fish oil intake increases, the antioxidants should also be increased to protect these double bonds from oxidation.

How Do Fish Oils Work?

The PUFAs in fish do their major good work in at least two different ways. The first is by lowering the blood's ability to clot. This is done by making the platelets less sticky and reducing fibrinogen, which, in turn, decreases the contribution of clotting to the plaque build-up and also helps prevent the clot that actually causes heart attacks.

The second benefit of the fish oils is in lowering triglycerides. The higher the triglycerides, the more they can be lowered by fish oils. If the triglycerides are seriously elevated, don't count on a few fish meals to correct them. You will have to do more. Weight loss, alcohol restriction, exercise, fat and sugar restriction, L-carnitine, and sometimes drugs will also be needed to lower triglycerides if they are seriously elevated.

A recent study showed that eating fatty fish or taking fish oil supplements had similar benefits on triglycerides and HDL-cholesterol. Fish oil and fish consumption both lowered triglycerides and raised HDL about the same amount. However, eating fatty fish had a more powerful impact on reducing the clotting factors than did fish oil supplements.

Other studies have not been consistent in showing positive changes in the LDL- and HDL-cholesterol with fish and fish oils. Some studies have shown increase and others have shown decreases in both the LDL and HDL.

Researchers from Harvard presented data very damaging to the hypothesis that fish is protective at the 1992 annual meeting of the American Heart Association. Fish intake was examined in over 21,000 men participating in the Physicians' Health Study. This is the same study that has shown benefits from vitamins E and C, beta-carotene, and aspirin. Dr. Hennekens was one of the principal investigators and when Dr. Hennekens speaks, I listen.

There was no benefit and essentially no difference in the number of heart attacks whether one, two to four, or more than five fish meals were eaten each week. If this research had been done by virtually any other investigator, I would tend to discount it, look for some reason not to believe it, or simply say that there was something fishy about it. However, because of the high esteem and regard that I have for Dr. Hennekens, I must now re-think my whole fish hypothesis.

Types of Fish

All fish are not equal. The fish from cold water contain much more fat than fish from warm water. The fat acts as insulation and helps the cold water fish maintain their body temperature. The more fat the fish has, the more potential benefit. The best fish are: salmon, tuna, halibut, sturgeon, cold lake trout, mackerel, sardines, anchovies, bluefish, sable fish, swordfish, and herring. The best sardines are those packed in SILD sardine oil. If you are trying to lose weight, drain off all the SILD sardine oil before eating the sardines. You will still get the good fish oil in the sardines.

Shellfish

Shrimp, crab, lobster, clams, scallops, muscles, and oysters are all low in fat, but do contain cholesterol. There is not much omega-3 fatty acid present. Cooked shellfish, on occasion, can be part of a healthy diet. Raw shellfish should be avoided because of pollution, contaminants, and the risk of hepatitis.

Precautions

Fish oils are polyunsaturated fatty acids (PUFAs), and PUFAs are easily oxidized. For this reason, increased intake of fish and fish oils should always be accompanied by increased antioxidant intake, especially vitamin E.

In one study, fish oil supplementation was shown to reduce the blood levels of vitamin E and weaken the immune system. Another study that showed a weakening of the immune system with fish oil supplementation found that this was totally reversed by vitamin E supplementation (200 IU per day).

None of the studies that showed decreased coronary heart disease mortality from increased fish consumption showed increased cancer mortality or any manifestations of immune system deficiency.

Over twenty years ago, a study at the Los Angeles VA Hospital showed that older men given large doses of corn oil (PUFA) had a lower rate of coronary disease deaths, but had increased cancer death rates. The question of PUFA causing cancer has haunted nutritionists ever since. It may well be that the corn oil weakened the immune system. In the study described above, the older women had the greatest immune weakening when given the PUFA fish oil. This work is still another argument for supplementing our diets with vitamin E and the other antioxidants.

Is Fish Safe?

Consumers Union did the definitive study on our fish supply and published the results of a six-month investigation in *Consumer Reports* (February, 1992). There are two major contaminants of our fish supply: bacteria and industrial toxins.

Bacteria

Consumers Union found that 30 percent of the fish tested was spoiled and another 9 percent was on the verge of spoiling. Nearly half the fish they tested was contaminated by human or animal feces. They got their fish samples from New York City and Chicago.

The good news is that the bacteria are killed by cooking. If the fish smells real fishy, chances are its bacterial count is high. A faint "seaweed" aroma is OK, but if it smells strong, sour, or like ammonia, chances are the bacteria count is high and you should pass it up.

Toxins

The *Consumer Reports* article explains:

> The waters where fish live are often dumping grounds for potentially harmful chemicals that have been on land.
>
> Once in water, these substances make their way into the sediments at the bottom and into aquatic plants and animals at the base of the food chain. Little fish eat plants and little animals, bigger fish eat the little fish, and so on up the food chain. Fish also absorb these substances directly from water that passes over their gills. Older fish, predatory fish, and fatty species of fish accumulate more such substances in their tissues than younger, smaller, or leaner ones do.

> Although the Environmental Protection Agency banned polychlorinated biphenyls (PCBs) and most chlorinated hydrocarbon pesticides in the 1970's, some residues that were released into the environment before these compounds were banned still remain. They do not decompose easily, so they linger in the water sediments and in the tissues of fish and humans for years.

Mercury. According to the article:

> Mercury is a poisonous metallic element that is released by burning fuels as well as by industrial and household wastes. Eventually it settles in waterways and oceans where it joins naturally occurring mercury. There, bacteria convert it to the toxic compound methylmercury.
>
> Methylmercury is a poison that affects the development of the nervous system. Unlike PCBs, which linger in the fatty tissues of humans for many years, mercury eventually leaves the body, usually within two years, provided you stop ingesting it.
>
> Mercury accumulates in large fish that live a long time, such as tuna, shark, and swordfish. Almost all of the mercury in fish is the compound methylmercury. The FDA has set an informal action level of 1 part per million for methylmercury in fish.
>
> Ninety percent of our swordfish samples had detectable levels of total mercury, ranging from 0.46 to 2.4 parts per million. The average of those samples was 1.14 parts per million. Forty percent contained mercury that exceeded the action level.
>
> The high levels of mercury we found in swordfish are not surprising, since mercury is present in oceans through-

out the world. There's no way to prevent swordfish from accumulating it in their tissues.

Since the *Consumer Reports* article was published, other reports have attested to continued pollution of our fish supply. The Great Lakes are full of PCB and, in my opinion, fish from the Great Lakes are not fit for human consumption. Swordfish are so highly contaminated with mercury that they should not be eaten. Pregnant women, nursing mothers, and young children should limit their fish intake because infants and developing children are extremely sensitive to these toxins. According to *Consumer Reports*, flounder and sole are virtually free of pollutants (they are not high in omega-3 fatty acids, however).

The bright side is canned tuna. The tuna does contain some mercury, but even if you ate a six-and-one-half ounce can every day, you would not ingest toxic amounts of mercury. Tuna fish is a great source of the healthy fish oils. For the past twenty years, tuna has been the most frequently eaten fish in this country. The average American consumer eats about ten six-and-one-half ounce cans each year.

Natural fish toxins. Ciguatera is a disease caused by toxins produced from fish eating on coral reefs. It occurs mainly in the Caribbean, South Pacific, Hawaii, and Florida. The fish most often associated with ciguatera are amber jack, barracuda, snapper, grouper, and goat fish.

Tuna, bluefish, and marlin have been associated with scombroid fish poisoning. This poisoning is caused by toxins produced from bacterial contamination and it is not abolished by cooking.

Shellfish poisoning comes from polluted shellfish—usually oysters, mussels, clams, and scallops. Raw shellfish are potentially dangerous and should not be eaten because of the risk of hepatitis.

Bottom line on fish:

Fish is one of the healthiest forms of animal protein. As little as two or three fish meals per week have been associated with decreased risk of developing coronary disease and decreased mortality after a heart attack. The Harvard study notwithstanding, I encourage you to incorporate fish into your diet.

A Favorite Recipe

The omega-3 fatty acids in fish will reduce platelet stickiness and retard clotting just like garlic and onion. Tuna fish packed in water is extremely low in fat and almost all the fat present is omega-3 fatty acids. Tuna is one of the best sources of omega-3 fatty acids. I make a tuna fish salad in my food processor. I put in a drained six-and-one-half ounce can of water-packed white albacore tuna, a thick slice of onion, a clove of garlic, a big teaspoon of Kraft Free Mayonnaise or Kraft Free Miracle Whip, one or two teaspoons of sweet pickle relish and process. When the concoction is about 80 percent processed, I add two hard-boiled egg whites and process a little more. I stop before the egg white pieces get too small. If you want it to be more moist, don't drain the tuna—use the water it is packed in as part of the recipe. This is an inexpensive, high-protein, lowfat, healthy, clot-preventing, cholesterol-lowering dish that is really tasty. Try it. You'll like it.

FOWL

All the fat in chicken and turkey is saturated fat and will raise LDL-cholesterol. Dark meat has more fat than white meat. The skin is very fatty and should always be removed along with all visible fat. **Skinless chicken breast and turkey breast is the best**. Ground turkey will often contain skin, raising its fat content. There is no advantage to ground turkey over Healthy Choice lean ground beef or ground flank steak. More often than not the Healthy Choice will have less fat than the ground turkey. Duck is too fatty. When you are at a restaurant, ordering a skinless, boneless, broiled chicken breast is usually a healthy option. A breast of turkey sandwich with mustard is another healthy option.

VEGETABLE PROTEIN SOURCES

Despite what you might have learned, complete protein can be made from pure vegetable sources. It's not nearly as efficient as from animal sources, but the resultant protein is just as good. Several million Americans call themselves vegetarians. Numerous studies have been done with Seventh-Day Adventists, many of whom are vegetarians for religious reasons. When Seventh-Day Adventist vegetarians are compared to their non-vegetarian counterparts, they are found to have lower LDL-cholesterol, lower triglycerides, lower blood pressures, less diabetes, and fewer heart attacks. A lowfat vegetarian diet can not only prevent coronary disease, it can be a powerful tool in reversing it.

Dr. Dean Ornish used an extremely lowfat vegetarian diet along with stress-reduction techniques to reverse coronary heart disease. A lowfat vegetarian diet means essentially no saturated fat and no cholesterol in the diet. These two factors will result in marked reductions in LDL-cholesterol, which will facilitate regression of the atherosclerotic plaque.

Vegetarian diets often will include liberal amounts of soy protein, which in itself has been shown to lower LDL-cholesterol and triglycerides. The soy protein contains vegetable sterols, like beta-sitosterol, which have been shown to help lower serum cholesterol levels (see Chapter 9). Whole grains (rice, wheat, barley, corn, buckwheat, millet, oats, rye, etc.) and legumes (peas, beans, lentils) will do the same thing as long as saturated fat and cholesterol are removed from the diet.

I am not now a vegetarian. I was a pure vegetarian for almost a year. My cholesterol fell to below 150, but I did not feel good on this diet. It's not for everyone. Adding small amounts of fish to my diet several times a week greatly improved my well-being. Today, I eat no animal products two or three days per week, fish two or three days per week, and chicken, turkey, or lean red meat one or two days per week. If I developed heart disease, I would once again become a pure vegetarian—only this time I would supplement my diet with cooked egg whites (cholesterol-free and saturated-fat free, high-quality protein) and I would take the supplements outlined in Part II, especially the antioxidants.

If you want to read a compelling argument for vegetarianism, try John Robbins' (the son of the founder of the Baskin Robbins ice cream chain) *Diet for a New America*. Just looking at the pictures in the book may be enough to convince you to become a vegetarian.

Dr. Ornish's books, the Pritikin books, the McDougall books, and *The New American Diet* books (by the Connors—not to be confused with the Robbins book) will all be helpful if you decide to move in the direction of vegetarianism by cutting back on your animal protein, cholesterol, and saturated fat.

14 *Carbohydrates, Sugar, and Fiber*

CARBOHYDRATES

Carbohydrate is the basic energy burned in the body. Carbohydrates come in different sizes, shapes, and forms and are totally free of fat and cholesterol. When chosen correctly, they may form the backbone of a heart-healthy diet.

Fruits, vegetables, sugars, grains, potatoes, yams, beans, and peas are all carbohydrates. There are basically two kinds of carbohydrates: simple sugars and complex carbohydrates. Complex carbohydrates are simple sugars that have been polymerized or attached to each other. Sugar is the basic fuel our bodies burn. Complex carbohydrates are time-released energy. The simple sugar in fruit and fruit juice is what may raise the triglycerides in some people. Simple sugars get into the bloodstream too fast and make the insulin go up too high. Since excess insulin is associated with an accelerated rate of atherosclerotic plaque formation, it is best to limit sugar intake and eat more complex carbohydrates, which do not raise insulin levels.

Fruits and Vegetables

You can improve your level of health by simply increasing your intake of fruits and vegetables. Fruits and vegetables are major sources of fiber and minerals such as potassium and magnesium. Low blood levels of potassium and magnesium have been associated with sudden death when a heart attack strikes. Increasing the fiber content of the diet has been shown to lower LDL-cholesterol levels. Whole grains are also a good source of fiber in the diet.

The National Cancer Institute has begun to investigate plant compounds that might prove to prevent or retard cancer. Cabbage, broccoli, cauliflower, and brussel sprouts appear to exert protective effects against cancer of the large intestine and maybe against cancer of the lung, prostate, stomach, breast, and esophagus as well. Celery, carrots, parsley, coriander, garlic, and onions have also been shown to reduce cancer risk. Lowfat, high-fiber diets also afford protection from cancer.

The more vegetables you eat, the more weight you will lose. This is so because the vegetables are not calorie dense. They contain a lot of water instead of calories. If you are overweight, losing weight will decrease your coronary risk. A good strategy is to eat more salad. A big salad before lunch and supper will fill you up with the fewest calories. Be sure to use nonfat salad dressing. The Kraft-Free line of salad dressings are essentially free of fat and cholesterol and are the tastiest reduced calorie dressings I have put in my mouth. The Pritikin line of salad dressings is healthier, lower in fat, but not as tasty to me.

If you have high blood pressure and you increase your intake of fruits and vegetables and in the process you lose a little weight, your blood pressure will come down. The weight loss plus the increased intake of potassium and magnesium in the vegetables are two of the most potent natural measures to attack and lower high blood pressure.

Precautions

If you are not overweight, eating huge quantities of vegetables will cause you to lose too much weight. A good alternative for people who are already slender is to increase your intake of whole grains and legumes. Like vegetables, whole grains (wheat, rye, barley, corn, millet, oats, buckwheat) and legumes (beans, lentils, peas) are fat-free, cholesterol-free, and loaded with minerals and fiber.

Another precaution is that drastically increasing your vegetable intake may cause gas. Raw broccoli and cauliflower are particularly bothersome to many people. If these vegetables are cooked, they become more digestible and cause less gas.

The only precaution about fruit is that in some people with high triglyceride levels, eating more than two pieces of fruit per day will raise the triglycerides even further. The same is true for diabetics. Excess fruit will elevate the blood sugar levels. Fruit juices will act the same way. So, if you have high triglycerides or diabetes, limit fruit intake to two per day and stay away from fruit juice.

Other Carbohydrates

Vegetables, grains, potatoes, beans, and peas are all excellent complex carbohydrate sources. The *Nutrition Action Health Letter* rated fifty-eight different vegetables based on their vitamin, mineral, and fiber content. The winner of the healthiest vegetable contest was the sweet potato. A medium large sweet potato (or yam) can be cooked in the microwave in under twenty minutes. It is one of the healthiest, most delicious snacks I know of and I cook one several times each week in my office microwave.

A diet based on complex carbohydrates will be low in saturated fat and cholesterol and will be helpful in preventing and reversing heart disease. Several times each week, I will cook brown rice or millet in my rice cooker at home. The automatic warmer keeps it warm overnight. A bowl of hot rice or millet for breakfast is a nice variation on the hot cereal routine. I'll then put the remainder of the rice or millet in a plastic container and take it to the office where I snack on it all day long. No fat, no cholesterol, complex carbohydrate for energy, and plenty of fiber—who could ask for anything more? Because it is extremely low in fat, you can pretty much eat all that you want and you won't gain weight.

The high complex carbohydrate foods are low in fat as long as you don't adulterate them with butter or margarine. If you need the buttery flavor, try Molly McButter. It's in the spice section of the grocery store and it only has four calories per serving. It tastes like butter and it is fat free. Great for anything you would put butter on. There is a sour cream and a cheese flavor that is delicious on baked potatoes.

PAINLESS Rx

As I said earlier, after almost forty years of trying to learn how to keep myself slender, it all boils down to two things: don't eat fat, and exercise regularly.

Pasta

Just the mention of the word pasta makes my mouth start to water. I could eat Italian food every day, and I often do. Pasta of all kinds topped with marinara sauce or made with olive oil and garlic is my idea of culinary paradise. Two brands of truly delicious lowfat pasta sauces are now available on the shelves of your supermarket. Ragu has a product line called *Today's Recipe*. These sauces have only one gram of fat and it is olive oil. Healthy Choice also has a delicious no-fat-added spaghetti sauce. They are both tasty and healthy.

Pasta, rice and other whole grains, and beans and peas are the backbone of a lowfat, low-cholesterol diet that can be very helpful in halting or reversing coronary artery disease.

SUGAR

Sugar will definitely raise triglyceride levels, but can it do other things to promote coronary heart disease? The answer is yes. As the triglycerides go up, HDL-cholesterol goes down, and you've lost some protection. The more sugar you eat, the more insulin you will produce to utilize the sugar. Insulin is a promoter of coronary heart disease—another strike against you. Other studies have shown a rise in LDL-cholesterol when sugar intake is increased. Three strikes, you're out! Eliminate as much sugar as possible from your diet. This includes fructose, which may even be worse than glucose or sucrose.

Dr. John Yudkin, an English physician, first postulated that sugar was in a large part responsible for coronary heart disease in his book, *Sweet and Dangerous*, in 1972. After twenty years of research, Dr. Yudkin hasn't changed his mind one iota. In fact, he is even more convinced. In a 1992 editorial in the *Journal of the Royal Society of Medicine,* Dr. Yudkin argues that sugar can produce all the findings that are found in coronary heart disease, including an increase in platelet stickiness. He asks, "Why blame fat?"

What's the answer? Sugar definitely plays an important role. By eating more whole foods and eliminating refined sugar, sucrose, glucose, and fructose, we will lower our risk of coronary heart disease.

The next question is: are artificial sweeteners healthy?

I can't answer that question with authority. My intuition tells me that both saccharin (Sweet'n Low) and aspartame (Equal and NutraSweet) are not that good for me. The science and the research do not support my intuition. I use the artificial sweeteners in moderation and that is my recommendation to you.

FIBER

Fiber is extremely important in achieving and maintaining good health. Not only will a high-fiber diet lower your LDL-cholesterol and reduce your risk of coronary heart disease, it will also lower your risk of colon cancer, hemorrhoids, varicose veins, and gallstones. If you have diabetes, additional fiber in your diet will often improve diabetic control and lower blood sugar.

Fiber can change your life. Fiber will often correct constipation and gas, inflammatory bowel disease, diverticulitis, and spastic colon. The fibers do their good work by adding bulk to the intestine and binding to substances and carrying them outside the body in the bowel movement. That's what dietary fiber does to cholesterol.

Fiber is a complex carbohydrate composed of many small simple sugar molecules that are joined together. However, these molecules cannot be broken down by digestive enzymes in the intestinal tract. Instead, they pass through the intestine and out in the bowel movement. Sometimes, bacterial enzymes from the bacteria in our large intestine will act on the fiber and partially break it down. When this happens, gas is formed, and I don't have to tell you what happens next.

Some cholesterol-lowering drugs bind to intestinal cholesterol in exactly the same way as the dietary fiber. These drugs, colestipol and cholestyramine, have both been used in studies that document regression of coronary artery disease. Although dietary fiber is not as potent as these drugs, it is much less expensive and you don't need a prescription from your doctor to use it.

Addition of modest amounts of fiber to your diet can lower your LDL-cholesterol 5 to 10 percent and substantially reduce your risk of coronary heart disease.

Types of Fiber

Basically, there are two types of fiber: soluble and insoluble. This refers to whether or not the fiber dissolves in water.

Soluble Fiber

Soluble fiber is fiber that dissolves in water. Oat bran, barley, psyllium, pectin, and guava and locust bean gums are all examples of soluble fiber.

Oat bran. A much-publicized study in the *New England Journal of Medicine* in 1990 purported to show that oat bran did not in and of itself lower cholesterol, but that it was the saturated fat that was eliminated from the diet and replaced by the oat bran that gave the cholesterol-lowering benefit.

A more recent study published in the *Journal of the American Medical Association* concluded in a meta-analysis of twenty studies that incorporating oat products into the diet causes a modest reduction in blood cholesterol levels.

A bowl of hot oatmeal for breakfast is an excellent way of increasing oat bran in your diet. But don't forget the *New England Journal of Medicine* article, either. Lowering your saturated fat intake is just as powerful a tool for lowering your blood LDL-cholesterol level as increasing the oat products in your diet. The combination of a lowfat, high-fiber diet is the best choice possible.

Barley is another whole grain that provides substantial amounts of soluble fiber. Increased barley intake has also been shown to lower LDL-cholesterol.

Psyllium. Several years ago, Kellogg introduced a cold cereal product called Heartwise. It was a high-fiber cereal containing psyllium (a soluble cereal grain fiber), oat bran, and whole wheat. Because numerous studies have shown that ingesting psyllium will lead to significant fall in LDL-cholesterol, Kellogg thought the name, Heartwise, was appropriate. The Texas attorney-general, however, thought the name implied an unfounded health claim, and Heartwise cereal was banned in Texas. Kellogg later changed the name to Fiberwise, but for several years it was not available in Texas. I had friends in Florida and Oklahoma send me a case of Fiberwise every six to eight weeks. It was my family's favorite cold cereal. Just when it had reappeared on the Texas grocery shelves, it disappeared again. The Texas attorney-general won out after all.

The long absence from the grocery shelves did in my favorite cereal. Kellogg's has another cereal, Bran Buds, which is a good substitute and which contains wheat bran and psyllium.

I find the psyllium less gassy than oats and the cholesterol lowering power is just as great. Psyllium is also available as Metamucil and Serutan in the drugstore and numerous psyllium products are available in the health food store.

It's worth noting that a very small number of people, especially nurses and people who work with psyllium dust, may develop an allergy to psyllium. Violent reactions have been reported.

Pectin. Pectin is a soluble fiber that comes from fruits and vegetables. Research so far has been mainly limited to animals, but we may be hearing more about pectin in the near future. In rats, pectin reduced colon cancer by 50 percent and reduced cholesterol levels by 25 to 30 percent. In addition, pectin has been shown to reduce platelet stickiness and decrease clotting. In guinea pigs, addition of pectin to the diet will lower serum cholesterol levels even when the animals are on a high cholesterol diet. One of the best sources of dietary pectin is apples. The old adage: "An apple a day will keep the doctor away," may have more substance than you ever imagined.

Guava and locust bean gums. These plant sources of soluble fiber have been shown to bind cholesterol in the intestine and lower serum cholesterol levels.

Insoluble Fiber

Insoluble fiber does not dissolve in water. Whole grains such as wheat, corn, rye, and rice are sources of insoluble fibers in the diet. Vegetables are also included in this category of fibers. The insoluble fibers add bulk to the bowel movement and reduce constipation and bowel diseases such as diverticulitis and hemorrhoids. The insoluble fibers are more strongly associated with decreased risk of colon cancer than soluble fiber. However, these insoluble bulking agents do not bind cholesterol in the intestine and carry it out of the body like the soluble fibers do. Brown rice, because of its rice bran oil, may result in lower levels of serum cholesterol, but the other insoluble fibers do not.

Insoluble fibers are healthy and should be incorporated into the diet along with soluble fiber. Whole grains and vegetables are your ticket to colon health and decreased cancer risk.

A recent article in the *Journal of the National Cancer Institute* titled "Evidence of Protective Effects of Wheat Fiber Grows" reported on the decreased potential risk of colon cancer as well as that of breast cancer when wheat fiber is regularly added to the diet. Millers wheat bran is available in the health food store and can be sprinkled on your salad, added to oat cereal or incorporated into other recipes. Kellogg's All-Bran and Bran Buds, General Mills' Fiber One, and Nabisco's 100% Bran are all excellent sources of wheat bran. If you make bran muffins, be sure and substitute olive oil for whatever fat/margarine/oil is called for in the recipe and bake at under 390 degrees (the smoke point of olive oil).

You could eat oat and wheat bran cereals on alternate days or you could mix them together. Some researchers recommend taking Metamucil as a dietary supplement not only to reduce constipation but to increase soluble fiber intake and lower serum cholesterol. Increasing whole grains—brown rice, oats, barley, and wheat—vegetables, and beans and peas in your diet is the natural, healthy way to do it.

Beans and Peas

Beans and peas cause gas because their fiber cannot be broken down and digested in the upper intestine. These fibers make it to the large intestine where they meet up with bacterial enzymes that are able to partially digest them. Gas is liberated in the process. Beans and peas are an excellent source of lowfat, no-cholesterol, high-fiber, high-protein food. Incorporating more beans and peas into your diet will be good for your heart.

Precautions

If you drastically increase your fiber intake all at once, you will in all likelihood fall victim to intestinal distention and excess gas. So, start slowly and gradually add extra fiber to your diet to minimize this potential side effect. Remember, extra fiber intake requires extra fluid intake to keep the bulk moving through the intestine.

Fiber and Diabetes

Dr. James W. Anderson, a professor of medicine at the University of Kentucky College of Medicine, has been using high-fiber, high-carbohydrate diet in the management of diabetes since 1974. He has found that many diabetic patients (both Type I and Type II) will have better glucose control on a high-fiber, high-carbohydrate, lowfat diet. In addition, this diet will often lower serum cholesterol levels, a problem that is all too common in diabetes.

Dr. Scott Grundy at the Center for Human Nutrition at the University of Texas Southwestern Medical School in Dallas has observed that many of the diabetics who are not benefitted by the high-carbohydrate, high-fiber diet will be benefitted by a

Mediterranean-type diet. By increasing the monounsaturated fat (olive oil) in the diet, the blood sugar and blood cholesterol will be better controlled.

Italian researchers from the University of Naples have shown that a diet high in soluble fiber (beans, peas, vegetables, fruits) in conjunction with monounsaturated fats (e.g., olive oil) will be of the greatest benefit to diabetic patients.

Oat Bran and Niacin

A few years ago, Robert E. Kowalski wrote a bestselling book called *The 8-Week Cholesterol Cure*, in which he advocated the use of oat bran and niacin. Both of these agents have been shown to be helpful in lowering serum cholesterol. Researchers at the University of Minnesota wanted to know if the combination of niacin and oat bran was synergistic. In other words, would the combination of the two agents do more than would be expected from the independent action of each agent? They confirmed that oat bran and niacin were both helpful and in about **10 percent** of the ninety-eight patients they studied, there was, in fact, a synergistic benefit from using the two together.

Therapeutic use of niacin to lower LDL-cholesterol and raise HDL-cholesterol requires monitoring liver functions with blood tests. Niacin can cause liver toxicity and in my opinion, **niacin should not be used except under the supervision of a physician**. Niacin may also worsen diabetes and gout. So, for now, go ahead and add the fiber to your diet, but **don't start niacin without your doctor's supervision.**

15 *Coffee, Tea, and Salt*

COFFEE

When I first made my outline for this book, I did not include coffee as a substance that needed to be addressed. I did not believe that it played an important role in coronary disease. As I began to review the medical literature on coronary heart disease, however, I saw a few articles on coffee and cholesterol. The paper that really got my attention was by Dr. Robert Superko at Stanford. He found that decaffeinated coffee raised LDL-cholesterol levels and caffeinated coffee did not. I thought this was a little strange, so I pursued the issue further. Dr. Superko explained that two different types of coffee beans are generally used in preparing caffeinated and decaffeinated coffee sold in the U.S. Arabica beans, which are mild, are usually used for caffeinated coffee, whereas the stronger, cheaper robust beans are used for decaf. In addition, the decaffeination process, with the exception of the European water method, uses volatile chemicals which may be in trace amounts in the decaf. At any rate, in this study, caffeine was not the culprit because it was the decaf that caused the elevation of LDL.

However, another study done at Johns Hopkins in Baltimore showed that filtered, caffeinated coffee leads to an increase in total cholesterol. The LDL goes up about twice as much as the HDL. Since the HDL is twice as effective in preventing coronary disease as LDL is in causing coronary disease, the changes cancel each other out. The authors conclude that coffee should not affect coronary risk.

The Johns Hopkins study used filtered coffee. This is important. A study from Finland and a Dutch study both showed that filtering the coffee removed whatever it is in the coffee that is responsible for raising the cholesterol.

In Italy, where most of the coffee is filtered, the more coffee consumed, the higher the total cholesterol. In Austria, there was no relationship between coffee drinking and cholesterol.

Are you confused? So was I, but I wanted to try to get to the bottom of this, so I kept on reading.

Coffee and Risk of Coronary Heart Disease

In one study, men who drank five or more cups of coffee per day had double the risk for heart disease and men who drank ten or more cups of coffee a day had a threefold risk. Another study in 45,000 Dutch men showed no link between coffee and heart disease. Still another Swedish study showed little or no adverse effect of coffee.

Coffee and Blood Pressure

I found several studies that examined the effects of coffee drinking on blood pressure. The effect is not great. At most there is a slight transient increase in blood pressure immediately after drinking the coffee with caffeine. This would make a difference if you were drinking coffee all day long.

What Should You Put in the Coffee?

Nonfat skim milk is the best whitener for your coffee if you choose to whiten it. The "lite" nondairy creamers, such as Cremora-lite and Coffeemate-lite, have taken most of the fat out and are acceptable, even though they do have a lot of additives and some fat. More than a few teaspoons a day could add up to quite a bit of fat.

What to use for a sweetener is a tough problem. I'm against white sugar, and I'm not sure the artificial sweeteners are entirely healthy, so it's a real dilemma for me. Honey, brown sugar, and molasses are a compromise, but they don't taste as good or as sweet. My solution to this problem is to use them all. I rotate. In this way, I won't get too much of whatever it is that is not good in any of them. I use raw or brown sugar, honey, Sweet'n Low, NutraSweet, and very rarely white sugar. The healthy alternative is to forego the sweetener all together, but this requires re-education of your taste buds and isn't easy.

Bottom line on coffee:

Since high coffee consumption may be associated with increased blood cholesterol, increased blood pressure, and increased coronary heart disease risk, it is best to limit your coffee intake to a maximum of two cups per day. Filtering the coffee will very probably remove whatever it is in the coffee that raises cholesterol. If you have uncontrolled hypertension or heart rhythm disturbances, I would stop coffee and all caffeine. Many people who are addicted to caffeine find they feel much better and entirely more relaxed when they stop it. If you stop caffeine, there is a good chance you will get a withdrawal headache. Whatever you use to treat the headache, it will be gone in a day or two.

TEA

There are only a few studies on the relationship of drinking black tea to cholesterol and coronary heart disease risk. Like coffee, regular black tea contains caffeine. Herbal tea and decaffeinated teas do not.

Green Tea

Green tea has been in the news lately because of studies showing that it can prevent cancer. This anticancer activity is probably due to its bioflavonoid content. Bioflavonoids account for about 30 percent of the dry weight of green tea leaves. Long before the health benefits of green tea were known, I began drinking it on a regular basis because I like the taste. You can find it in the oriental section of your grocery store or organic green teas are available in the health food store. Also, Twinlab makes a product called Wine & Tea Polyphenols, which is a concentrate of the bioflavonoids found in green tea and red wine. Some people are allergic, so go slowly if you decide to try this product.

Look for more research on the healthful benefits of green tea in the near future.

SALT

Not everyone needs to restrict salt. The main heart condition that responds to salt restriction is congestive heart failure (CHF). CHF is the result of a weakened heart muscle and this results in salt and fluid retention. One of the main treatments for CHF is diuretics. Diuretics force the kidneys to get rid of salt. Not eating salt would make the work of the diuretics much easier and maybe decrease the need for diuretics altogether.

Somewhere between 30 and 50 percent of the population have blood pressures that are sensitive to salt. So 50 percent to 70 percent of people with high blood pressure will **not** respond to salt restriction. If you are one of the 30 to 50 percent who are sensitive to salt and you are overweight, you have the best chance of correcting your blood pressure with weight loss and salt restriction. When exercise is added to this regimen, it is the best proven natural treatment for hypertension.

Part IV

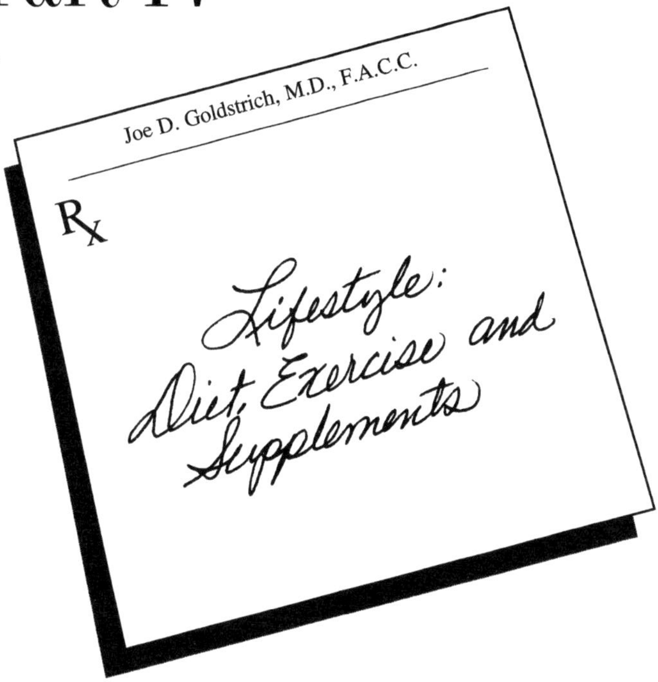

In the final analysis, the lifestyle that we adopt will determine our success or failure in preventing or reversing heart disease. To me, lifestyle means how I live my life on a day-to-day basis. It means having a set of guidelines to follow.

I can't tell you how to style your life. The best I can do is to have a healthy lifestyle for myself and share that with you. Hopefully, I can inspire you to take better care of yourself. If I can do that in some way, then I consider myself successful.

In this section, we will look at diet, stress management, exercise, and supplements.

16 *Diet and Stress Management*

DIET

I recently treated a patient who had a bypass operation a few years ago. He hadn't taken good care of himself and had gained a lot of excess weight. In the process, he had acquired diabetes, hypertension, and congestive heart failure. His internist was concerned that he wasn't even in good enough shape to be a candidate for a heart transplant. I put him on a lowfat diet and a full measure of vitamin and mineral supplements—including chromium for the diabetes, CoQ10 and L-carnitine for the heart failure, and hefty doses of all the antioxidants. In a matter of a few days, he was feeling better. His ankle-swelling improved, and he was able to do more exercise without getting short of breath. At the time this diet and supplement program was begun, he was already on full doses of the conventional drugs from his internist, but he wasn't getting better. The addition of a painless prescription of diet and vitamins turned his condition around. Hopefully, now he won't even need to be a candidate for a heart transplant.

For myself, I always choose the lowest fat option. I eschew saturated fat and trans-fatty acids. I use moderate amounts of olive oil and other monounsaturated fatty acids without feeling guilty. I choose fish over fowl, white meat over dark, and I occasionally eat lean red meat. I enjoy a glass of wine with my dinner. I limit salt and sugar. I seek out fruits, vegetables, and fiber. I drink green tea.

STRESS MANAGEMENT

Life is full of stress. When the stress is gone, we are dead. I try to forgive and let anger roll off my back. Carrying around negative emotions is toxic for me. I look to see the glass half-full instead of half-empty. Comparison and judgment tend to bring unhappiness and so I also eschew them. I have tried meditation and yoga, but my most effective stress reducer is exercise.

17 *Exercise*

The American Heart Association (AHA) now recognizes the lack of exercise to be a major risk factor for coronary heart disease. Failure to exercise is on the same list as elevated LDL-cholesterol, high blood pressure, and smoking. Exercise can definitely make a difference in the state of a person's health. Recent studies have shown that substantial benefits can accrue from relatively modest amounts of exercise. Exercise plays an important role in improving other risk factors for heart disease. It helps control obesity, lower blood pressure, and reduces the blood's clotting tendency. Exercise is vital to your health!

I have been trying to figure out the most painless prescription I could give you about exercise. After much deliberation I have decided that the Nike slogan, **Just Do It,** *is the best prescription I have to offer.*

It doesn't matter so much what you do, as long as you just do it. Golf, tennis, basketball, walking, stair climbing, running, bicycling, swimming, weight training, even bowling is better than sitting in front of the TV and being a couch potato.

WALKING

Walking is perhaps the best exercise for the average person. It doesn't require any special equipment, although a good pair of walking shoes is an extremely worthwhile investment. Recent studies have confirmed the value of walking and have demonstrated the powerful cardiovascular benefits of this incredibly simple and effective exercise. Not only can walking improve the cardiovascular system, it can even raise the HDL-cholesterol.

A surgeon friend of mine recently told me about one of his patients—an eighty-five-year-old lady whom he had just operated on. He said she had the body of a woman in her fifties. When he asked her about her exercise habits, suspecting that exercise might have contributed to her youthful appearance, she told him the following story:

Sixty years earlier, as a young mother, she was under a lot of stress, and often by the end of the day she would find that her children were really getting on her nerves. She started a lifelong habit of taking thirty minutes after dinner to walk. She found that this routine not only gave her physical release but was also mentally relaxing. Sixty years later, she not only had the body of a much younger woman, she had also learned a powerful technique for releasing stress.

My grandmother walked daily into her early nineties. She had a spryness in her step that many younger people envied. A lifelong habit of exercise will pay off. Find an activity that you can enjoy and just do it. It will be painless and it will be your prescription for a healthier heart and a longer life.

OTHER TYPES OF EXERCISE

I have found that stair climbing machines, like the Stairmaster and the Tectrix Climb Max, are extremely effective exercise tools. I use one of these devices about three times a week. I wear a pulse monitor, so I can keep my heart rate exactly where I want it throughout my exercise. The stair climbing machines are great for many people with knee, hip, back, or foot problems because the exercise is essentially free of the impact trauma of running, and it is just as good as running from a cardiovascular conditioning perspective.

Another device that I use on a regular basis is an upper body ergometer. This contraption is basically a bicycle for the arms. It was developed so people with severe problems with their legs—people who couldn't walk, run, or use the stair climbing machines—could get an aerobic workout. Several studies have shown that exercising with an upper body ergometer provides cardiovascular fitness and relieves angina pectoris just as well as other forms of aerobic exercise using the legs. After much experimentation, I have settled on the upper body ergometer as my method of choice for an upper body workout. It gives me an aerobic workout and it develops upper body strength at the same time—an ideal combination found no where else that I am aware of. As the benefits of this remarkable device are becoming more widely appreciated, an increasing number of health clubs and gyms are installing them.

CARDIOVASCULAR BENEFITS OF EXERCISE

German researchers have found that spending 2,400 calories or more exercising each week, in conjunction with a heart-healthy diet, will result in reversal of blockages in the coronary arteries. The stair climbing devices, many stationary bicycles and treadmills, and the high-end upper body ergometers all count the calories during exercise. Twenty-four hundred calories a week translates to 400 calories six days a week (it's always a good idea to take off at least one day each week). This will require from thirty minutes to about two hours a day, depending on your body weight and the intensity of your work-out.

HOW MUCH SHOULD YOU EXERCISE?

I make time for exercise at least four days each week. Sometimes I exercise five or six days a week. I enjoy my exercise time. It makes me feel good and is one of my most effective stress reducers.

I began running at age forty when I stopped smoking. Today, I run on the average three times weekly.

PRECAUTIONS

If you are over thirty-five years old or have any risk factors for coronary disease, including a family history of heart disease, you will want to get a physician-supervised exercise test before beginning any exercise program. This procedure will not only insure that the exercise will be safe, it will also give you a target heart rate. The target heart rate is the heart rate that you can shoot for during exercise to achieve the maximum benefits with the minimum chance of adverse effects. I can't emphasize enough the importance of this physician-supervised exercise test.

When beginning an exercise program, no matter what the exercise, always begin slowly and build up the level and intensity of the exercise slowly. When beginning, **you can't do too little!** Doing too much, too soon, is the surest way to sabotage your exercise program and it could be dangerous. Strenuous exertion in untrained individuals has been associated with sudden death. Start slowly and build up your exercise level slowly. Be safe. Exercise is a lifelong activity. Don't try to do too much too fast.

We can all be like the eighty-five-year-old lady who looked a lot younger after 60 years of exercise. If done properly, it's painless, and we can all do it.

18 *Supplements*

I take my nutritional supplements and aspirin every day. It's not always convenient, especially when I travel. The supplements are a very important part of my lifestyle. I feel that they protect me, and I definitely feel better and stronger since I began using them. I do not delude myself into thinking that I can be indiscriminate in my eating habits because I am protected by the supplements. The real protection comes from a combination of heart-healthy nutrition and intelligent supplementation.

Part V

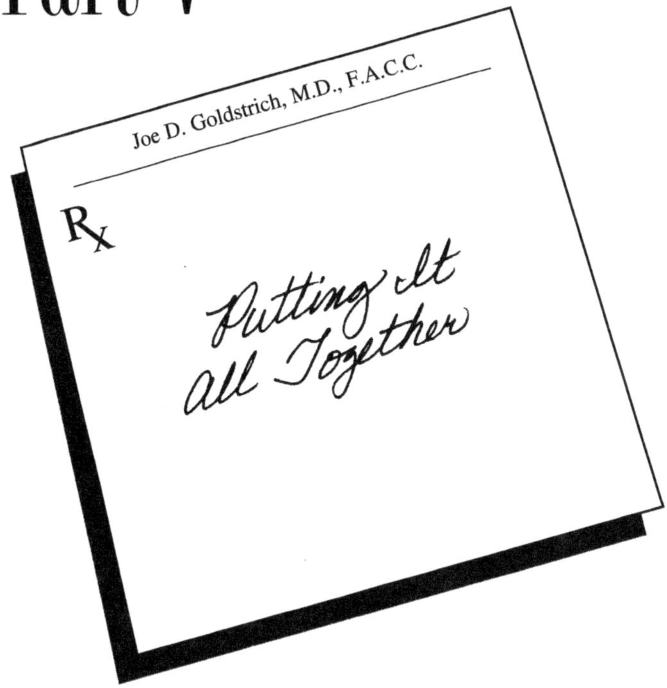

To get the most out of this book requires action in at least three areas. Nutritional supplements alone could substantially lower your risk of, or the progression of, heart disease. If you add exercise and the dietary changes that I have spelled out, you will be well along the path to a healthier heart and a longer life.

In Chapter 19, I will suggest ways for you to get started living your life according to the Painless Prescription program, while reviewing what you have already learned. In Chapter 20, I will show you specific treatments for specific cardiac conditions that you or your friends and loved ones may need help with.

19 *The Painless Prescription*

SUPPLEMENTS

If you haven't started taking your vitamins yet, a trip to the health food store is definitely in order. Translating the information in this book into the actual selection of your vitamin and mineral supplements is no easy matter. There are very few products on the market that actually contain the optimum ratios and amounts of all the nutrients that you will want to take.

When you start reading the label on a bottle of vitamins, and you find that there is 400 IU of vitamin E in each capsule, and you have decided that you want to take 1,200 IU of vitamin E daily, would it be reasonable to take three of these capsules each day? The answer depends on what else is in the capsule. If it only had 10,000 IU of beta-carotene in each capsule, three a day wouldn't be enough to get you to the desired 50,000 IU of beta-carotene each day.

If each capsule also contained 200 micrograms of selenium or 400 IU of vitamin D, three caps a day would be way too much of both selenium and vitamin D. Unfortunately, very few of the vitamin and mineral supplement companies actually formulate their products based on optimum ratios or the very latest information in the scientific literature.

I postponed writing this chapter for several weeks because I wasn't sure how to tell you the best way to select your supplements without having to make specific product recommendations. While I don't want to endorse any one vitamin company over another, I do want to make it as easy as possible for you to find the products that will best fill your needs and give you the results you desire.

I have gone through the exercise of reading all the labels in the health food stores in order to decide what I will take. I am simply going to tell you what supplements I use on a daily basis. Some of you will choose to take a lesser dose, some will want to take more. At the time of this writing, I have no arrangement with any vitamin company and I get no kickback or compensation of any sort. Hopefully, knowing what I take will make your job easier. I am also including a few variations that I prescribe for my patients.

I take my supplements in two doses during the day, half immediately after breakfast and half immediately after lunch. The fat-soluble vitamins that I take (E, beta-carotene, and CoQ10) are best absorbed when taken with a little fat in the diet. That's one of the reasons for taking them immediately after meals.

I have been insuring a little healthy fat in my breakfast by eating whole wheat toast spread with crunchy, natural almond butter and topped with a little jelly. The almond butter contains healthy monounsaturated fat and is probably healthier than peanut butter because peanuts are subject to contamination with aflatoxin, a liver poison.

Oatmeal also contains enough fat to insure absorption of the fat-soluble vitamins.

If I eat eggs for breakfast, it's either an egg-white omelet or the reduced saturated fat eggs (e.g. Good News Eggs) fried in olive oil. If I'm eating the egg yolks, I will precede the meal with three capsules of Blockaid 200 (Solaray).

Since I take the bulk of my fat-soluble vitamins in the morning, I make no special attempt to incorporate fat into my diet at lunch time.

My current morning regimen is:

1. one B-50 Caps (Twinlab)
2. six super C, E, & Carotene (Twinlab)
3. four Allergy-C Caps (Twinlab)
4. one Wine & Tea Polyphenol (Twinlab)
5. two Super Garlic 3X (Metagenics)
6. one Ultra CoQ10 (Twinlab)
7. two CellMins Multi Mineral (without iron) (Twinlab)
8. one adult low strength enteric-coated aspirin (Bayer)

This provides 1,200 IU of vitamin E; 6,000 mg of vitamin C; 45 mg (75,000 IU) of beta-carotene; 100 mg of CoQ10; 50 mg of each B-vitamin; one half of my daily dose of minerals; all of my aspirin (81 mg); and half of my garlic, wine, and tea intake.

My current noontime regimen is:

1. eight Maximum Nutrition Caps without iron (Twinlab)
2. four Allergy-C Caps (Twinlab)
3. one Wine & Tea Polyphenol (Twinlab)
4. two Super Garlic 3X (Metagenics)

This gives me another 500 IU of vitamin E, 4,500 mg of vitamin C, 15 mg (25,000 IU) of beta-carotene, the other half of my minerals, 25 mg more of the B-vitamins, and another dose of garlic, tea, and wine.

Many of my patients take sixteen capsules a day of the Maximum Nutrition Caps without iron product because this provides 1,000 IU of vitamin E, 50,000 IU of beta-carotene, 3,000 mg of vitamin C, all the essential minerals in the proper dosage, and 50 mg of the B-vitamins. If you just added the CoQ10, garlic, and perhaps the wine and tea polyphenols, you would have all the bases covered with reasonable amounts of all the essential nutrients and the minimum number of bottles and products. Those that prefer to take 100 mg of the B-vitamins simply add an extra B-50 cap.

Sixteen Maximum Nutrition Caps without iron can be divided into two doses of eight each, or five or six caps can be taken with each meal. This regimen is not inexpensive. At this time, sixteen capsules a day of the Maximum Nutrition Caps without iron will cost about $68 a month. The CoQ10 costs about $33 a month for 100 mg a day and the wine, tea, and garlic will add another $40 or so to the cost. In my opinion, it's still a bargain.

If the above plan is too expensive for you, there are some alternatives. Four Super C, E, & Carotene capsules a day will provide 800 IU of vitamin E, 50,000 IU (30 mg) of beta-carotene, and 2,000 mg of vitamin C, and cost less than $30 a month. The aspirin and 50 mg of the B-vitamins will add another few pennies. A dollar a day will probably give you at least 50 percent of the full protection which costs about five times that much.

DIET

As you now know, the people who live in the Mediterranean countries have some of the lowest rates of cardiovascular disease in the world. Their diets contain lots of fruits, vegetables, pasta, rice, beans, and peas. They don't eat red meat on a daily basis. Olive oil is the primary fat in their diet. Garlic and herbs are eaten regularly. This translates to lots of natural antioxidants in the fruits and vegetables and plenty of fiber in the beans, peas, rice, and pasta. The saturated fat intake is low, and there are generous amounts of nonoxidizable olive oil in their diets. The garlic has numerous beneficial effects.

This is a diet definitely worth emulating! Eat lots of fruits and vegetables and other high fiber foods, limit fat intake, and eliminate saturated and partially hydrogenated oils or trans-fatty acids from your diet. Use olive oil for everything. Canola is a close second choice.

Fish, skinless chicken or turkey breast, whole grains, and pasta will round out this healthy Mediterranean diet. Whole grain bread without added cholesterol or fat is also an integral part of this diet. Butter and margarine are not. If the bread must be spread with something, use olive oil like they do in the countries with the lowest incidence of heart disease.

Soy bean products, while not part of the Mediterranean diet, are an excellent choice because they help lower LDL-cholesterol and are low in saturated fat. Antioxidants are required, however, to protect from the polyunsaturated fatty acids in the soy beans. But, antioxidants are essential anyway.

Added fiber, over and above the whole grains, fruits, and vegetables can be helpful in the form of wheat bran, oat bran, psyllium, and pectin.

Re-read the section on alcohol to help you decide about this potentially useful addition to your diet.

EXERCISE

I can't emphasize enough the importance of exercise. An average of thirty minutes a day, or about three and a half hours per week, seems to be sufficient. Both weight training and aerobic exercise are beneficial. Just walking briskly for thirty minutes a day will be a big step in the right direction. If you are over thirty-five years old, have one or more risk factors for coronary heart disease, or if you have known heart disease, definitely check with your doctor before beginning any exercise program. Always start your exercise program slowly and build up slowly. That's the safe way to do it.

20 *Specific Treatments*

This chapter is organized differently than the rest of the book. The rest of the book lays out the information in terms of each nutrient or food category, and then tells which conditions or diseases are benefitted or adversely effected by the nutrient or food.

In this chapter, the diseases and conditions are categorized, and the nutrients and foodstuffs that will benefit each of these conditions are discussed all together. You can use this chapter as a clinical therapeutic index—simply look up an individual clinical problem and find the treatments for the problem together in one place.

The material here is more clinical and medical. This chapter can be read and consulted by itself, but in my opinion it will be much more useful after the background material in the rest of the book has already been digested. You can also use this chapter as a quick reference guide to the major conditions that are discussed in this book.

LOWERING LDL-CHOLESTEROL

Diet

The most important dietary maneuver for lowering LDL is reducing the intake of saturated fat. Trans-fatty acids from partially hydrogenated sources must also be eliminated. Substituting monounsaturated fats, such as olive oil and canola oil, for the saturated and trans-fatty acids may make the task easier and also provide other benefits. Reducing total fat intake will help even more. Limiting cholesterol in the diet and moving toward or to a vegetarian diet will lower LDL faster than anything else. Increasing the fiber in your diet will help remove the LDL from the body in the bowel movement. Diet is the cornerstone of all therapy to lower LDL.

Drugs

Cholesterol-lowering drugs will mainly target LDL. Zocor, Mevacor, and Pravachol are the three most potent drugs for lowering LDL-cholesterol. When coronary disease is unequivocally present, the use of these drugs, along with niacin and the cholesterol-binding resins Questran and Colestid, is definitely helpful. In my opinion, these drugs can be a real asset, with the benefits far outweighing the risks when advanced coronary artery disease is present. When combined with a lowfat, low-cholesterol diet and the antioxidant and vitamin and mineral supplements, including CoQ10, these drugs are extremely useful in reversing coronary heart disease and preventing heart attacks.

One of the causes of elevated LDL that is often missed is a low level of thyroid hormone. I always check the thyroid function of my patients to make sure they do not need thyroid hormone replacement.

Supplements

The supplement with the most proven power to substantially lower LDL-cholesterol is niacin. Niacin works synergistically with the drugs listed above. Many other supplements have shown some lowering of LDL (vitamin C, magnesium, calcium, garlic, beta-sitosterol, and the bioflavonoids). The amino acid arginine has also been shown to block the build-up of blockages without lowering LDL. In my opinion, it would be a mistake to rely solely on these supplements as the main way to lower LDL. They can be used as adjuncts. You will get much more punch in your LDL-lowering program from using the dietary approaches outlined above and adding the supplements as an accessory. There is also a definite place for cholesterol-lowering drugs in a program to maximally lower LDL.

The effect of the antioxidant supplements on LDL is another story altogether. In my opinion, the antioxidants (vitamins E and C, beta-carotene, selenium, bioflavonoids, and CoQ10) will, to a significant degree, neutralize and protect against the adverse effects of LDL without lowering it. Supplementing with vitamin E and C together has been shown to protect up to 50 percent of the LDL from oxidation. LDL that is not oxidized cannot be incorporated into arterial blockages. If LDL has been neutralized and **rendered ineffective** in creating blockages in the arteries, a big step has been taken toward **preventing** coronary heart disease. When LDL has been **lowered and rendered ineffective**, a giant leap has been taken to **prevent and possibly reverse** coronary disease. This is real heart protection!

Other

In the 1960's, surgeons at the University of Minnesota School of Medicine began doing a surgical procedure to bypass the part of the small intestine where cholesterol is absorbed. In the early 1980's, they began a controlled scientific study to evaluate the effectiveness of this procedure. The procedure is effective for those with serious coronary disease who can't lower their LDL with diet and/or drugs.

Another procedure that has been used for extremely high levels of LDL when diet and/or drugs don't work is called LDL apheresis. This is a technique that removes LDL from the body similar to the way a kidney dialysis machine removes waste products. This technique is also effective.

On the Horizon

Recently genetic material has been injected into people who do not have the genes to make the receptors that remove LDL from the bloodstream. This technique has worked and holds hope for those who would otherwise die because nothing else could be done. And, finally, one last research tool on the horizon is an implant of enzymes to help breakdown the LDL and get it out of the bloodstream.

LOWERING TRIGLYCERIDES

Diet and Exercise

Triglycerides are often difficult to lower by diet alone. If a person is overweight, weight loss is a proven therapy and should be the first step in any triglyceride-lowering program. Most people will only be able to lower their triglycerides by severely limiting their carbohydrate intake. This includes complex carbohydrates, all simple sugars, fruits, and fruit juices. In order to do this you would have to increase your intake of lean protein foods. The first choice in this category is fish, because the fish oils may help push the triglycerides down even further. Other choices are skinned chicken and turkey breast, skimmed milk products, and egg whites.

Eating plenty of cooked and raw vegetables will help both the weight loss and the triglyceride lowering. Most will also respond to reductions in their fat intake. When fat is eaten, it should be a monounsaturate such as olive oil or canola oil. Almost everyone with elevated triglycerides will lower them with alcohol restriction and exercise. A relatively low-carbohydrate, high-vegetable, high-fiber, high-protein, lowfat diet, exercise, and alcohol restriction are the cornerstones of triglyceride lowering. Sometimes the fat intake can be liberalized as long as it is monounsaturated fat.

Drugs

Lopid is the only prescription drug on the market at this time that acts specifically on triglycerides. Mevacor, Pravachol, and Zocor will lower triglycerides when this elevation is accompanied by a raised LDL level, which is often the case. Because the dose of niacin required to lower triglycerides is so high (way out of the range of its role as a vitamin supplement), I think of it as a drug. Niacin is very effective in lowering triglycerides. It should only be used under the supervision of a physician, in my opinion.

Supplements

A supplement that I have had some initial success with in lowering triglycerides is L-carnitine. L-carnitine has other beneficial actions on the heart which make it a desirable supplement in coronary heart disease.

The medical literature is replete with articles on the use of fish oil supplements to lower triglycerides. My experience has been that often when the triglycerides come down, the LDL goes up. For this reason, I only rarely use fish oil supplements to treat elevated triglycerides. Extra antioxidants need to be used with the fish oils, because they are polyunsaturated fatty acids and as such are subject to easy oxidation.

LOWERING Lp(a)

Supplements and Drugs

Diet will have absolutely no effect in lowering Lp(a) levels. Trans-fatty acids (margarine, partially hydrogenated fats) will raise Lp(a). The only agent that has been useful in lowering Lp(a) with any consistency at all is niacin. As I have said many times, therapeutic doses of niacin require a physician's supervision. Estrogen replacement in post-menopausal women has also lowered Lp(a). Antioxidants will protect against the LDL part of the Lp(a) molecule. Dr. Linus Pauling believes that vitamin C will protect against the adverse effects of Lp(a), without necessarily lowering it.

RAISING HDL-CHOLESTEROL

Diet and Exercise

The diet that lowers triglycerides will also raise HDL. HDL goes down as triglyceride goes up and vice-versa. It is not easy to raise HDL by diet alone unless the triglycerides are elevated and the person is also overweight. In this situation weight loss plus regular exercise can raise the HDL as much as 10 to 20 percent.

We now have some idea as to the minimum amount of exercise necessary to raise HDL. One study in middle-aged men found that it was necessary to jog at least 11.5 miles per week in order to raise HDL levels. Pre-menopausal women who walked about fifteen miles per week—as slow as three miles per hour—were also able to raise their HDL. So it looks like your perambulatory goal is in the neighborhood of fifteen miles a week at whatever pace you choose.

Several studies have shown that monounsaturated fatty acids, such as olive oil, nuts, and avocados, lower LDL while maintaining HDL levels. In effect, this is a rise in HDL relative to LDL. A few other studies have shown that olive oil can raise HDL while LDL stays the same.

Alcohol will usually raise HDL levels. Because alcohol can also raise triglycerides, it sometimes has a paradoxical effect on HDL. If alcohol raises the triglycerides, there is a chance that the HDL level will not go up and it could go down. The only way to know for sure is by doing a blood test and then adding or subtracting the alcohol and seeing what happens.

Smoking

Tobacco smoking and passive smoke will lower HDL. Smoking cessation and removal of environmental smoke will raise HDL. Smokers will not be able to raise their HDL with exercise. More good reasons to quit smoking.

Drugs

Useful drugs for raising HDL are niacin; the HMG-CoA reductase inhibitors—Pravachol, Zocor, Mevacor (if the LDL is elevated), and Lopid (if the triglycerides are elevated); and estrogen replacement after the menopause in women. Niacin is my first choice of the drugs to raise HDL.

Supplements

Vitamin E inconsistently raises HDL levels. Vitamin C and beta-carotene will raise HDL modestly. Chromium seems to be even better than these two vitamins in raising HDL. My current regimen to raise HDL with nutritional supplements is to give chromium (600 mcg per day), full doses of vitamins E, C, and beta-carotene, and to use niacin. My preliminary experience is that it doesn't take as much niacin to get the HDL up when it is used in conjunction with the other vitamins and chromium. Garlic has also been shown to have some HDL-raising properties. I always include a balanced B-complex supplement and minerals with this regimen.

RETARDING CLOTTING

Clotting not only contributes to the growth of the obstructing plaques, it is also the ultimate cause of heart attacks. I currently recommend an enteric-coated, low-strength (81 mg) aspirin tablet for prevention for all my patients over 50 years of age, unless there is some specific reason not to do so. If coronary artery disease is present, I will recommend this same aspirin regimen no matter what the age is, unless there is some very compelling reason not to use aspirin.

Chewing an adult-sized aspirin (325 mg) at the first sign of a heart attack will help halt the propagation of the clot that is causing the heart attack and will improve the chances of surviving the heart attack.

Other useful supplements in a primary or secondary prevention program to retard clotting include: vitamin E, garlic, bioflavonoids, alcohol—especially red wine, magnesium, along with the balancing minerals calcium and potassium, selenium, vitamin C, and beta-carotene. Others would add fish oils to this list.

I use vitamins B_6, B_{12}, and folic acid to cover homocysteine and its influence on clotting in all my patients.

Exercise will increase fibrinolysis and lower fibrinogen levels and help retard the clotting process.

LOWERING HIGH BLOOD PRESSURE

I first became interested in and started prescribing so-called hygienic or natural nondrug treatments for high blood pressure over twenty years ago. My experience is that the milder the pressure, the more likely these measures are to be effective. When the blood pressure is very high and has been elevated for a long time, the natural measures may help reduce the amount of prescription medicine needed to control the pressure, but they are not likely to totally eliminate the need for drug therapy. Again, calling on my experience, those people who employ these hygienic measures as part of their lifestyle are much less likely to develop high blood pressure in the first place.

Bottom line on blood pressure control:

It must be controlled to reduce the risk of coronary heart disease. If you can't lower it by natural means, then drug therapy may be beneficial for you. There are many useful drugs available to treat high blood pressure. It is beyond the purpose and scope of this book to describe them in any detail. I have chosen to focus in on the natural therapies that I have been using and studying for the past two decades.

Diet and Exercise

Weight reduction and exercise are the two best proven natural methods to lower high blood pressure. If you are overweight and you have high blood pressure, your chances of improving your blood pressure through weight loss are great. If you also begin an exercise program in conjunction with your weight-loss program, your chances get even better. The exercise doesn't even have to be vigorous to be beneficial. A walking program is a good place to start and it will help.

Alcohol consumption has been highly associated with high blood pressure. In most people, if alcohol intake is restricted to no more than two drinks a day, there will be no problem with blood pressure. More than two drinks a day in alcohol-sensitive people will raise the blood pressure.

Thirty to 50 percent of the population is "salt sensitive" and will lower their blood pressure by drastically lowering salt intake. The only way to find out if you are a member of the "30-50" club is to severely limit your salt intake for a period of at least six weeks and see what happens to your pressure. If you have done a good job of restricting the salt and your blood pressure hasn't budged, then you are probably not a member of the club and severe salt restriction won't help you.

In societies where salt intake is low, hypertension is uncommon. Where salt intake is high, so is the blood pressure.

At the Pritikin Longevity Center, we found that many people were able to lower their blood pressure by natural means. Pritikin maintained that eating a vegetable-based, high-fiber, lowfat diet had a lot to do with it. Others have argued that it was due entirely to the weight loss, exercise, and salt restriction. There is definitely truth in both assertions. The no-smoking policy at the Pritikin center may have also played a role, because smoking will raise blood pressure.

High-fiber diets are associated with lower blood pressures. The exact mechanism whereby fiber lowers blood pressure is not known for sure. The fiber associated with fruit consumption was more protective than the fiber from vegetables or grains. This could mean that the extra potassium and magnesium in the fruits contributed to the beneficial effects.

Magic Minerals

Calcium, potassium, and magnesium have all been studied and shown to have a relationship to blood pressure. There are studies that show that one or the other of these minerals will lower blood pressure. There are about an equal number of studies showing that these minerals don't lower blood pressure. Over the years, I have generally been disappointed when I have prescribed these minerals to try to lower blood pressure. Weight loss, exercise, reducing excessive alcohol intake, and salt restriction have all been more powerful tools in my hands. More recently, I have used these minerals as part of a more comprehensive vitamin and mineral supplement program, and I believe I am seeing more positive results. The results are even better when combined with weight loss, exercise, alcohol reduction, and salt restriction in those sensitive to salt and alcohol.

Specific Supplements

Two recent studies have provided evidence that vitamin C may be important in controlling blood pressure. The first study found that those with higher blood levels of vitamin C had lower pressures and the second study showed that vitamin C supplementation resulted in lower blood pressures. At least four other recent articles have shown a beneficial relationship between vitamin C and blood pressure.

Another supplement with significant pressure-lowering properties is CoQ10. Several animal studies have shown an antihypertensive action of CoQ10. The first research that I could find showing that CoQ10 lowered blood pressure in human beings appeared in the medical literature in 1992. The study was conducted in Italy and the blood pressure reductions achieved with 50 mg of CoQ10 twice daily were quite impressive.

L-arginine stimulates the artery wall to produce a relaxing factor, which is showing great promise as an antihypertension supplement.

Relaxation Therapy

There is no question that a tense lifestyle will contribute to high blood pressure in many people. In the early 1980's, I routinely recommended some form of relaxation therapy for most of my hypertensive patients. This included meditation, yoga, biofeedback, and sometimes psychotherapy. These interventions seemed to help while the person was doing them, but the results were not lasting. I encourage people to do anything they can to help themselves relax, but I no longer actively refer my patients for these therapies.

Use weight loss, exercise, alcohol restriction to not more than two drinks a day, high-fiber, lowfat, high-fruit diet, salt restriction if sensitive, smoking cessation, and vitamin and mineral supplements to include but not limited to CoQ10, vitamin C, potassium, magnesium, and calcium. If you still have elevated blood pressure, you will need the help of your physician and possible drug therapy. Remember, the real bottom line on blood pressure is that the pressure is controlled, not what supplements you take.

SMOKING AND ENVIRONMENTAL SMOKE

Smokers tend to get shortchanged by the medical system. Many physicians are afraid to advise smokers about how to protect themselves from tobacco smoke for fear this will be interpreted as covert permission to smoke. For those of you who choose not to stop smoking, or for those who are exposed to passive or environmental smoke that is beyond your control, here is some information that will help you shield yourself from the adverse effects of the smoke. Please do not interpret this in any way as permission to smoke and remember that the specific and ultimate treatment for smoking is to stop.

Tobacco smoke contains many compounds emitted as gasses and condensed tar particles that are capable of producing free radicals inside the body. The organ that receives the highest concentrations of these inhaled noxious substances is the lungs. For this reason it has been postulated that oxidative damage may play a major role in initiating lung cancer.

Government funded studies are currently underway to see if beta-carotene can prevent lung cancer.

In addition to the direct oxidative damage to the lung by inhaled tobacco smoke, these oxidative byproducts are absorbed directly into the bloodstream from the lungs. They then travel throughout the body where they produce free radicals and wreck havoc on a multitude of tissues. They also oxidize LDL. Blood levels of beta-carotene, as well as vitamins E and C, are decreased in smokers.

These lower levels of circulating antioxidants more readily allow the oxidation of LDL-cholesterol. The lower blood levels of protective antioxidants is one of the major reasons why smokers have a higher risk of coronary heart disease and heart attack.

Selenium, a mineral necessary for the production of the important antioxidant glutathione peroxidase, has also been found to be deficient in smokers. Japanese investigators have found that a combined deficiency of vitamins E and A, beta-carotene, and selenium will predispose to the development of lung cancer.

Male smokers with the highest beta-carotene intake (greater than 14,000 IU per day) had a 70 percent reduction in coronary risk when compared to smokers with very low beta-carotene intake in the Harvard male health care professionals' follow-up study. Even beta-carotene intake at the level of about a half a carrot a day provided some protection from coronary disease in this study!

Both beta-carotene and vitamin A appear to act somewhat independently in their ability to prevent lung cancer. For this reason, supplementation with both nutrients may be helpful.

Several of the B-vitamins have been found to be reduced in the bloodstream of smokers. This is of particular importance, because supplementation of smokers with folic acid and vitamin B_{12} has partially reversed some of the cellular changes that are thought to be precursors of lung cancer.

Smoking increases platelet stickiness and raises fibrinogen levels—two of the major clotting risk factors. Supplementation with garlic and aspirin will help neutralize these adverse actions of tobacco smoke. The bioflavonoids will also help with the platelet stickiness and provide additional antioxidant protection.

PAINLESS Rx

Here is my regimen to protect smokers and those exposed to environmental smoke. This is one example of what you can do when you can't do what you should do: a full measure of all the antioxidants—including beta-carotene, vitamins C and E, selenium, CoQ10, and bioflavonoids; garlic, aspirin, and 25,000 IU of vitamin A daily, plus 50 mg to 100 mg of the B-complex vitamins, including vitamin B_{12} and 800 mcg of folic acid.

ANGINA

Sometimes, angina persists despite full doses of traditional cardiac medicines. In this situation, a dietary change and supplements will very often turn off this incapacitating pain. An extremely lowfat diet based on vegetables, fruits, grains, beans, and peas will often stop the pain in several days to a few weeks. This was my experience at the Pritikin center, and it is what Dr. Dean Ornish has reported from his research. What I have learned recently is that adding L-carnitine, L-arginine, CoQ10, NAC, aspirin, vitamins E and C, and the B-complex vitamins to the very lowfat diet will often make the angina retreat in few days or even sooner. Progressive, supervised exercise will also be beneficial.

While working at the Pritikin center, I learned of two catastrophes possibly caused by a dietary-induced abatement of angina. Two men who had significant angina prior to going on the Pritikin diet became pain-free on this extremely lowfat, near-vegetarian diet. One gentleman after about six months of no pain offered to help his sixteen-year-old son chop wood. It became competitive and the older gentleman tried to keep up with his young son. He died suddenly without having angina.

The second tragedy was also in a very competitive man who was a tennis player. When he got angina, he began to only play doubles tennis. After his treatment at the Pritikin center and again after about six months of no angina, he decided to play singles tennis on a very hot day against a younger man—another case where strong competition came into play. He had a massive heart attack and survived, but so much of his heart muscle was damaged that he was never able to play tennis again.

I tell you these two cases to impress upon you that just because the angina goes away quickly doesn't mean that the arteries are any less narrow. The fact that the angina abates implies that blood flow is more streamlined and the metabolism of the heart muscle has improved. The lowfat diet probably does more to improve blood flow, while the supplements help blood flow and improve heart muscle metabolism.

CONGESTIVE HEART FAILURE AND CARDIOMYOPATHY

In my research for this book, I came across several reports on two supplements, L-carnitine and CoQ10, that could improve heart muscle metabolism and actually make the heart stronger. My own experience is limited to less than a dozen patients, but I have not been disappointed by these two wonderful supplements.

INTERMITTENT CLAUDICATION

This condition is to the lower legs what angina is to the heart. Exercise and the increased demand for blood flow through narrowed arteries causes pain in the leg, usually the calf. The same diet and supplement regimen given for angina will also be helpful here. In addition, exercise will play a big role improving circulation.

OBESITY

I wish I could give you a big list of supplements that would melt the pounds away. Unfortunately, there is no such list. The only two things of importance that I have learned in almost 40 years of studying and struggling with the weight-loss problem are: don't eat fat, and exercise. If you don't eat fat, your body can burn the fat that is stored, and if you exercise, you'll burn more stored fat.

Clinical References

The clinical references that follow were collected over a period of about seven years. As the clinical information on nutrition and nutritional supplements began to mushroom, it became harder and harder for me to keep up with the medical literature. In 1992 I subscribed to the computer-based Medline from the National Library of Medicine. A single CD will hold **all** the articles published and indexed by the National Library of Medicine over a two-year period. The excellent search program, Knowledge Finder [supplied by Aries Systems of North Andover, MA (508-975-7570)] enables me to find any article on a given topic, with its abstract, in a matter of minutes.

I have read the abstracts of virtually all the articles that follow. I have read the entire article of many of these references. I was able to use my computer to cross index the references into over a hundred categories. Frequently a reference is listed in more than one place because it deals with more than one subject. For example, the reference on chromium raising HDL is listed under both chromium and HDL.

Before beginning my final editing for this book, I had over 4,000 references from the mid 1980's through the summer of 1993, and the clinical reference section was bigger than the entire book! Needless to say, I had to do some editing. It caused me great pain to cut even one reference. In the final analysis, I decided to give you the most current references available. There are a few important articles from the 1980's and the early 1990's, but over 80 percent of the clinical references are from 1992 and 1993.

The scientific literature on nutritional supplements continues to mushroom. I plan on keeping up with it and hopefully I'll be able to pass it on to you.

The topic groups are arranged in alphabetical order. Within each group the references are arranged chronologically with the most recent listed first. Within each year the references are listed alphabetically by the first author's last name.

Alcohol

Bjorneboe, A. and G. E. Bjorneboe (1993). "Antioxidant status and alcohol-related diseases." Alcohol Alcohol **28**(1): 111-6.

Cullen, K. J., M. W. Knuiman, et al. (1993). "Alcohol and mortality in Busselton, Western Australia." Am J Epidemiol **137**(2): 242-8.

Garg, R., D. K. Wagener, et al. (1993). "Alcohol consumption and risk of ischemic heart disease in women." Arch Int Med **153**: 1211-1216.

Giovannucci, E., M. J. Stampfer, et al. (1993). "Folate, methionine, and alcohol intake and risk of colorectal adenoma [see comments]." J Natl Cancer Inst **85**(11): 875-84.

Klatsky, A. L. and M. A. Armstrong (1993). "Alcoholic beverage choice and risk of coronary artery disease mortality: do red wine drinkers fare best?" Am J Cardiol **71**(5): 467-9.

Reichman, M. E., J. T. Judd, et al. (1993). "Effects of alcohol consumption on plasma and urinary hormone concentrations in premenopausal women." J Natl Cancer Inst **9**: 722-726.

Rimm, E. and G. Colditz (1993). "Smoking, alcohol, and plasma levels of carotenes and vitamin E." Ann N Y Acad Sci **686**(1): 323-33.

Schonwetter, D. J., J. M. Gerrard, et al. (1993). "Type A behavior and alcohol consumption: effects on resting and post-exercise bleeding time thromboxane and prostacyclin metabolites." Prostaglandins Leukot Essent Fatty Acids **48**(2): 143-8.

Stampfer, M. J., E. B. Rimm, et al. (1993). "Commentary: alcohol, the heart, and public policy." Am J Public Health **83**(6): 801-4.

Thorogood, M., J. Mann, et al. (1993). "Alcohol intake and the U-shaped curve: do non-drinkers have a higher prevalence of cardiovascular-related disease?" J Public Health Med **15**(1): 61-8.

Ueshima, H., K. Mikawa, et al. (1993). "Effect of reduced alcohol consumption on blood pressure in untreated hypertensive men." Hypertension **21**(2): 248-52.

Beilin, L. J. and I. B. Puddey (1992). "Alcohol and hypertension." Clin Exp Hypertens [a] **14**(1-2): 119-38.

Ben-Shlomo, Y., H. Markowe, et al. (1992). "Stroke risk from alcohol consumption using different control groups." Stroke **23**(8): 1093-8.

de Labry, L. O., R. J. Glynn, et al. (1992). "Alcohol consumption and mortality in an American male population: recovering the U-shaped curve—findings from the normative Aging Study." J Stud Alcohol **53**(1): 25-32.

Dufour, M. C., L. Archer, et al. (1992). "Alcohol and the elderly." Clin Geriatr Med **8**(1): 127-41.

Farchi, G., F. Fidanza, et al. (1992). "Alcohol and mortality in the Italian rural cohorts of the Seven Countries Study." Int J Epidemiol **21**(1): 74-81.

Gavaler, J. S. and D. H. Van Thiel (1992). "The association between moderate alcoholic beverage consumption and serum estradiol and testosterone levels in normal postmenopausal women: relationship to the literature." Alcohol Clin Exp Res **16**(1): 87-92.

Hojnacki, J. L., J. E. Cluette-Brown, et al. (1992). "Alcohol delays clearance of lipoproteins from the circulation." Metabolism **41**(11): 1151-3.

Hojnacki, J. L., J. E. Cluette-Brown, et al. (1992). "Alcohol dose and low density lipoprotein heterogeneity in squirrel monkeys (Saimiri sciureus)." Atherosclerosis **94**(2-3): 249-61.

Hsieh, S. T., H. Sano, et al. (1992). "Magnesium supplementation prevents the development of alcohol-induced hypertension." Hypertension **19**(2): 175-82.

Jackson, R., R. Scragg, et al. (1992). "Does recent alcohol consumption reduce the risk of acute myocardial infarction and coronary death in regular drinkers?" Am J Epidemiol **136**(7): 819-24.

Klatsky, A. L. and M. A. Armstrong (1992). "Alcohol, smoking, coffee, and cirrhosis." Am J Epidemiol **136**(10): 1248-57.

Klatsky, A. L., M. A. Armstrong, et al. (1992). "Alcohol and mortality." Ann Intern Med **117**(8): 646-54.

Kune, G. A., S. Bannerman, et al. (1992). "Diet, alcohol, smoking, serum beta-carotene, and vitamin A in male nonmelanocytic skin cancer patients and controls." Nutr Cancer **18**(3): 237-44.

Kune, G. A., S. Bannerman, et al. (1992). "Attributable risk for diet, alcohol, and family history in the Melbourne Colorectal Cancer Study." Nutr Cancer **18**(3): 231-5.

Kune, G. A. and L. Vitetta (1992). "Alcohol consumption and the etiology of colorectal cancer: a review of the scientific evidence from 1957 to 1991." Nutr Cancer **18**(2): 97-111.

Langer, R. D., M. H. Criqui, et al. (1992). "Lipoproteins and blood pressure as biological pathways for effect of moderate alcohol consumption on coronary heart disease." Circulation **85**(3): 910-5.

Leo, M. A., C. Kim, et al. (1992). "Interaction of ethanol with beta-carotene: delayed blood clearance and enhanced hepatotoxicity." Hepatology **15**(5): 883-91.

Maheswaran, R., M. Beevers, et al. (1992). "Effectiveness of advice to reduce alcohol consumption in hypertensive patients." Hypertension **19**(1): 79-84.

Morse, R. M. and D. K. Flavin (1992). "The definition of alcoholism. The Joint Committee of the National Council on Alcoholism and Drug Dependence and the American Society of Addiction Medicine to Study the Definition and Criteria for the Diagnosis of Alcoholism." Jama **268**(8): 1012-4.

Odeleye, O. E., C. D. Eskelson, et al. (1992). "Vitamin E inhibition of lipid peroxidation and ethanol-mediated promotion of esophageal tumorigenesis." Nutr Cancer **17**(3): 223-34.

Puddey, I. B., M. Parker, et al. (1992). "Effects of alcohol and caloric restrictions on blood pressure and serum lipids in overweight men." Hypertension **20**(4): 533-41.

Rand, M. L., P. L. Gross, et al. (1992). "Acute in vitro effects of ethanol on responses of platelets from cholesterol-fed and Watanabe heritable hyperlipidemic rabbits." Arterioscler Thromb **12**(4): 437-45.

Razay, G., K. W. Heaton, et al. (1992). "Alcohol consumption and its relation to cardiovascular risk factors in British women." Bmj **304**(6819): 80-3.

Renaud, S. and M. de Lorgeril (1992). "Wine, alcohol, platelets, and the French paradox for coronary heart disease." Lancet **339**(8808): 1523-6.

Renaud, S. C., A. D. Beswick, et al. (1992). "Alcohol and platelet aggregation: the Caerphilly Prospective Heart Disease Study." Am J Clin Nutr **55**(5): 1012-7.

Rutledge, R. and W. J. Messick (1992). "The association of trauma death and alcohol use in a rural state." J Trauma **33**(5): 737-42.

Scherr, P. A., A. Z. La Croix, et al. (1992). "Light to moderate alcohol consumption and mortality in the elderly." J Am Geriatr Soc **40**(7): 651-7.

Schnall, P. L., J. E. Schwartz, et al. (1992). "Relation between job strain, alcohol, and ambulatory blood pressure." Hypertension **19**(5): 488-94.

Seppa, K., P. Sillanaukee, et al. (1992). "Moderate and heavy alcohol consumption have no favorable effect on lipid values [see comments]." Arch Intern Med **152**(2): 297-300.

Sheehy, T. W. (1992). "Alcohol and the heart. How it helps, how it harms." Postgrad Med **91**(5): 271-7.

Suh, I., B. J. Shaten, et al. (1992). "Alcohol use and mortality from coronary heart disease: the role of high-density lipoprotein cholesterol. The Multiple Risk Factor Intervention Trial Research Group." Ann Intern Med **116**(11): 881-7.

Superko, H. R. (1992). "Effects of acute and chronic alcohol consumption on postprandial lipemia in healthy normotriglyceridemic men." Am J Cardiol **69**(6): 701-4.

Ahlawat, S., S. B. Siwach, et al. (1991). "Indirect assessment of acute effects of ethyl alcohol on coronary circulation in patients with chronic stable angina." Int J Cardiol **33**(3): 385-91.

Blackburn, H., A. Wagenaar, et al. (1991). "Alcohol: good for your health?" Epidemiology **2**(3): 230-1.

Colditz, G. A., E. Giovannucci, et al. (1991). "Alcohol intake in relation to diet and obesity in women and men [see comments]." Am J Clin Nutr **54**(1): 49-55.

Giovannucci, E., G. Colditz, et al. (1991). "The assessment of alcohol consumption by a simple self-administered questionnaire." Am J Epidemiol **133**(8): 810-7.

Hamet, P., E. Mongeau, et al. (1991). "Interactions among calcium, sodium, and alcohol intake as determinants of blood pressure." Hypertension **17**(1 Suppl): I150-4.

Howe, G., T. Rohan, et al. (1991). "The association between alcohol and breast cancer risk: evidence from the combined analysis of six dietary case-control studies." Int J Cancer **47**(5): 707-10.

Jackson, R., R. Scragg, et al. (1991). "Alcohol consumption and risk of coronary heart disease [see comments]." Bmj **303**(6796): 211-6.

Kaplan, N. M. (1991). "Bashing booze: the danger of losing the benefits of moderate alcohol consumption [editorial]." Am Heart J **121**(6 Pt 1): 1854-6.

Numminen, H., M. Hillbom, et al. (1991). "Effects of exercise and ethanol ingestion on platelet thromboxane release in healthy men." Metabolism **40**(7): 695-701.

Rimm, E. B., E. L. Giovannucci, et al. (1991). "Prospective study of alcohol consumption and risk of coronary disease in men [see comments]." Lancet **338**(8765): 464-8.

Steinberg, D., T. A. Pearson, et al. (1991). "Alcohol and atherosclerosis." Ann Intern Med **114**(11): 967-76.

Angina

Boesgaard, S., H. E. Poulsen, et al. (1993). "Acute effects of nitroglycerin depend on both plasma and intracellular sulfhydryl compound levels in vivo. Effect of agents with different sulfhydryl-modulating properties." Circulation **87**(2): 547-53.

Jackson, G. (1993). "The management of stable angina." Hosp Pract **28**(1): 59-63.

(1992). Optimizing antianginal therapy: a consensus conference. Am J Cardiology.

(1992). A symposium: Third North American conference on nitroglycerine therapy. AM J Cardiology.

Boesgaard, S., J. Aldershvile, et al. (1992). "Preventive administration of intravenous N-acetyl-cysteine and development of tolerance to isosorbide dinitrate in patients with angina pectoris." Circulation **85**(1): 143-9.

Grambow, D. W. and E. J. Topol (1992). "Effect of maximal medical therapy on refractoriness of unstable angina pectoris." Am J Cardiol **70**(6): 577-81.

Horowitz, J. D. (1992). "Role of nitrates in unstable angina pectoris." Am J Cardiol **70**(8): 64B-71B.

Jayakumari, N., V. Ambikakumari, et al. (1992). "Antioxidant status in relation to free radical production during stable and unstable anginal syndromes." Atherosclerosis **94**(2-3): 183-90.

Juul-Moller, S., N. Edvardsson, et al. (1992). "Double-blind trial of aspirin in primary prevention of myocardial infarction in patients with stable chronic angina pectoris. The Swedish Angina Pectoris Aspirin Trial (SAPAT) Group." Lancet **340**(8833): 1421-5.

Lagioia, R., D. Scrutinio, et al. (1992). "Propionyl-L-carnitine: a new compound in the metabolic approach to the treatment of effort angina." Int J Cardiol **34**(2): 167-72.

McMurray, J., M. Chopra, et al. (1992). "Evidence for oxidative stress in unstable angina." Br Heart J **68**(5): 454-7.

Sakata, K., T. Hoshino, et al. (1992). "Circadian fluctuations of tissue plasminogen activator antigen and plasminogen activator inhibitor-1 antigens in vasospastic angina." Am Heart J **124**(4): 854-60.

Waters, D. and J. Y. Lam (1992). "Is thrombolytic therapy striking out in unstable angina? [editorial; comment]." Circulation **86**(5): 1642-4.

Riemersma, R. A., D. A. Wood, et al. (1991). "Risk of angina pectoris and plasma concentrations of vitamins A, C, and E and carotene [see comments]." Lancet **337**(8732): 1-5.

Antioxidants

(1993). "Antioxidants and Heart Disease. Symposium proceedings." Clin Cardiol **16**(4 Suppl 1): I1-26.

Bjorneboe, A. and G. E. Bjorneboe (1993). "Antioxidant status and alcohol-related diseases." Alcohol Alcohol **28**(1): 111-6.

Block, G. (1993). "Micronutrients and cancer: time for action? [editorial; comment]." J Natl Cancer Inst **85**(11): 846-8.

Buettner, G. R. (1993). "The pecking order of free radicals and antioxidants: lipid peroxidation, alpha-tocopherol, and ascorbate." Arch Biochem Biophys **300**(2): 535-43.

Bulkley, G. B. (1993). "Free radicals and other reactive oxygen metabolites: clinical relevance and the therapeutic efficacy of antioxidant therapy." Surgery **113**(5): 479-83.

Bunce, G. E. (1993). "Antioxidant nutrition and cataract in women: a prospective study." Nutr Rev **51**(3): 84-6.

Cleland, J. G. and D. M. Krikler (1993). "Modification of atherosclerosis by agents that do not lower cholesterol." Br Heart J **69**(1 Suppl): S54-62.

Cross, C. E., C. A. O'Neill, et al. (1993). "Cigarette smoke oxidation of human plasma constituents." Ann N Y Acad Sci **686**(1): 72-89.

Davidson, M. H. (1993). "Antioxidants and lipid metabolism. Implications for the present and direction for the future." Am J Cardiol **71**(6): 32B-36B.

Duthie, G. G., J. R. Arthur, et al. (1993). "Cigarette smoking, antioxidants, lipid peroxidation, and coronary heart disease." Ann N Y Acad Sci **686**(1): 120-9.

Freyschuss, A., A. Stiko-Rahm, et al. (1993). "Antioxidant treatment inhibits the development of intimal thickening after balloon injury of the aorta in hypercholesterolemic rabbits." J Clin Invest **91**(4): 1282-8.

Gey, K. F., U. K. Moser, et al. (1993). "Increased risk of cardiovascular disease at suboptimal plasma concentrations of essential antioxidants: an epidemiological update with special attention to carotene and vitamin C." Am J Clin Nutr **57**(5 Suppl): 787S-797S.

Godin, D. V. and D. M. Dahlman (1993). "Effects of hypercholesterolemia on tissue antioxidant status in two species differing in susceptibility to atherosclerosis." Res Commun Chem Pathol Pharmacol **79**(2): 151-66.

Halliwell, B. (1993). "The role of oxygen radicals in human disease, with particular reference to the vascular system." Haemostasis **23**(1): 118-26.

Hennekens, C. H. and J. M. Gaziano (1993). "Antioxidants and heart disease: epidemiology and clinical evidence." Clin Cardiol **16**(4 Suppl 1): I13-5.

Jialal, I. and C. J. Fuller (1993). "Oxidized LDL and antioxidants." Clin Cardiol **16**(4 Suppl 1): I6-9.

Kahl, R. and H. Kappus (1993). "[Toxicology of the synthetic antioxidants BHA and BHT in comparison with the natural antioxidant vitamin E]." Z Lebensm Unters Forsch **196**(4): 329-38.

Kahler, W., B. Kuklinski, et al. (1993). "[Diabetes mellitus—a free radical-associated disease. Results of adjuvant antioxidant supplementation]." Z Gesamte Inn Med **48**(5): 223-32.

Kanter, M. M., L. A. Nolte, et al. (1993). "Effects of an antioxidant vitamin mixture on lipid peroxidation at rest and postexercise." J Appl Physiol **74**(2): 965-9.

Klimov, A. N., V. S. Gurevich, et al. (1993). "Antioxidative activity of high density lipoproteins in vivo." Atherosclerosis **100**(1): 13-8.

Kuzuya, M. and F. Kuzuya (1993). "Probucol as an antioxidant and antiatherogenic drug." Free Radic Biol Med **14**(1): 67-77.

Maxwell, S. R. (1993). "Can anti-oxidants prevent ischaemic heart disease?" J Clin Pharm Ther **18**(2): 85-95.

Morel, I., G. Lescoat, et al. (1993). "Antioxidant and iron-chelating activities of the flavonoids catechin, quercetin and diosmetin on iron-loaded rat hepatocyte cultures." Biochem Pharmacol **45**(1): 13-9.

Rabl, H., G. Khoschsorur, et al. (1993). "A multivitamin infusion prevents lipid peroxidation and improves transplantation performance." Kidney Int **43**(4): 912-7.

Reaven, P. D., A. Khouw, et al. (1993). "Effect of dietary antioxidant combinations in humans. Protection of LDL by vitamin E but not by beta-carotene." Arterioscler Thromb **13**(4): 590-600.

Retsky, K. L., M. W. Freeman, et al. (1993). "Ascorbic acid oxidation product(s) protect human low density lipoprotein against atherogenic modification. Anti- rather than prooxidant activity of vitamin C in the presence of transition metal ions." J Biol Chem **268**(2): 1304-9.

Rimm, E. B., M. J. Stampfer, et al. (1993). "Vitamin E consumption and the risk of coronary heart disease in men [see comments]." N Engl J Med **328**(20): 1450-6.

Steinberg, D. (1993). "Antioxidant vitamins and coronary heart disease [editorial; comment]." N Engl J Med **328**(20): 1487-9.

Steiner, M. (1993). "Vitamin E: more than an antioxidant." Clin Cardiol **16**(4 Suppl 1): I16-8.

Walldius, G., J. Regnstrom, et al. (1993). "The role of lipids and antioxidative factors for development of atherosclerosis. The Probucol Quantitative Regression Swedish Trial (PQRST)." Am J Cardiol **71**(6): 15B-19B.

Arduini, A. (1992). "Carnitine and its acyl esters as secondary antioxidants? [letter]." Am Heart J **123**(6): 1726-7.

Beyer, R. E. (1992). "An analysis of the role of coenzyme Q in free radical generation and as an antioxidant." Biochem Cell Biol **70**(6): 390-403.

Bocan, T. M., S. B. Mueller, et al. (1992). "Antiatherosclerotic effects of antioxidants are lesion-specific when evaluated in hypercholesterolemic New Zealand white rabbits." Exp Mol Pathol **57**(1): 70-83.

Bolton-Smith, C., M. Woodward, et al. (1992). "The Scottish Heart Health Study. Dietary intake by food frequency questionnaire and odds ratios for coronary heart disease risk. II. The antioxidant vitamins and fibre." Eur J Clin Nutr **46**(2): 85-93.

Bunker, V. (1992). "Free radicals, antioxidants, and ageing." Med Lab Sci **49**: 299-312.

Cabre, E., J. L. Periago, et al. (1992). "Factors related to the plasma fatty acid profile in healthy subjects, with special reference to antioxidant micronutrient status: a multivariate analysis." Am J Clin Nutr **55**(4): 831-7.

Canfield, L. M., J. W. Forage, et al. (1992). "Carotenoids as cellular antioxidants." Proc Soc Exp Biol Med **200**(2): 260-5.

Chen, J., C. Geissler, et al. (1992). "Antioxidant status and cancer mortality in China." Int J Epidemiol **21**(4): 625-35.

Clausen, J. (1992). "The influence of antioxidants on the enhanced respiratory burst reaction in smokers." Ann N Y Acad Sci **669**(1): 337-41.

Cotelle, N., J. L. Bernier, et al. (1992). "Scavenger and antioxidant properties of ten synthetic flavones." Free Radic Biol Med **13**(3): 211-9.

Dargel, R. (1992). "Lipid peroxidation—a common pathogenetic mechanism?" Exp Toxicol Pathol **44**(4): 169-81.

Deucher, G. P. (1992). "Antioxidant therapy in the aging process." Exs **62**(1): 428-37.

Diplock, A. T. (1992). "Theoretical basis for antioxidant action in disease prevention." J Nutr Sci Vitaminol **1**(7): 545-7.

Dzhavad-zade, M. D., K. K. Selimkhanova, et al. (1992). "[Disorders of pulmonary hemodynamics in patients with diabetic nephroangiopathy and its correction with antioxidants]." Probl Endokrinol **38**(2): 20-2.

Eichholzer, M., H. B. Stahelin, et al. (1992). "Inverse correlation between essential antioxidants in plasma and subsequent risk to develop cancer, ischemic heart disease and stroke respectively: 12-year follow-up of the Prospective Basel Study." Exs **62**(1): 398-410.

Ernster, L., P. Forsmark, et al. (1992). "The mode of action of lipid-soluble antioxidants in biological membranes: relationship between the effects of ubiquinol and vitamin E as inhibitors of lipid peroxidation in submitochondrial particles." Biofactors **3**(4): 241-8.

Esterbauer, H., J. Gebicki, et al. (1992). "The role of lipid peroxidation and antioxidants in oxidative modification of LDL." Free Radic Biol Med **13**(4): 341-90.

Esterbauer, H., G. Waeg, et al. (1992). "Inhibition of LDL oxidation by antioxidants." Exs **62**(1): 145-57.

Garewal, H. S. (1992). "Potential role of beta-carotene and antioxidant vitamins in the prevention of oral cancer." Ann N Y Acad Sci **669**(1): 260-7.

Gaziano, J. M., J. E. Manson, et al. (1992). "Dietary antioxidants and cardiovascular disease." Ann N Y Acad Sci **669**(1): 249-58.

Halliwell, B., J. M. Gutteridge, et al. (1992). "Free radicals, antioxidants, and human disease: where are we now?" J Lab Clin Med **119**(6): 598-620.

Harris, W. S. (1992). "The prevention of atherosclerosis with antioxidants." Clin Cardiol **15**(9): 636-40.

Ho, C. T., Q. Chen, et al. (1992). "Antioxidative effect of polyphenol extract prepared from various Chinese teas." Prev Med **21**(4): 520-5.

Jayakumari, N., V. Ambikakumari, et al. (1992). "Antioxidant status in relation to free radical production during stable and unstable anginal syndromes." Atherosclerosis **94**(2-3): 183-90.

Jialal, I. and S. M. Grundy (1992). "Influence of antioxidant vitamins on LDL oxidation." Ann N Y Acad Sci **669**(1): 237-47.

Kalyanaraman, B., U. V. Darley, et al. (1992). "Synergistic interaction between the probucol phenoxyl radical and ascorbic acid in inhibiting the oxidation of low density lipoprotein." J Biol Chem **267**(10): 6789-95.

Kawasaki, T. (1992). "Antioxidant function of coenzyme Q." J Nutr Sci Vitaminol **1**(5): 552-5.

Khan, S. G., S. K. Katiyar, et al. (1992). "Enhancement of antioxidant and phase II enzymes by oral feeding of green tea polyphenols in drinking water to SKH-1 hairless mice: possible role in cancer chemoprevention." Cancer Res **52**(14): 4050-2.

Kita, T., M. Yokode, et al. (1992). "The role of oxidized lipoproteins in the pathogenesis of atherosclerosis." Clin Exp Pharmacol Physiol Suppl **20**(1): 37-42.

Knekt, P., M. Heliovaara, et al. (1992). "Serum antioxidant vitamins and risk of cataract." Bmj **305**(6866): 1392-4.

Krinsky, N. I. (1992). "Mechanism of action of biological antioxidants." Proc Soc Exp Biol Med **200**(2): 248-54.

Menzel, D. B. (1992). "Antioxidant vitamins and prevention of lung disease." Ann N Y Acad Sci **669**(1): 141-55.

Merati, G., P. Pasquali, et al. (1992). "Antioxidant activity of ubiquinone-3 in human low density lipoprotein." Free Radic Res Commun **16**(1): 11-7.

Meydani, M. (1992). "Vitamin E requirement in relation to dietary fish oil and oxidative stress in elderly." Exs **62**(1): 411-8.

Minnunni, M., U. Wolleb, et al. (1992). "Natural antioxidants as inhibitors of oxygen species induced mutagenicity." Mutat Res **269**(2): 193-200.

Mogelvang, B. (1992). "[Can arteriosclerosis be prevented by antioxidants?]." Nord Med **107**(2): 53-6.

Murphy, M. E., R. Kolvenbach, et al. (1992). "Antioxidant depletion in aortic crossclamping ischemia: increase of the plasma alpha-tocopheryl quinone/alpha-tocopherol ratio." Free Radic Biol Med **13**(2): 95-100.

Murthy, V. K., J. C. Shipp, et al. (1992). "Delayed onset and decreased incidence of diabetes in BB rats fed free radical scavengers." Diabetes Res Clin Pract **18**(1): 11-6.

Negre-Salvayre, A. and R. Salvayre (1992). "Protection by Ca2+ channel blockers (nifedipine, diltiazem and verapamil) against the toxicity of oxidized low density lipoprotein to cultured lymphoid cells." Br J Pharmacol **107**(3): 738-44.

Negre-Salvayre, A. and R. Salvayre (1992). "Quercetin prevents the cytotoxicity of oxidized LDL on lymphoid cell lines." Free Radic Biol Med **12**(2): 101-6.

Niki, E. (1992). "Free radical pathology and antioxidants: overview." J Nutr Sci Vitaminol **1**(40): 538-40.

Nilsson, J., J. Regnstrom, et al. (1992). "Lipid oxidation and atherosclerosis." Herz **17**(5): 263-9.

Olson, J. A. and S. Kobayashi (1992). "Antioxidants in health and disease: overview." Proc Soc Exp Biol Med **200**(2): 245-7.

Packer, L. (1992). "Interactions among antioxidants in health and disease: vitamin E and its redox cycle." Proc Soc Exp Biol Med **200**(2): 271-6.

Palozza, P. and N. I. Krinsky (1992). "beta-Carotene and alpha-tocopherol are synergistic antioxidants." Arch Biochem Biophys **297**(1): 184-7.

Parthasarathy, S. (1992). "Evidence for an additional intracellular site of action of probucol in the prevention of oxidative modification of low density lipoprotein. Use of a new water-soluble probucol derivative." J Clin Invest **89**(5): 1618-21.

Parthasarathy, S. (1992). "Role of lipid peroxidation and antioxidants in atherogenesis." J Nutr Sci Vitaminol **1**(6): 183-6.

Parthasarathy, S. and S. M. Rankin (1992). "Role of oxidized low density lipoprotein in atherogenesis." Prog Lipid Res **31**(2): 127-43.

Parthasarathy, S., D. Steinberg, et al. (1992). "The role of oxidized low-density lipoproteins in the pathogenesis of atherosclerosis." Annu Rev Med **43**(1): 219-25.

Reddy, A. C. and B. R. Lokesh (1992). "Studies on spice principles as antioxidants in the inhibition of lipid peroxidation of rat liver microsomes." Mol Cell Biochem **111**(1-2): 117-24.

Reznick, A. Z., V. E. Kagan, et al. (1992). "Antiradical effects in L-propionyl carnitine protection of the heart against ischemia-reperfusion injury: the possible role of iron chelation." Arch Biochem Biophys **296**(2): 394-401.

Reznick, A. Z., E. H. Witt, et al. (1992). "The threshold of age in exercise and antioxidants action." Exs **62**(1): 423-7.

Santiago, L. A., M. Hiramatsu, et al. (1992). "Japanese soybean paste miso scavenges free radicals and inhibits lipid peroxidation." J Nutr Sci Vitaminol **38**(3): 297-304.

Sies, H. (1992). "Carotenoids and tocopherols as antioxidants and singlet oxygen quenchers." J Nutr Sci Vitaminol **1**(33): 27-33.

Sies, H., W. Stahl, et al. (1992). "Antioxidant functions of vitamins. Vitamins E and C, beta-carotene, and other carotenoids." Ann N Y Acad Sci **669**(1): 7-20.

Simonoff, M., C. Sergeant, et al. (1992). "Antioxidant status (selenium, vitamins A and E) and aging." Exs **62**(1): 368-97.

Steinberg, D. (1992). "Antioxidants in the prevention of human atherosclerosis. Summary of the proceedings of a National Heart, Lung, and Blood Institute Workshop: September 5-6, 1991, Bethesda, Maryland." Circulation **85**(6): 2337-44.

Taylor, A. (1992). "Effect of photooxidation on the eye lens and role of nutrients in delaying cataract." Exs **62**(1): 266-79.

Taylor, A. (1992). "Role of nutrients in delaying cataracts." Ann N Y Acad Sci **669**(1): 111-23.

Tsang, N. C., P. L. Penfold, et al. (1992). "Serum levels of antioxidants and age-related macular degeneration." Doc Ophthalmol **81**(4): 387-400.

Vericel, E., C. Rey, et al. (1992). "Age-related changes in arachidonic acid peroxidation and glutathione-peroxidase activity in human platelets." Prostaglandins **43**(1): 75-85.

Weglicki, W. B., S. Bloom, et al. (1992). "Antioxidants and the cardiomyopathy of Mg-deficiency." Am J Cardiovasc Pathol **4**(3): 210-5.

Witt, E. H., A. Z. Reznick, et al. (1992). "Exercise, oxidative damage and effects of antioxidant manipulation." J Nutr **122**(3 Suppl): 766-73.

Yamamoto, Y., K. Wakabayashi, et al. (1992). "Comparison of plasma levels of lipid hydroperoxides and antioxidants in hyperlipidemic Nagase analbuminemic rats, Sprague-Dawley rats, and humans." Biochem Biophys Res Commun **189**(1): 518-23.

Anderson, R. (1991). "Assessment of the roles of vitamin C, vitamin E, and beta-carotene in the modulation of oxidant stress mediated by cigarette smoke-activated phagocytes." Am J Clin Nutr **53**(1 Suppl): 358S-361S.

Bast, A., G. R. Haenen, et al. (1991). "Oxidants and antioxidants: state of the art." Am J Med **91**(3C): 2S-13S.

Bjorkhem, I., A. Henriksson-Freyschuss, et al. (1991). "The antioxidant butylated hydroxytoluene protects against atherosclerosis." Arterioscler Thromb **11**(1): 15-22.

Ceriello, A., D. Giugliano, et al. (1991). "Anti-oxidants show an anti-hypertensive effect in diabetic and hypertensive subjects." Clin Sci **81**(6): 739-42.

Chisolm, G. 3. (1991). "Antioxidants and atherosclerosis: a current assessment." Clin Cardiol **14**(2 Suppl 1): I25-30.

Cutler, R. G. (1991). "Antioxidants and aging." Am J Clin Nutr **53**(1 Suppl): 373S-379S.

Di Mascio, P., M. E. Murphy, et al. (1991). "Antioxidant defense systems: the role of carotenoids, tocopherols, and thiols." Am J Clin Nutr **53**(1 Suppl): 194S-200S.

Diplock, A. T. (1991). "Antioxidant nutrients and disease prevention: an overview." Am J Clin Nutr **53**(1 Suppl): 189S-193S.

Dorgan, J. F. and A. Schatzkin (1991). "Antioxidant micronutrients in cancer prevention." Hematol Oncol Clin North Am **5**(1): 43-68.

Esterbauer, H., H. Puhl, et al. (1991). "Effect of antioxidants on oxidative modification of LDL." Ann Med **23**(5): 573-81.

Flaherty, J. T. (1991). "Myocardial injury mediated by oxygen free radicals." Am J Med **91**(3C): 79S-85S.

Frei, B. (1991). "Ascorbic acid protects lipids in human plasma and low-density lipoprotein against oxidative damage." Am J Clin Nutr **54**(6 Suppl): 1113S-1118S.

Ganguly, P. K. (1991). "Antioxidant therapy in congestive heart failure: is there any advantage? [editorial] [see comments]." J Intern Med **229**(3): 205-8.

Halliwell, B. (1991). "Drug antioxidant effects. A basis for drug selection?" Drugs **42**(4): 569-605.

Halliwell, B. (1991). "Reactive oxygen species in living systems: source, biochemistry, and role in human disease." Am J Med **91**(3C): 14S-22S.

Halliwell, B. and C. E. Cross (1991). "Reactive oxygen species, antioxidants, and acquired immunodeficiency syndrome. Sense or speculation?" Arch Intern Med **151**(1): 29-31.

Hearse, D. J. (1991). "Prospects for antioxidant therapy in cardiovascular medicine." Am J Med **91**(3C): 118S-121S.

Henning, S. M., J. Z. Zhang, et al. (1991). "Glutathione blood levels and other oxidant defense indices in men fed diets low in vitamin C." J Nutr **121**(12): 1969-75.

Henry, P. D. (1991). "Antiperoxidative actions of calcium antagonists and atherogenesis." J Cardiovasc Pharmacol **18**(1): S6-10.

Jacob, R. A., D. S. Kelley, et al. (1991). "Immunocompetence and oxidant defense during ascorbate depletion of healthy men." Am J Clin Nutr **54**(6 Suppl): 1302S-1309S.

Jacques, P. F. and L. Chylack Jr. (1991). "Epidemiologic evidence of a role for the antioxidant vitamins and carotenoids in cataract prevention." Am J Clin Nutr **53**(1 Suppl): 352S-355S.

Jialal, I. and S. M. Grundy (1991). "Preservation of the endogenous antioxidants in low density lipoprotein by ascorbate but not probucol during oxidative modification." J Clin Invest **87**(2): 597-601.

Knekt, P., R. Jarvinen, et al. (1991). "Dietary antioxidants and the risk of lung cancer." Am J Epidemiol **134**(5): 471-9.

Kok, F. J., G. van Poppel, et al. (1991). "Do antioxidants and polyunsaturated fatty acids have a combined association with coronary atherosclerosis?" Atherosclerosis **86**(1): 85-90.

Kuzuya, M., M. Naito, et al. (1991). "Probucol prevents oxidative injury to endothelial cells." J Lipid Res **32**(2): 197-204.

Malone, W. F. (1991). "Studies evaluating antioxidants and beta-carotene as chemopreventives." Am J Clin Nutr **53**(1 Suppl): 305S-313S.

Mao, S. J., M. T. Yates, et al. (1991). "Antioxidant activity of probucol and its analogues in hypercholesterolemic Watanabe rabbits." J Med Chem **34**(1): 298-302.

Mulholland, C. W. and J. J. Strain (1991). "Serum total free radical trapping ability in acute myocardial infarction." Clin Biochem **24**(5): 437-41.

Nagano, Y., H. Arai, et al. (1991). "High density lipoprotein loses its effect to stimulate efflux of cholesterol from foam cells after oxidative modification." Proc Natl Acad Sci U S A **88**(15): 6457-61.

Niki, E., Y. Yamamoto, et al. (1991). "Membrane damage due to lipid oxidation." Am J Clin Nutr **53**(1 Suppl): 201S-205S.

Noronha-Dutra, A. A., E. M. Steen-Dutra, et al. (1991). "An antioxidant role for calcium antagonists in the prevention of adrenaline mediated myocardial and endothelial damage." Br Heart J **65**(6): 322-5.

Packer, L. (1991). "Protective role of vitamin E in biological systems." Am J Clin Nutr **53**(4 Suppl): 1050S-1055S.

Pryor, W. A. (1991). "The antioxidant nutrients and disease prevention—what do we know and what do we need to find out?" Am J Clin Nutr **53**(1 Suppl): 391S-393S.

Riemersma, R. A., D. A. Wood, et al. (1991). "Risk of angina pectoris and plasma concentrations of vitamins A, C, and E and carotene [see comments]." Lancet **337**(8732): 1-5.

Salonen, J. T. (1991). "Dietary fats, antioxidants and blood pressure." Ann Med **23**(3): 295-8.

Salonen, J. T., R. Salonen, et al. (1991). "Effects of antioxidant supplementation on platelet function: a randomized pair-matched, placebo-controlled, double-blind trial in men with low antioxidant status [see comments]." Am J Clin Nutr **53**(5): 1222-9.

Santamaria, L. and A. Bianchi-Santamaria (1991). "Free radicals as carcinogens and their quenchers as anticarcinogens." Med Oncol Tumor Pharmacother **8**(3): 121-40.

Schmidt, K. (1991). "Antioxidant vitamins and beta-carotene: effects on immunocompetence." Am J Clin Nutr **53**(1 Suppl): 383S-385S.

Sies, H. (1991). "Oxidative stress: from basic research to clinical application." Am J Med **91**(3C): 31S-38S.

Sies, H. (1991). "Role of reactive oxygen species in biological processes." Klin Wochenschr **69**(21-23): 965-8.

Singh, V. N. and S. K. Gaby (1991). "Premalignant lesions: role of antioxidant vitamins and beta-carotene in risk reduction and prevention of malignant transformation." Am J Clin Nutr **53**(1 Suppl): 386S-390S.

Stahelin, H. B., K. F. Gey, et al. (1991). "Plasma antioxidant vitamins and subsequent cancer mortality in the 12-year follow-up of the prospective Basel Study [see comments]." Am J Epidemiol **133**(8): 766-75.

Steinberg, D. (1991). "Antioxidants and atherosclerosis. A current assessment [editorial]." Circulation **84**(3): 1420-5.

Stocker, R., V. W. Bowry, et al. (1991). "Ubiquinol-10 protects human low density lipoprotein more efficiently against lipid peroxidation than does alpha-tocopherol." Proc Natl Acad Sci U S A **88**(5): 1646-50.

Strain, J. J. (1991). "Disturbances of micronutrient and antioxidant status in diabetes." Proc Nutr Soc **50**(3): 591-604.

Vaage, J. and G. Valen (1991). "Could treatment with scavengers of oxygen free radicals minimize complications in cardiac surgery?" Klin Wochenschr **69**(21-23): 1066-72.

Varma, S. D. (1991). "Scientific basis for medical therapy of cataracts by antioxidants [published erratum appears in Am J Clin Nutr 1992 Jan; 55(1):iv]." Am J Clin Nutr **53**(1 Suppl): 335S-345S.

Weisburger, J. H. (1991). "Nutritional approach to cancer prevention with emphasis on vitamins, antioxidants, and carotenoids." Am J Clin Nutr **53**(1 Suppl):

Zamora, R., F. J. Hidalgo, et al. (1991). "Comparative antioxidant effectiveness of dietary beta-carotene, vitamin E, selenium and coenzyme Q10 in rat erythrocytes and plasma." J Nutr **121**(1): 50-6.

Frei, B., M. C. Kim, et al. (1990). "Ubiquinol-10 is an effective lipid-soluble antioxidant at physiological concentrations." Proc Natl Acad Sci U S A **87**(12): 4879-83.

Riemersma, R. A., M. Oliver, et al. (1990). "Plasma antioxidants and coronary heart disease: vitamins C and E, and selenium." Eur J Clin Nutr **44**(2): 143-50.

Salonen, J. T., R. Salonen, et al. (1988). "Relationship of serum selenium and antioxidants to plasma lipoproteins, platelet aggregability and prevalent ischaemic heart disease in Eastern Finnish men." Atherosclerosis **70**(1-2): 155-60.

Salonen, J. T., R. Salonen, et al. (1985). "Serum fatty acids, apolipoproteins, selenium and vitamin antioxidants and the risk of death from coronary artery disease." Am J Cardiol **56**(4): 226-31.

Aspirin

Altman, J. D., D. Dulas, et al. (1993). "Effect of aspirin on coronary collateral blood flow." Circulation **87**(2): 583-9.

Budd, J. S., K. Allen, et al. (1993). "The effectiveness of low dose slow release aspirin as an antiplatelet agent." J R Soc Med **86**(5): 261-3.

Fetkovska, N., Z. Jakubovska, et al. (1993). "Treatment of hypertension with calcium antagonists and aspirin. Effects on 24-h platelet activity." Am J Hypertens **6**(3 Pt 2): 98S-101S.

Fremes, S. E., C. Levinton, et al. (1993). "Optimal antithrombotic therapy following aorto-coronary bypass: a meta-analysis." Eur J Cardiothorac Surg **7**(4): 169-80.

Fuster, V., M. L. Dyken, et al. (1993). "Aspirin as a therapeutic agent in cardiovascular disease. Special Writing Group." Circulation **87**(2): 659-75.

Greenberg, E. R., J. A. Baron, et al. (1993). "Reduced risk of large-bowel adenomas among aspirin users. The Polyp Prevention Study Group." J Natl Cancer Inst **85**(11): 912-6.

Helgason, C. M., K. L. Tortorice, et al. (1993). "Aspirin response and failure in cerebral infarction." Stroke **24**(3): 345-50.

Huang, Z. S., C. M. Teng, et al. (1993). "Combined use of aspirin and heparin inhibits in vivo acute carotid thrombosis." Stroke **24**(6): 829-36.

Karlberg, K. E., J. Ahlner, et al. (1993). "Effects of nitroglycerin on platelet aggregation beyond the effects of acetylsalicylic acid in healthy subjects." Am J Cardiol **71**(4): 361-4.

Kearon, C. and J. Hirsh (1993). "Optimal dose for starting and maintaining low-dose aspirin." Arch Intern Med **153**(6): 700-2.

Kelly, R. (1993). "Selections from current literature: using aspirin for primary or secondary prevention." Fam Pract **10**(1): 88-92.

Meijer, A., F. W. Verheugt, et al. (1993). "Aspirin versus coumadin in the prevention of reocclusion and recurrent ischemia after successful thrombolysis: a prospective placebo-controlled angiographic study. Results of the APRICOT Study [see comments]." Circulation **87**(5): 1524-30.

Mickelson, J. K., P. T. Hoff, et al. (1993). "High dose intravenous aspirin, not low dose intravenous or oral aspirin, inhibits thrombus formation and stabilizes blood flow in experimental coronary vascular injury [see comments]." J Am Coll Cardiol **21**(2): 502-10.

Mohri, H. and T. Ohkubo (1993). "Single-dose effect of enteric-coated aspirin on platelet function and thromboxane generation in middle-aged men." Ann Pharmacother **27**(4): 405-10.

Prager, N. A., S. R. Torr-Brown, et al. (1993). "Maintenance of patency after thrombolysis in stenotic coronary arteries requires combined inhibition of thrombin and platelets." J Am Coll Cardiol **22**(1): 296-301.

Ranke, C., H. Hecker, et al. (1993). "Dose-dependent effect of aspirin on carotid atherosclerosis." Circulation **87**(6): 1873-9.

Sivenius, J., P. J. Riekkinen, et al. (1993). "European Stroke Prevention Study (ESPS): antithrombotic therapy is also effective in the elderly." Acta Neurol Scand **87**(2): 111-4.

Sun, Y. P., B. Q. Zhu, et al. (1993). "Aspirin inhibits platelet activity but does not attenuate experimental atherosclerosis." Am Heart J **125**(1): 79-86.

Thun, M. J., M. M. Namboodiri, et al. (1993). "Aspirin use and risk of fatal cancer." Cancer Res **53**(6): 1322-7.

(1992). "Aspirin effects on mortality and morbidity in patients with diabetes mellitus. Early Treatment Diabetic Retinopathy Study report 14. ETDRS Investigators." Jama **268**(10): 1292-300.

(1992). "Results of a randomized controlled trial of carotid endarterectomy for asymptomatic carotid stenosis. Mayo Asymptomatic Carotid Endarterectomy Study Group [see comments]." Mayo Clin Proc **67**(6): 513-8.

Blache, D., D. Bouthillier, et al. (1992). "Acute influence of smoking on platelet behaviour, endothelium and plasma lipids and normalization by aspirin." Atherosclerosis **93**(3): 179-88.

Dalen, J. E. and R. J. Goldberg (1992). "Prophylactic aspirin and the elderly population." Clin Geriatr Med **8**(1): 119-26.

Dalen, J. E. and J. Hirsh (1992). "Antithrombotic therapy. Introduction." Chest **102**(4 Suppl): 303S-304S.

Goldhaber, S. Z., J. E. Manson, et al. (1992). "Low-dose aspirin and subsequent peripheral arterial surgery in the Physicians' Health Study." Lancet **340**(8812): 143-5.

Grines, C. L. (1992). "Thrombolytic, antiplatelet, and antithrombotic agents." Am J Cardiol **70**(21): 18I-26I.

Hirsh, J., J. E. Dalen, et al. (1992). "Aspirin and other platelet-active drugs. The relationship between dose, effectiveness, and side effects." Chest **102**(4 Suppl): 327S-336S.

Iacoviello, L., C. Amore, et al. (1992). "Modulation of fibrinolytic response to venous occlusion in humans by a combination of low-dose aspirin and n-3 polyunsaturated fatty acids." Arterioscler Thromb **12**(10): 1191-7.

Jimenez, A. H., M. E. Stubbs, et al. (1992). "Rapidity and duration of platelet suppression by enteric-coated aspirin in healthy young men." Am J Cardiol **69**(3): 258-62.

Johnson, W. D., K. L. Kayser, et al. (1992). "Aspirin use and survival after coronary bypass surgery." Am Heart J **123**(3): 603-8.

Juul-Moller, S., N. Edvardsson, et al. (1992). "Double-blind trial of aspirin in primary prevention of myocardial infarction in patients with stable chronic angina pectoris. The Swedish Angina Pectoris Aspirin Trial (SAPAT) Group." Lancet **340**(8833): 1421-5.

McAnally, L. E., C. R. Corn, et al. (1992). "Aspirin for the prevention of vascular death in women." Ann Pharmacother **26**(12): 1530-4.

Meade, T. W., P. J. Roderick, et al. (1992). "Extra-cranial bleeding and other symptoms due to low dose aspirin and low intensity oral anticoagulation." Thromb Haemost **68**(1): 1-6.

Mori, T. A., R. Vandongen, et al. (1992). "Differential effect of aspirin on platelet aggregation in IDDM." Diabetes **41**(3): 261-6.

Nyman, I., H. Larsson, et al. (1992). "Prevention of serious cardiac events by low-dose aspirin in patients with silent myocardial ischaemia. The Research Group on Instability in Coronary Artery Disease in Southeast Sweden." Lancet **340**(8818): 497-501.

Paganini-Hill, A., G. Hsu, et al. (1992). "Aspirin use and reduced risk of fatal colon cancer [letter]." N Engl J Med **326**(19): 1290-1.

Ratnatunga, C. P., S. F. Edmondson, et al. (1992). "High-dose aspirin inhibits shear-induced platelet reaction involving thrombin generation." Circulation **85**(3): 1077-82.

Sivenius, J., M. Laakso, et al. (1992). "European stroke prevention study: effectiveness of antiplatelet therapy in diabetic patients in secondary prevention of stroke." Stroke **23**(6): 851-4.

Terres, W., C. W. Hamm, et al. (1992). "Residual platelet function under acetylsalicylic acid and the risk of restenosis after coronary angioplasty." J Cardiovasc Pharmacol **19**(2): 190-3.

Thun, M. J., E. E. Calle, et al. (1992). "Risk factors for fatal colon cancer in a large prospective study." J Natl Cancer Inst **84**(19): 1491-500.

Tohgi, H., S. Konno, et al. (1992). "Effects of low-to-high doses of aspirin on platelet aggregability and metabolites of thromboxane A2 and prostacyclin." Stroke **23**(10): 1400-3.

van Gijn, J. (1992). "Aspirin: dose and indications in modern stroke prevention." Neurol Clin **10**(1): 193-207.

Whelan, A. M., S. O. Price, et al. (1992). "The effect of aspirin on niacin-induced cutaneous reactions [see comments]." J Fam Pract **34**(2): 165-8.

Willard, J. E., R. A. Lange, et al. (1992). "The use of aspirin in ischemic heart disease [see comments]." N Engl J Med **327**(3): 175-81.

(1991). "Carotid surgery versus medical therapy in asymptomatic carotid stenosis. The CASANOVA Study Group [see comments]." Stroke **22**(10): 1229-35.

(1991). "A comparison of two doses of aspirin (30 mg vs. 283 mg a day) in patients after a transient ischemic attack or minor ischemic stroke. The Dutch TIA Trial Study Group [see comments]." N Engl J Med **325**(18): 1261-6.

(1991). "Swedish Aspirin Low-Dose Trial (SALT) of 75 mg aspirin as secondary prophylaxis after cerebrovascular ischaemic events. The SALT Collaborative Group [see comments]." Lancet **338**(8779): 1345-9.

Appel, L. J. and T. Bush (1991). "Preventing heart disease in women. Another role for aspirin? [editorial; comment]." Jama **266**(4): 565-6.

Baron, J. A. and E. R. Greenberg (1991). "Could aspirin really prevent colon cancer? [editorial; comment]." N Engl J Med **325**(23): 1644-6.

Berglund, U. and L. Wallentin (1991). "Persistent inhibition of platelet function during long-term treatment with 75 mg acetylsalicylic acid daily in men with unstable coronary artery disease." Eur Heart J **12**(3): 428-33.

Braden, G. A., H. R. Knapp, et al. (1991). "Suppression of eicosanoid biosynthesis during coronary angioplasty by fish oil and aspirin." Circulation **84**(2): 679-85.

Clarke, R. J., G. Mayo, et al. (1991). "Combined administration of aspirin and a specific thrombin inhibitor in man [see comments]." Circulation **83**(5): 1510-8.

Clarke, R. J., G. Mayo, et al. (1991). "Suppression of thromboxane A2 but not of systemic prostacyclin by controlled-release aspirin." N Engl J Med **325**(16): 1137-41.

Cohen, M., A. Merino, et al. (1991). "Clinical and angiographic characteristics and outcome of patients with rest-unstable angina occurring during regular aspirin use." J Am Coll Cardiol **18**(6): 1458-62.

Dalen, J. E. (1991). "An apple a day or an aspirin a day? [see comments]." Arch Intern Med **151**(6): 1066-9.

Force, T., R. Milani, et al. (1991). "Aspirin-induced decline in prostacyclin production in patients with coronary artery disease is due to decreased endoperoxide shift. Analysis of the effects of a combination of aspirin and n-3 fatty acids on the eicosanoid profile [see comments]." Circulation **84**(6): 2286-93.

Grotemeyer, K. H. (1991). "Effects of acetylsalicylic acid in stroke patients. Evidence of nonresponders in a subpopulation of treated patients." Thromb Res **63**(6): 587-93.

Lassila, R., M. Lepantalo, et al. (1991). "The effect of acetylsalicylic acid on the outcome after lower limb arterial surgery with special reference to cigarette smoking." World J Surg **15**(3): 378-82.

Mahon, J., K. Steel, et al. (1991). "Use of acetylsalicylic acid by physicians and in the community." Can Med Assoc J **145**(9): 1107-16.

Manson, J. E., M. J. Stampfer, et al. (1991). "A prospective study of aspirin use and primary prevention of cardiovascular disease in women [see comments]." Jama **266**(4): 521-7.

McCall, N. T., G. H. Tofler, et al. (1991). "The effect of enteric-coated aspirin on the morning increase in platelet activity." Am Heart J **121**(5): 1382-8.

Mehrotra, T. N. and R. Katira (1991). "Aspirin and coronary artery disease [editorial]." J Indian Med Assoc **89**(8): 215-6.

Mills, J. A. (1991). "Aspirin, the ageless remedy? [editorial; comment]." N Engl J Med **325**(18): 1303-4.

Mueller, B. A., R. L. Talbert, et al. (1991). "The bleeding time effects of a single dose of aspirin in subjects receiving omega-3 fatty acid dietary supplementation." J Clin Pharmacol **31**(2): 185-90.

Ridker, P. M., J. E. Manson, et al. (1991). "Clinical characteristics of nonfatal myocardial infarction among individuals on prophylactic low-dose aspirin therapy." Circulation **84**(2): 708-11.

Ridker, P. M., J. E. Manson, et al. (1991). "The effect of chronic platelet inhibition with low-dose aspirin on atherosclerotic progression and acute thrombosis: clinical evidence from the Physicians' Health Study." Am Heart J **122**(6): 1588-92.

Ridker, P. M., J. E. Manson, et al. (1991). "Low-dose aspirin therapy for chronic stable angina. A randomized, placebo-controlled clinical trial." Ann Intern Med **114**(10): 835-9.

Ridker, P. M., S. N. Willich, et al. (1991). "Aspirin, platelet aggregation, and the circadian variation of acute thrombotic events." Chronobiol Int **8**(5): 327-35.

Seddon, J. M., W. G. Christen, et al. (1991). "Low-dose aspirin and risks of cataract in a randomized trial of US physicians [see comments]." Arch Ophthalmol **109**(2): 252-5.

Singh, R. B., R. Verma, et al. (1991). "The effect of diet and aspirin on patient outcome after myocardial infarction." Nutrition **7**(2): 125-9.

Taylor, R. R., F. A. Gibbons, et al. (1991). "Effects of low-dose aspirin on restenosis after coronary angioplasty." Am J Cardiol **68**(9): 874-8.

Thun, M. J., M. M. Namboodiri, et al. (1991). "Aspirin use and reduced risk of fatal colon cancer [see comments]." N Engl J Med **325**(23): 1593-6.

Vane, J. R. and R. M. Botting (1991). "Heart disease, aspirin, and fish oil [editorial; comment]." Circulation **84**(6): 2588-90.

Verstraete, M. (1991). "Risk factors, interventions and therapeutic agents in the prevention of atherosclerosis-related ischaemic diseases." Drugs **42**(1): 22-38.

Wallentin, L. C. (1991). "Aspirin (75 mg/day) after an episode of unstable coronary artery disease: long-term effects on the risk for myocardial infarction, occurrence of severe angina and the need for revascularization. Research Group on Instability in Coronary Artery Disease in Southeast Sweden [comment]." J Am Coll Cardiol **18**(7): 1587-93.

(1990). "Risk of myocardial infarction and death during treatment with low dose aspirin and intravenous heparin in men with unstable coronary artery disease. The RISC Group [see comments]." Lancet **336**(8719): 827-30.

Manson, J. E., D. E. Grobbee, et al. (1990). "Aspirin in the primary prevention of angina pectoris in a randomized trial of United States physicians." Am J Med **89**(6): 772-6.

Ridker, P. M., J. E. Manson, et al. (1990). "Circadian variation of acute myocardial infarction and the effect of low-dose aspirin in a randomized trial of physicians." Circulation **82**(3): 897-902.

(1989). "Final report on the aspirin component of the ongoing Physicians' Health Study. Steering Committee of the Physicians' Health Study Research Group [see comments]." N Engl J Med **321**(3): 129-35.

B-vitamins

Manna, R., A. Migliore, et al. (1992). "Nicotinamide treatment in subjects at high risk of developing IDDM improves insulin secretion." Br J Clin Pract **46**(3): 177-9.

Mason, J. B. and J. W. Miller (1992). "The effects of vitamins B12, B6, and folate on blood homocysteine levels." Ann N Y Acad Sci **669**(1): 197-203.

Heimburger, D. C., C. B. Alexander, et al. (1988). "Improvement in bronchial squamous metaplasia in smokers treated with folate and vitamin B12. Report of a preliminary randomized, double-blind intervention trial [published erratum appears in JAMA 1988 Jun 27;259(23):3410]." Jama **259**(10): 1525-30.

Manna, R., A. Migliore, et al. (1992). "Nicotinamide treatment in subjects at high risk of developing IDDM improves insulin secretion." Br J Clin Pract **46**(3): 177-9.

Mason, J. B. and J. W. Miller (1992). "The effects of vitamins B12, B6, and folate on blood homocysteine levels." Ann N Y Acad Sci **669**(1): 197-203.

Heimburger, D. C., C. B. Alexander, et al. (1988). "Improvement in bronchial squamous metaplasia in smokers treated with folate and vitamin B12. Report of a preliminary randomized, double-blind intervention trial [published erratum appears in JAMA 1988 Jun 27;259(23):3410]." Jama **259**(10): 1525-30.

Beta-blockers

Croft, K. D., S. B. Dimmitt, et al. (1992). "Low density lipoprotein composition and oxidizability in coronary disease—apparent favourable effect of beta blockers." Atherosclerosis **97**(2-3): 123-30.

Pitt, B. (1992). "The role of beta-adrenergic blocking agents in preventing sudden cardiac death." Circulation **85**(1 Suppl): I107-11.

Roeback, J. J., K. M. Hla, et al. (1991). "Effects of chromium supplementation on serum high-density lipoprotein cholesterol levels in men taking beta-blockers. A randomized, controlled trial [see comments]." Ann Intern Med **115**(12): 917-24.

Beta-carotene

Chug-Ahuja, J. K., J. M. Holden, et al. (1993). "The development and application of a carotenoid database for fruits, vegetables, and selected multicomponent foods." J Am Diet Assoc **93**(3): 318-23.

Fujii, Y., S. Sakamoto, et al. (1993). "Effects of beta-carotene-rich algae Dunaliella bardawil on the dynamic changes of normal and neoplastic mammary cells and general metabolism in mice." Anticancer Res **13**(2): 389-93.

Gey, K. F., U. K. Moser, et al. (1993). "Increased risk of cardiovascular disease at suboptimal plasma concentrations of essential antioxidants: an epidemiological update with special attention to carotene and vitamin C." Am J Clin Nutr **57**(5 Suppl): 787S-797S.

Gey, K. F., H. B. Stahelin, et al. (1993). "Poor plasma status of carotene and vitamin C is associated with higher mortality from ischemic heart disease and stroke: Basel Prospective Study." Clin Investig **71**(1): 3-6.

Gottlieb, K., E. J. Zarling, et al. (1993). "Beta-carotene decreases markers of lipid peroxidation in healthy volunteers." Nutr Cancer **19**(2): 207-12.

Lavy, A., A. Ben Amotz, et al. (1993). "Preferential inhibition of LDL oxidation by the all-trans isomer of beta-carotene in comparison with 9-cis beta-carotene." Eur J Clin Chem Clin Biochem **31**(2): 83-90.

Mangels, A. R., J. M. Holden, et al. (1993). "Carotenoid content of fruits and vegetables: an evaluation of analytic data." J Am Diet Assoc **93**(3): 284-96.

Prince, M. R. and J. K. Frisoli (1993). "Beta-carotene accumulation in serum and skin." Am J Clin Nutr **57**(2): 175-81.

Rimm, E. and G. Colditz (1993). "Smoking, alcohol, and plasma levels of carotenes and vitamin E." Ann N Y Acad Sci **686**(1): 323-33.

van Poppel, G., S. Spanhaak, et al. (1993). "Effect of beta-carotene on immunological indexes in healthy male smokers." Am J Clin Nutr **57**(3): 402-7.

Zheng, W., W. J. Blot, et al. (1993). "Serum micronutrients and the subsequent risk of oral and pharyngeal cancer." Cancer Res **53**(4): 795-8.

Albanes, D., J. Virtamo, et al. (1992). "Serum beta-carotene before and after beta-carotene supplementation." Eur J Clin Nutr **46**(1): 15-24.

Ascherio, A., M. J. Stampfer, et al. (1992). "Correlations of vitamin A and E intakes with the plasma concentrations of carotenoids and tocopherols among American men and women." J Nutr **122**(9): 1792-801.

Bos, R. P., G. van Poppel, et al. (1992). "Decreased excretion of thioethers in urine of smokers after the use of beta-carotene." Int Arch Occup Environ Health **64**(3): 189-93.

Byers, T. and G. Perry (1992). "Dietary carotenes, vitamin C, and vitamin E as protective antioxidants in human cancers." Annu Rev Nutr **12**(1): 139-59.

Canfield, L. M., J. W. Forage, et al. (1992). "Carotenoids as cellular antioxidants." Proc Soc Exp Biol Med **200**(2): 260-5.

Comstock, G. W., T. L. Bush, et al. (1992). "Serum retinol, beta-carotene, vitamin E, and selenium as related to subsequent cancer of specific sites." Am J Epidemiol **135**(2): 115-21.

Garewal, H. S. (1992). "Potential role of beta-carotene and antioxidant vitamins in the prevention of oral cancer." Ann N Y Acad Sci **669**(1): 260-7.

Goodman, G. E. and G. S. Omenn (1992). "Carotene and retinol efficacy trial: lung cancer chemoprevention trial in heavy cigarette smokers and asbestos-exposed workers. CARET Coinvestigators and Staff." Adv Exp Med Biol **320**(1): 137-40.

Johnson, E. J. and R. M. Russell (1992). "Distribution of orally administered beta-carotene among lipoproteins in healthy men." Am J Clin Nutr **56**(1): 128-35.

Leo, M. A., C. Kim, et al. (1992). "Interaction of ethanol with beta-carotene: delayed blood clearance and enhanced hepatotoxicity." Hepatology **15**(5): 883-91.

Muggli, R. (1992). "beta-Carotene and disease prevention." J Nutr Sci Vitaminol **1**(3): 560-3.

Naruszewicz, M., E. Selinger, et al. (1992). "Oxidative modification of lipoprotein(a) and the effect of beta-carotene." Metabolism **41**(11): 1215-24.

Palozza, P. and N. I. Krinsky (1992). "beta-Carotene and alpha-tocopherol are synergistic antioxidants." Arch Biochem Biophys **297**(1): 184-7.

Rock, C. L. and M. E. Swendseid (1992). "Plasma beta-carotene response in humans after meals supplemented with dietary pectin." Am J Clin Nutr **55**(1): 96-9.

Santamaria, L. and A. Bianchi-Santamaria (1992). "Carotenoids in cancer chemoprevention and therapeutic interventions." J Nutr Sci Vitaminol **1**(6): 321-6.

Shibata, A., A. Paganini-Hill, et al. (1992). "Dietary beta-carotene, cigarette smoking, and lung cancer in men." Cancer Causes Control **3**(3): 207-14.

Sies, H. (1992). "Carotenoids and tocopherols as antioxidants and singlet oxygen quenchers." J Nutr Sci Vitaminol **1**(33): 27-33.

Sies, H., W. Stahl, et al. (1992). "Antioxidant functions of vitamins. Vitamins E and C, beta-carotene, and other carotenoids." Ann N Y Acad Sci **669**(1): 7-20.

Tee, E. S. (1992). "Carotenoids and retinoids in human nutrition." Crit Rev Food Sci Nutr **31**(1-2): 103-63.

Toma, S., S. Benso, et al. (1992). "Treatment of oral leukoplakia with beta-carotene." Oncology **49**(2): 77-81.

Tominaga, K., Y. Saito, et al. (1992). "An evaluation of serum microelement concentrations in lung cancer and matched non-cancer patients to determine the risk of developing lung cancer: a preliminary study." Jpn J Clin Oncol **22**(2): 96-101.

van Poppel, G., F. J. Kok, et al. (1992). "Beta-carotene supplementation in smokers reduces the frequency of micronuclei in sputum." Br J Cancer **66**(6): 1164-8.

Comstock, G. W., K. J. Helzlsouer, et al. (1991). "Prediagnostic serum levels of carotenoids and vitamin E as related to subsequent cancer in Washington County, Maryland." Am J Clin Nutr **53**(1 Suppl): 260S-264S.

Di Mascio, P., M. E. Murphy, et al. (1991). "Antioxidant defense systems: the role of carotenoids, tocopherols, and thiols." Am J Clin Nutr **53**(1 Suppl): 194S-200S.

Engle, A., J. E. Muscat, et al. (1991). "Nutritional risk factors and ovarian cancer." Nutr Cancer **15**(3-4): 239-47.

Garewal, H. S. (1991). "Potential role of beta-carotene in prevention of oral cancer [see comments]." Am J Clin Nutr **53**(1 Suppl): 294S-297S.

Gerster, H. (1991). "Potential role of beta-carotene in the prevention of cardiovascular disease." Int J Vitam Nutr Res **61**(4): 277-91.

Harris, R. W., T. J. Key, et al. (1991). "A case-control study of dietary carotene in men with lung cancer and in men with other epithelial cancers." Nutr Cancer **15**(1): 63-8.

Jacques, P. F. and L. Chylack Jr. (1991). "Epidemiologic evidence of a role for the antioxidant vitamins and carotenoids in cataract prevention." Am J Clin Nutr **53**(1 Suppl): 352S-355S.

Jialal, I., E. P. Norkus, et al. (1991). "Beta-Carotene inhibits the oxidative modification of low-density lipoprotein." Biochim Biophys Acta **1086**(1): 134-8.

Malone, W. F. (1991). "Studies evaluating antioxidants and beta-carotene as chemopreventives." Am J Clin Nutr **53**(1 Suppl): 305S-313S.

Mathews-Roth, M. M., N. Lausen, et al. (1991). "Effects of carotenoid administration on bladder cancer prevention." Oncology **48**(3): 177-9.

Nierenberg, D. W., G. T. Bayrd, et al. (1991). "Lack of effect of chronic administration of oral beta-carotene on serum cholesterol and triglyceride concentrations." Am J Clin Nutr **53**(3): 652-4.

Omenn, G. S. (1991). "CARET, the beta-carotene and retinol efficacy trial to prevent lung cancer in high-risk populations." Public Health Rev **19**(1-4): 205-8.

Omenn, G. S., G. Goodman, et al. (1991). "CARET, the beta-carotene and retinol efficacy trial to prevent lung cancer in asbestos-exposed workers and in smokers." Anticancer Drugs **2**(1): 79-86.

Riemersma, R. A., D. A. Wood, et al. (1991). "Risk of angina pectoris and plasma concentrations of vitamins A, C, and E and carotene [see comments]." Lancet **337**(8732): 1-5.

Ringer, T. V., M. J. De Loof, et al. (1991). "Beta-carotene's effects on serum lipoproteins and immunologic indices in humans [see comments]." Am J Clin Nutr **53**(3): 688-94.

Schmidt, K. (1991). "Antioxidant vitamins and beta-carotene: effects on immunocompetence." Am J Clin Nutr **53**(1 Suppl): 383S-385S.

Singh, V. N. and S. K. Gaby (1991). "Premalignant lesions: role of antioxidant vitamins and beta-carotene in risk reduction and prevention of malignant transformation." Am J Clin Nutr **53**(1 Suppl): 386S-390S.

Stahelin, H. B., K. F. Gey, et al. (1991). "Beta-carotene and cancer prevention: the Basel Study." Am J Clin Nutr **53**(1 Suppl): 265S-269S.

Weisburger, J. H. (1991). "Nutritional approach to cancer prevention with emphasis on vitamins, antioxidants, and carotenoids." Am J Clin Nutr **53**(1 Suppl):

Zamora, R., F. J. Hidalgo, et al. (1991). "Comparative antioxidant effectiveness of dietary beta-carotene, vitamin E, selenium and coenzyme Q10 in rat erythrocytes and plasma." J Nutr **121**(1): 50-6.

Ziegler, R. G. (1991). "Vegetables, fruits, and carotenoids and the risk of cancer." Am J Clin Nutr **53**(1 Suppl): 251S-259S.

Leibovitz, B., M. L. Hu, et al. (1990). "Dietary supplements of vitamin E, beta-carotene, coenzyme Q10 and selenium protect tissues against lipid peroxidation in rat tissue slices." J Nutr **120**(1): 97-104.

Connett, J. E., L. H. Kuller, et al. (1989). "Relationship between carotenoids and cancer. The Multiple Risk Factor Intervention Trial (MRFIT) Study." Cancer **64**(1): 126-34.

Ziegler, R. G. (1989). "A review of epidemiologic evidence that carotenoids reduce the risk of cancer." J Nutr **119**(1): 116-22.

Beta-sitosterol

Becker, M., D. Staab, et al. (1993). "Treatment of severe familial hypercholesterolemia in childhood with sitosterol and sitostanol." J Pediatr **122**(2): 292-6.

Becker, M., D. Staab, et al. (1992). "Long-term treatment of severe familial hypercholesterolemia in children: effect of sitosterol and bezafibrate." Pediatrics **89**(1): 138-42.

Rao, A. V. and S. A. Janezic (1992). "The role of dietary phytosterols in colon carcinogenesis." Nutr Cancer **18**(1): 43-52.

Salen, G., S. Shefer, et al. (1992). "Sitosterolemia." J Lipid Res **33**(7): 945-55.

Sutherland, W. H., E. R. Nye, et al. (1992). "Cholesterol metabolism in distance runners." Clin Physiol **12**(1): 29-37.

Vanhanen, H. T. and T. A. Miettinen (1992). "Effects of unsaturated and saturated dietary plant sterols on their serum contents." Clin Chim Acta **205**(1-2): 97-107.

Day, C. E. (1991). "Hypocholesterolemic activity of beta-sitosterol in cholesterol fed sea quail." Artery **18**(3): 125-32.

Heinemann, T., G. A. Kullak-Ublick, et al. (1991). "Mechanisms of action of plant sterols on inhibition of cholesterol absorption. Comparison of sitosterol and sitostanol." Eur J Clin Pharmacol **40**(1): S59-63.

Sutherland, W. H., M. C. Robertson, et al. (1991). "Plasma noncholesterol sterols in male distance runners and sedentary men." Eur J Appl Physiol **63**(2): 119-23.

Mattson, F. H., S. M. Grundy, et al. (1982). "Optimizing the effect of plant sterols on cholesterol absorption in man." Am J Clin Nutr **35**: 697-700.

Bioflavonoids

Frankel, E. N., J. Kanner, et al. (1993). "Inhibition of oxidation of human low-density lipoprotein by phenolic substances in red wine." Lancet **341**(8843): 454-7.

Morel, I., G. Lescoat, et al. (1993). "Antioxidant and iron-chelating activities of the flavonoids catechin, quercetin and diosmetin on iron-loaded rat hepatocyte cultures." Biochem Pharmacol **45**(1): 13-9.

Cotelle, N., J. L. Bernier, et al. (1992). "Scavenger and antioxidant properties of ten synthetic flavones." Free Radic Biol Med **13**(3): 211-9.

Ho, C. T., Q. Chen, et al. (1992). "Antioxidative effect of polyphenol extract prepared from various Chinese teas." Prev Med **21**(4): 520-5.

Mangiapane, H., J. Thomson, et al. (1992). "The inhibition of the oxidation of low density lipoprotein by (+)-catechin, a naturally occurring flavonoid." Biochem Pharmacol **43**(3): 445-50.

Middleton, E., Jr. and C. Kandaswami (1992). "Effects of flavonoids on immune and inflammatory cell functions." Biochem Pharmacol **43**(6): 1167-79.

Negre-Salvayre, A. and R. Salvayre (1992). "Quercetin prevents the cytotoxicity of oxidized LDL on lymphoid cell lines." Free Radic Biol Med **12**(2): 101-6.

Post, J. F. and R. S. Varma (1992). "Growth inhibitory effects of bioflavonoids and related compounds on human leukemic CEM-C1 and CEM-C7 cells." Cancer Lett **67**(2-3): 207-13.

Bracke, M., B. Vyncke, et al. (1991). "Effect of catechins and citrus flavonoids on invasion in vitro." Clin Exp Metastasis **9**(1): 13-25.

Calcium

Bostick, R. M., J. D. Potter, et al. (1993). "Calcium and colorectal epithelial cell proliferation: a preliminary randomized, double-blinded, placebo-controlled clinical trial." J Natl Cancer Inst **85**(2): 132-41.

Curhan, G. C., W. C. Willett, et al. (1993). "A prospective study of dietary calcium and other nutrients and the risk of symptomatic kidney stones [see comments]." N Engl J Med **328**(12): 833-8.

Galloe, A. M., N. Graudal, et al. (1993). "Effect of oral calcium supplementation on blood pressure in patients with previously untreated hypertension: a randomised, double-blind, placebo-controlled, crossover study." J Hum Hypertens **7**(1): 43-5.

Hatton, D. C., K. E. Scrogin, et al. (1993). "Dietary calcium modulates blood pressure through alpha 1-adrenergic receptors." Am J Physiol **264**(2 Pt 2): F234-8.

Kleibeuker, J. H., J. W. Welberg, et al. (1993). "Epithelial cell proliferation in the sigmoid colon of patients with adenomatous polyps increases during oral calcium supplementation." Br J Cancer **67**(3): 500-3.

Lind, L., H. Lithell, et al. (1993). "Calcium metabolism and sodium sensitivity in hypertensive subjects." J Hum Hypertens **7**(1): 53-7.

(1992). "Calcium supplementation prevents hypertensive disorders of pregnancy." Nutr Rev **50**(8): 233-6.

Appleton, G. V., R. W. Owen, et al. (1992). "The effect of dietary calcium supplementation on intestinal lipid metabolism." J Steroid Biochem Mol Biol **42**(3-4): 383-7.

Arbman, G., O. Axelson, et al. (1992). "Cereal fiber, calcium, and colorectal cancer." Cancer **69**(8): 2042-8.

Atkinson, J. (1992). "Vascular calcium overload. Physiological and pharmacological consequences." Drugs **44**(1): 111-8.

Bell, L., C. E. Halstenson, et al. (1992). "Cholesterol-lowering effects of calcium carbonate in patients with mild to moderate hypercholesterolemia." Arch Intern Med **152**(12): 2441-4.

Gillman, M. W., S. A. Oliveria, et al. (1992). "Inverse association of dietary calcium with systolic blood pressure in young children." Jama **267**(17): 2340-3.

Hamet, P., M. Daignault-Gelinas, et al. (1992). "Epidemiological evidence of an interaction between calcium and sodium intake impacting on blood pressure. A Montreal study." Am J Hypertens **5**(6 Pt 1): 378-85.

Knight, K. B. and R. E. Keith (1992). "Calcium supplementation on normotensive and hypertensive pregnant women." Am J Clin Nutr **55**(4): 891-5.

Laragh, J. H. (1992). "Lewis K. Dahl Memorial Lecture. The renin system and four lines fo hypertension research. Nephron heterogeneity, the calcium connection, the prorenin vasodilator limb, and plasma renin and heart attack." Hypertension **20**(3): 267-79.

Morris, C. D. and D. A. McCarron (1992). "Effect of calcium supplementation in an older population with mildly increased blood pressure." Am J Hypertens **5**(4 Pt 1): 230-7.

Newmark, H. L. and M. Lipkin (1992). "Calcium, vitamin D, and colon cancer." Cancer Res **52**(7 Suppl): 2067s-2070s.

Resnick, L. M. (1992). "Cellular calcium and magnesium metabolism in the pathophysiology and treatment of hypertension and related metabolic disorders." Am J Med **93**(2A): 11S-20S.

Resnick, L. M. (1992). "Cellular ions in hypertension, insulin resistance, obesity, and diabetes: a unifying theme." J Am Soc Nephrol **3**(4 Suppl): S78-85.

Wargovich, M. J., G. Isbell, et al. (1992). "Calcium supplementation decreases rectal epithelial cell proliferation in subjects with sporadic adenoma." Gastroenterology **103**(1): 92-7.

Appleton, G. V., R. W. Owen, et al. (1991). "Effect of dietary calcium on the colonic luminal environment." Gut **32**(11): 1374-7.

Garland, C. F., F. C. Garland, et al. (1991). "Can colon cancer incidence and death rates be reduced with calcium and vitamin D?" Am J Clin Nutr **54**(1 Suppl): 193S-201S.

McCarron, D. A. (1991). "Epidemiological evidence and clinical trials of dietary calcium's effect on blood pressure." Contrib Nephrol **90**(1): 2-10.

McCarron, D. A., C. D. Morris, et al. (1991). "Dietary calcium and blood pressure: modifying factors in specific populations." Am J Clin Nutr **54**(1 Suppl): 215S-219S.

Calcium Channel Blockers

Ali, K., M. Morimoto, et al. (1993). "Improvement of cardiac function impaired by repeated ischemic arrests in isolated rat hearts." Ann Thorac Surg **55**(4): 902-7.

Fetkovska, N., Z. Jakubovska, et al. (1993). "Treatment of hypertension with calcium antagonists and aspirin. Effects on 24-h platelet activity." Am J Hypertens **6**(3 Pt 2): 98S-101S.

Fleckenstein-Grun, G., M. Frey, et al. (1992). "Calcium overload—an important cellular mechanism in hypertension and arteriosclerosis." Drugs **44**(1): 23-30.

Negre-Salvayre, A. and R. Salvayre (1992). "Protection by Ca2+ channel blockers (nifedipine, diltiazem and verapamil) against the toxicity of oxidized low density lipoprotein to cultured lymphoid cells." Br J Pharmacol **107**(3): 738-44.

Vanhoutte, P. M. (1992). "Role of calcium and endothelium in hypertension, cardiovascular disease, and subsequent vascular events." J Cardiovasc Pharmacol **19**(1): S6-10.

Waters, D. and J. Lesperance (1992). "Interventions that beneficially influence the evolution of coronary atherosclerosis. The case for calcium channel blockers." Circulation **86**(6 Suppl): III111-6.

Breugnot, C., C. Maziere, et al. (1991). "Calcium antagonists prevent monocyte and endothelial cell-induced modification of low density lipoproteins." Free Radic Res Commun **15**(2): 91-100.

Cummings, D. M., P. Amadio Jr., et al. (1991). "The role of calcium channel blockers in the treatment of essential hypertension." Arch Intern Med **151**(2): 250-9.

Henry, P. D. (1991). "Antiperoxidative actions of calcium antagonists and atherogenesis." J Cardiovasc Pharmacol **18**(1): S6-10.

Noronha-Dutra, A. A., E. M. Steen-Dutra, et al. (1991). "An antioxidant role for calcium antagonists in the prevention of adrenaline mediated myocardial and endothelial damage." Br Heart J **65**(6): 322-5.

Touyz, R. M. (1991). "Magnesium supplementation as an adjuvant to synthetic calcium channel antagonists in the treatment of hypertension." Med Hypotheses **36**(2): 140-1.

Gotto, A., Jr. (1990). "Calcium channel blockers and the prevention of atherosclerosis." Am J Hypertens **3**(12 Pt 2): 342S-346S.

Cancer

(1993). "Report of the Council on Scientific Affairs. Diet and cancer: where do matters stand?" Arch Intern Med **153**(1): 50-6.

Bayerdorffer, E., G. A. Mannes, et al. (1993). "Decreased high-density lipoprotein cholesterol and increased low-density cholesterol levels in patients with colorectal adenomas." Ann Intern Med **118**(7): 481-7.

Benner, S. E., R. J. Winn, et al. (1993). "Regression of oral leukoplakia with alpha-tocopherol: a community clinical oncology program chemoprevention study." J Natl Cancer Inst **85**(1): 44-7.

Bjorneboe, A. and G. E. Bjorneboe (1993). "Antioxidant status and alcohol-related diseases." Alcohol Alcohol **28**(1): 111-6.

Block, G. (1993). "Micronutrients and cancer: time for action? [editorial; comment]." J Natl Cancer Inst **85**(11): 846-8.

Bostick, R. M., J. D. Potter, et al. (1993). "Calcium and colorectal epithelial cell proliferation: a preliminary randomized, double-blinded, placebo-controlled clinical trial." J Natl Cancer Inst **85**(2): 132-41.

Boyd, N. F. (1993). "Nutrition and breast cancer [editorial]." J Natl Cancer Inst **85**(1): 6-7.

Chung, F. L., M. A. Morse, et al. (1993). "Inhibition of tobacco-specific nitrosamine-induced lung tumorigenesis by compounds derived from cruciferous vegetables and green tea." Ann N Y Acad Sci **686**(1): 186-201.

Clark, L. C., L. J. Hixson, et al. (1993). "Plasma selenium concentration predicts the prevalence of colorectal adenomatous polyps." Cancer Epidemiol Biomarkers Prev **2**(1): 41-6.

Colditz, G. A. (1993). "Epidemiology of breast cancer. Findings from the nurses' health study." Cancer **71**(4 Suppl): 1480-9.

Dorant, E., P. A. van den Brandt, et al. (1993). "Garlic and its significance for the prevention of cancer in humans: a critical view." Br J Cancer **67**(3): 424-9.

Dragsted, L. O., M. Strube, et al. (1993). "Cancer-protective factors in fruits and vegetables: biochemical and biological background." Pharmacol Toxicol **72**(1): 116-35.

Folkers, K., R. Brown, et al. (1993). "Survival of cancer patients on therapy with coenzyme Q10." Biochem Biophys Res Commun **192**(1): 241-5.

Fujii, Y., S. Sakamoto, et al. (1993). "Effects of beta-carotene-rich algae Dunaliella bardawil on the dynamic changes of normal and neoplastic mammary cells and general metabolism in mice." Anticancer Res **13**(2): 389-93.

Gerrish, K. E. and H. L. Gensler (1993). "Prevention of photocarcinogenesis by dietary vitamin E." Nutr Cancer **19**(2): 125-33.

Giovannucci, E., M. J. Stampfer, et al. (1993). "A comparison of prospective and retrospective assessments of diet in the study of breast cancer." Am J Epidemiol **137**(5): 502-11.

Giovannucci, E., M. J. Stampfer, et al. (1993). "Folate, methionine, and alcohol intake and risk of colorectal adenoma [see comments]." J Natl Cancer Inst **85**(11): 875-84.

Gordon, G. B., K. J. Helzlsouer, et al. (1993). "Serum levels of dehydroepiandrosterone and dehydroepiandrosterone sulfate and the risk of developing gastric cancer." Cancer Epidemiol Biomarkers Prev **2**(1): 33-5.

Greenberg, E. R., J. A. Baron, et al. (1993). "Reduced risk of large-bowel adenomas among aspirin users. The Polyp Prevention Study Group." J Natl Cancer Inst **85**(11): 912-6.

Harlan, L. C., R. J. Coates, et al. (1993). "Estrogen receptor status and dietary intakes in breast cancer patients." Epidemiology **4**(1): 25-31.

Hoffmann, D., A. Rivenson, et al. (1993). "Potential inhibitors of tobacco carcinogenesis." Ann N Y Acad Sci **686**(1): 140-60.

Hunter, D. J., J. E. Manson, et al. (1993). "A prospective study of the intake of vitamins C, E, and A and the risk of breast cancer." N Engl J Med **329**(4): 234-40.

Jacobson, E. L. and M. K. Jacobson (1993). "A biomarker for the assessment of niacin nutriture as a potential preventive factor in carcinogenesis." J Intern Med **233**(1): 59-62.

Kleibeuker, J. H., J. W. Welberg, et al. (1993). "Epithelial cell proliferation in the sigmoid colon of patients with adenomatous polyps increases during oral calcium supplementation." Br J Cancer **67**(3): 500-3.

Knekt, P. (1993). "Vitamin E and smoking and the risk of lung cancer." Ann N Y Acad Sci **686**(1): 280-7.

Krinsky, N. I. (1993). "Micronutrients and their influence on mutagenicity and malignant transformation." Ann N Y Acad Sci **686**(1): 229-42.

Levi, F., S. Franceschi, et al. (1993). "Dietary factors and the risk of endometrial cancer." Cancer **71**(11): 3575-81.

Pastorino, U., M. Infante, et al. (1993). "Adjuvant treatment of stage I lung cancer with high-dose vitamin A [see comments]." J Clin Oncol **11**(7): 1216-22.

Reichman, M. E., J. T. Judd, et al. (1993). "Effects of alcohol consumption on plasma and urinary hormone concentrations in premenopausal women." J Natl Cancer Inst **9**: 722-726.

Rohan, T. E., G. R. Howe, et al. (1993). "Dietary fiber, vitamins A, C, and E, and risk of breast cancer: a cohort study." Cancer Causes Control **4**(1): 29-37.

Tanaka, N., K. Ochi, et al. (1993). "[Clinical application of vitamin A, D and E against malignant tumor in humans]." Nippon Rinsho **51**(4): 989-96.

Thun, M. J., M. M. Namboodiri, et al. (1993). "Aspirin use and risk of fatal cancer." Cancer Res **53**(6): 1322-7.

Yang, C. S. and Z. Y. Wang (1993). "Tea and cancer." J Natl Cancer Inst **85**(13): 1038-49.

Yano, T., G. Ishikawa, et al. (1993). "Is vitamin E a useful agent to protect against oxy radical-promoted lung tumorigenesis in ddY mice?" Carcinogenesis **14**(6): 1133-6.

Zheng, W., W. J. Blot, et al. (1993). "Serum micronutrients and the subsequent risk of oral and pharyngeal cancer." Cancer Res **53**(4): 795-8.

Canola Oil

Corboy, J., W. H. Sutherland, et al. (1993). "Fatty acid composition and the oxidation of low-density lipoproteins." Biochem Med Metab Biol **49**(1): 25-35.

Valsta, L. M., M. Jauhiainen, et al. (1992). "Effects of a monounsaturated rapeseed oil and a polyunsaturated sunflower oil diet on lipoprotein levels in humans." Arterioscler Thromb **12**(1): 50-7.

Bierenbaum, M. L., R. P. Reichstein, et al. (1991). "Effects of canola oil on serum lipids in humans." J Am Coll Nutr **10**(3): 228-33.

Kwon, J. S., J. T. Snook, et al. (1991). "Effects of diets high in saturated fatty acids, canola oil, or safflower oil on platelet function, thromboxane B2 formation, and fatty acid composition of platelet phospholipids." Am J Clin Nutr **54**(2): 351-8.

Wardlaw, G. M., J. T. Snook, et al. (1991). "Serum lipid and apolipoprotein concentrations in healthy men on diets enriched in either canola oil or safflower oil." Am J Clin Nutr **54**(1): 104-10.

Carbohydrates

Berry, E. M., S. Eisenberg, et al. (1992). "Effects of diets rich in monounsaturated fatty acids on plasma lipoproteins—the Jerusalem Nutrition Study. II. Monounsaturated fatty acids vs carbohydrates." Am J Clin Nutr **56**(2): 394-403.

Colquhoun, D. M., D. Moores, et al. (1992). "Comparison of the effects on lipoproteins and apolipoproteins of a diet high in monounsaturated fatty acids, enriched with avocado, and a high-carbohydrate diet." Am J Clin Nutr **56**(4): 671-7.

Garg, A. and S. M. Grundy (1992). "High-carbohydrate, low-fat diet? Negative [comment]." Hosp Pract (Off Ed) **27**(1): 11-4.

Garg, A., S. M. Grundy, et al. (1992). "Comparison of effects of high and low carbohydrate diets on plasma lipoproteins and insulin sensitivity in patients with mild NIDDM." Diabetes **41**(10): 1278-85.

Parillo, M., A. A. Rivellese, et al. (1992). "A high-monounsaturated-fat/low-carbohydrate diet improves peripheral insulin sensitivity in non-insulin-dependent diabetic patients." Metabolism **41**(12): 1373-8.

Hollenbeck, C. B. and A. M. Coulston (1991). "Effects of dietary carbohydrate and fat intake on glucose and lipoprotein metabolism in individuals with diabetes mellitus." Diabetes Care **14**(9): 774-85.

Riccardi, G. and A. A. Rivellese (1991). "Effects of dietary fiber and carbohydrate on glucose and lipoprotein metabolism in diabetic patients." Diabetes Care **14**(12): 1115-25.

Stacpoole, P. W., K. von Bergmann, et al. (1991). "Nutritional regulation of cholesterol synthesis and apolipoprotein B kinetics: studies in patients with familial hypercholesterolemia and normal subjects treated with a high carbohydrate, low fat diet." J Lipid Res **32**(11): 1837-48.

Ullmann, D., W. E. Connor, et al. (1991). "Will a high-carbohydrate, low-fat diet lower plasma lipids and lipoproteins without producing hypertriglyceridemia?" Arterioscler Thromb **11**(4): 1059-67.

Fukagawa, N. K., J. W. Anderson, et al. (1990). "High-carbohydrate, high-fiber diets increase peripheral insulin sensitivity in healthy young and old adults." Am J Clin Nutr **52**(3): 524-8.

Cataract

Bunce, G. E. (1993). "Antioxidant nutrition and cataract in women: a prospective study." Nutr Rev **51**(3): 84-6.

Taylor, A. (1993). "Cataract: relationship between nutrition and oxidation." J Am Coll Nutr **12**(2): 138-46.

Taylor, A., P. F. Jacques, et al. (1993). "Oxidation and aging: impact on vision." Toxicol Ind Health **9**(1-2): 349-71.

Vitale, S., S. West, et al. (1993). "Plasma antioxidants and risk of cortical and nuclear cataract [see comments]." Epidemiology **4**(3): 195-203.

Christen, W. G., J. E. Manson, et al. (1992). "A prospective study of cigarette smoking and risk of cataract in men [see comments]." Jama **268**(8): 989-93.

Hankinson, S. E., M. J. Stampfer, et al. (1992). "Nutrient intake and cataract extraction in women: a prospective study." Bmj **305**(6849): 335-9.

Knekt, P., M. Heliovaara, et al. (1992). "Serum antioxidant vitamins and risk of cataract." Bmj **305**(6866): 1392-4.

Taylor, A. (1992). "Effect of photooxidation on the eye lens and role of nutrients in delaying cataract." Exs **62**(1): 266-79.

Taylor, A. (1992). "Role of nutrients in delaying cataracts." Ann N Y Acad Sci **669**(1): 111-23.

Tsang, N. C., P. L. Penfold, et al. (1992). "Serum levels of antioxidants and age-related macular degeneration." Doc Ophthalmol **81**(4): 387-400.

Devamanoharan, P. S., M. Henein, et al. (1991). "Prevention of selenite cataract by vitamin C." Exp Eye Res **52**(5): 563-8.

Jacques, P. F. and L. Chylack Jr. (1991). "Epidemiologic evidence of a role for the antioxidant vitamins and carotenoids in cataract prevention." Am J Clin Nutr **53**(1 Suppl): 352S-355S.

Robertson, J. M., A. P. Donner, et al. (1991). "A possible role for vitamins C and E in cataract prevention." Am J Clin Nutr **53**(1 Suppl): 346S-351S.

Seddon, J. M., W. G. Christen, et al. (1991). "Low-dose aspirin and risks of cataract in a randomized trial of US physicians [see comments]." Arch Ophthalmol **109**(2): 252-5.

Taylor, A., P. F. Jacques, et al. (1991). "Relationship in humans between ascorbic acid consumption and levels of total and reduced ascorbic acid in lens, aqueous humor, and plasma." Curr Eye Res **10**(8): 751-9.

Varma, S. D. (1991). "Scientific basis for medical therapy of cataracts by antioxidants [published erratum appears in Am J Clin Nutr 1992 Jan; 55(1):iv]." Am J Clin Nutr **53**(1 Suppl): 335S-345S.

Chocolate

Denke, M. A. and S. M. Grundy (1991). "Effects of fats high in stearic acid on lipid and lipoprotein concentrations in men." Am J Clin Nutr **54**(6): 1036-40.

Cholesterol-Lowering Drugs

(1993). "Choice of cholesterol-lowering drugs." Med Lett Drugs Ther **35**(891): 19-22.

Brown, B. G., X.-Q. Zhao, et al. (1993). "Lipid lowering and plaque regression. New insights into prevention of plaque disruption and clinical events in coronary disease." Circulation **87**(6): 1781-1791.

Brown, B. G., X. Q. Zhao, et al. (1993). "Atherosclerosis regression, plaque disruption, and cardiovascular events: a rationale for lipid lowering in coronary artery disease." Annu Rev Med **44**(1): 365-76.

D'Agostino, R. B., W. B. Kannel, et al. (1993). "Efficacy and tolerability of lovastatin in hypercholesterolemia in patients with systemic hypertension." Am J Cardiol **71**(1): 82-7.

Franceschini, G. and R. Paoletti (1993). "Drugs controlling triglyceride metabolism." Med Res Rev **13**(2): 125-38.

Ghirlanda, G., A. Oradei, et al. (1993). "Evidence of plasma CoQ10-lowering effect by HMG-CoA reductase inhibitors: a double-blind, placebo-controlled study." J Clin Pharmacol **33**(3): 226-9.

Giroux, L. M., J. Davignon, et al. (1993). "Simvastatin inhibits the oxidation of low-density lipoproteins by activated human monocyte-derived macrophages." Biochim Biophys Acta **1165**(3): 335-8.

Gotto, A., Jr. (1993). "Overview of current issues in management of dyslipidemia." Am J Cardiol **71**(6): 3B-8B.

McGovern, M. E. and M. J. Mellies (1993). "Long-term experience with pravastatin in clinical research trials." Clin Ther **15**(1): 57-64.

Roberts, W. C. (1993). "The best anti-heart failure agent will be a lipid-lowering agent [editorial]." Am J Cardiol **71**(7): 628.

Schectman, G., J. Hiatt, et al. (1993). "Evaluation of the effectiveness of lipid-lowering therapy (bile acid sequestrants, niacin, psyllium and lovastatin) for treating hypercholesterolemia in veterans." Am J Cardiol **71**(10): 759-65.

Schmidt, E. B., D. R. Illingworth, et al. (1993). "Hypolipidemic effects of nicotinic acid in patients with familial defective apolipoprotein B-100." Metabolism **42**(2): 137-9.

(1992). "Efficacy and tolerability of simvastatin and pravastatin in patients with primary hypercholesterolemia (multicountry comparative study). The European Study Group." Am J Cardiol **70**(15): 1281-6.

Aviram, M., G. Dankner, et al. (1992). "Lovastatin inhibits low-density lipoprotein oxidation and alters its fluidity and uptake by macrophages: in vitro and in vivo studies." Metabolism **41**(3): 229-35.

Becker, M., D. Staab, et al. (1992). "Long-term treatment of severe familial hypercholesterolemia in children: effect of sitosterol and bezafibrate." Pediatrics **89**(1): 138-42.

Betteridge, D. J., D. Bhatnager, et al. (1992). "Treatment of familial hypercholesterolaemia. United Kingdom lipid clinics study of pravastatin and cholestyramine." Bmj **304**(6838): 1335-8.

Brown, B. G. (1992). "Effect of lovastatin or niacin combined with colestipol and regression of coronary atherosclerosis." Eur Heart J **13**(1): 17-20.

Brown, W. V. (1992). "When do we treat hypercholesterolemia?" Clin Cardiol **15**(11): III15-7.

Clifton, P. M., M. B. Wight, et al. (1992). "Is fat restriction needed with HMGCoA reductase inhibitor treatment?" Atherosclerosis **93**(1-2): 59-70.

D'Agostino, R. B., W. B. Kannel, et al. (1992). "A comparison between lovastatin and gemfibrozil in the treatment of primary hypercholesterolemia." Am J Cardiol **69**(1): 28-34.

Davey Smith, G. and J. Pekkanen (1992). "Should there be a moratorium on the use of cholesterol lowering drugs? [see comments]." Bmj **304**(6824): 431-4.

Fowkes, F. G., G. C. Leng, et al. (1992). "Serum cholesterol, triglycerides, and aggression in the general population." Lancet **340**(8826): 995-8.

Fujii, S. and B. E. Sobel (1992). "Direct effects of gemfibrozil on the fibrinolytic system. Diminution of synthesis of plasminogen activator inhibitor type 1." Circulation **85**(5): 1888-93.

Gotto, A., Jr. (1992). "Therapeutic intervention for hypercholesterolemia." Clin Cardiol **15**(11): III22-4.

Grover, S. A., M. Abrahamowicz, et al. (1992). "The benefits of treating hyperlipidemia to prevent coronary heart disease. Estimating changes in life expectancy and morbidity." Jama **267**(6): 816-22.

Grundy, S. M. (1992). "Cholesterol-lowering drugs as cardioprotective agents." Am J Cardiol **70**(21): 27I-32I.

Hoffman, R., G. J. Brook, et al. (1992). "Hypolipidemic drugs reduce lipoprotein susceptibility to undergo lipid peroxidation: in vitro and ex vivo studies." Atherosclerosis **93**(1-2): 105-13.

Holzgartner, H., U. Schmidt, et al. (1992). "Comparison of the efficacy and tolerance of a garlic preparation vs. bezafibrate." Arzneimittelforschung **42**(12): 1473-7.

Hulley, S. B., J. M. Walsh, et al. (1992). "Health policy on blood cholesterol. Time to change directions [editorial]." Circulation **86**(3): 1026-9.

Kaplan, N. M. (1992). "Lipid intervention trials in primary prevention: a critical review." Clin Exp Hypertens [a] **14**(1-2): 109-18.

La Rosa, J. C. (1992). "Cholesterol and cardiovascular disease: how strong is the evidence?" Clin Cardiol **15**(11 Suppl 3): III8-9.

La Rosa, J. C. and J. I. Cleeman (1992). "Cholesterol lowering as a treatment for established coronary heart disease." Circulation **85**(3): 1229-35.

Leren, T. P., I. Hjermann, et al. (1992). "Long-term effect of lovastatin alone and in combination with cholestyramine on lipoprotein (a) level in familial hypercholesterolemic subjects." Clin Investig **70**(8): 711-8.

McKenney, J. M., M. D. Barnett, et al. (1992). "Comparison of gemfibrozil and lovastatin in patients with high low-density lipoprotein and low high-density lipoprotein cholesterol levels." Arch Intern Med **152**(9): 1781-7.

Prihoda, J. S. and D. R. Illingworth (1992). "Drug therapy of hyperlipidemia." Curr Probl Cardiol **17**(9): 545-605.

Quiney, J., G. F. Watts, et al. (1992). "One year experience in the treatment of familial hypercholesterolaemia with simvastatin." Postgrad Med J **68**(801): 575-80.

Savica, V., G. Bellinghieri, et al. (1992). "[The hypotriglyceridemic action of the combination of L-carnitine + simvastatin vs. L-carnitine and vs. simvastatin]." Clin Ter **140**(1 Pt 2): 17-22.

Shear, C. L., F. A. Franklin, et al. (1992). "Expanded Clinical Evaluation of Lovastatin (EXCEL) study results. Effect of patient characteristics on lovastatin-induced changes in plasma concentrations of lipids and lipoproteins." Circulation **85**(4): 1293-303.

Slunga, L., O. Johnson, et al. (1992). "Changes in Lp(a) lipoprotein levels during the treatment of hypercholesterolaemia with simvastatin." Eur J Clin Pharmacol **43**(4): 369-73.

Superko, H. R., P. Greenland, et al. (1992). "Effectiveness of low-dose colestipol therapy in patients with moderate hypercholesterolemia." Am J Cardiol **70**(2): 135-40.

Tatami, R., N. Inoue, et al. (1992). "Regression of coronary atherosclerosis by combined LDL-apheresis and lipid-lowering drug therapy in patients with familial hypercholesterolemia: a multicenter study. The LARS Investigators." Atherosclerosis **95**(1): 1-13.

Vanhanen, H. and T. A. Miettinen (1992). "Pravastatin and lovastatin similarly reduce serum cholesterol and its precursor levels in familial hypercholesterolaemia." Eur J Clin Pharmacol **42**(2): 127-30.

Watts, G. F., B. Lewis, et al. (1992). "Effects on coronary artery disease of lipid-lowering diet, or diet plus cholestyramine, in the St Thomas' Atherosclerosis Regression Study (STARS) [see comments]." Lancet **339**(8793): 563-9.

Beigel, Y., J. Fuchs, et al. (1991). "Lovastatin therapy in heterozygous familial hypercholesterolaemic patients: effect on blood rheology and fibrinogen levels." J Intern Med **230**(1): 23-7.

Blankenhorn, D. H. (1991). "Regression of atherosclerosis: what does it mean?" Am J Med **90**(2A): 42S-47S.

Blankenhorn, D. H., S. P. Azen, et al. (1991). "Effects of colestipol-niacin therapy on human femoral atherosclerosis [see comments]." Circulation **83**(2): 438-47.

Blankenhorn, D. H. and H. N. Hodis (1991). "Treating serum lipid abnormalities in high-priority patients." Postgrad Med **89**(1): 81-2.

Superko, H. R. (1991). "Prevention and regression of atherosclerosis with drug therapy." Clin Cardiol **14**(2 Suppl 1): I40-7.

Uusitupa, M., T. Ebeling, et al. (1991). "Combination therapy with lovastatin and guar gum versus lovastatin and cholestyramine in treatment of hypercholesterolemia." J Cardiovasc Pharmacol **18**(4): 496-503.

Vega, G. L. and S. M. Grundy (1991). "Influence of lovastatin therapy on metabolism of low density lipoproteins in mixed hyperlipidaemia." J Intern Med **230**(4): 341-50.

Blankenhorn, D. H. (1990). "Can atherosclerotic lesions regress? Angiographic evidence in humans." Am J Cardiol **65**(12): 41F-43F.

Blankenhorn, D. H., P. Alaupovic, et al. (1990). "Prediction of angiographic change in native human coronary arteries and aortocoronary bypass grafts. Lipid and nonlipid factors [see comments]." Circulation **81**(2): 470-6.

Blankenhorn, D. H., R. L. Johnson, et al. (1990). "The influence of diet on the appearance of new lesions in human coronary arteries [see comments]." Jama **263**(12): 1646-52.

Brown, G., J. J. Albers, et al. (1990). "Regression of coronary artery disease as a result of intensive lipid-lowering therapy in men with high levels of apolipoprotein B [see comments]." N Engl J Med **323**(19): 1289-98.

Cashin-Hemphill, L., W. J. Mack, et al. (1990). "Beneficial effects of colestipol-niacin on coronary atherosclerosis. A 4-year follow-up [see comments]." Jama **264**(23): 3013-7.

Folkers, K., P. Langsjoen, et al. (1990). "Lovastatin decreases coenzyme Q levels in humans." Proc Natl Acad Sci U S A **87**(22): 8931-4.

Kane, J. P., M. J. Malloy, et al. (1990). "Regression of coronary atherosclerosis during treatment of familial hypercholesterolemia with combined drug regimens [see comments]." Jama **264**(23): 3007-12.

Blankenhorn, D. H. (1989). "Prevention or reversal of atherosclerosis: review of current evidence." Am J Cardiol **63**(16): 38H-41H.

Blankenhorn, D. H. and D. M. Kramsch (1989). "Reversal of atherosis and sclerosis. The two components of atherosclerosis." Circulation **79**(1): 1-7.

Kostner, G. M., D. Gavish, et al. (1989). "HMG CoA reductase inhibitors lower LDL cholesterol without reducing Lp(a) levels." Circulation **80**(5): 1313-9.

Blankenhorn, D. H., S. A. Nessim, et al. (1987). "Beneficial effects of combined colestipol-niacin therapy on coronary atherosclerosis and coronary venous bypass grafts [published erratum appears in JAMA 1988 May 13; 259(18):2698]." Jama **257**(23): 3233-40.

Malloy, M. J., J. P. Kane, et al. (1987). "Complementarity of colestipol, niacin, and lovastatin in treatment of severe familial hypercholesterolemia." Ann Intern Med **107**(5): 616-23.

Chromium

Anderson, R. A. (1993). "Recent advances in the clinical and biochemical effects of chromium deficiency." Prog Clin Biol Res **380**(1): 221-34.

Abraham, A. S., B. A. Brooks, et al. (1992). "The effects of chromium supplementation on serum glucose and lipids in patients with and without non-insulin-dependent diabetes." Metabolism **41**(7): 768-71.

Anderson, R. A. (1992). "Chromium, glucose tolerance, and diabetes." Biol Trace Elem Res **32**(1): 19-24.

Anderson, R. A., N. A. Bryden, et al. (1992). "Dietary chromium intake. Freely chosen diets, institutional diet, and individual foods." Biol Trace Elem Res **32**(1): 117-21.

Ani, M. and A. A. Moshtaghie (1992). "The effect of chromium on parameters related to iron metabolism." Biol Trace Elem Res **32**(1): 57-64.

Baruthio, F. (1992). "Toxic effects of chromium and its compounds." Biol Trace Elem Res **32**(1): 145-53.

Ducros, V. (1992). "Chromium metabolism. A literature review." Biol Trace Elem Res **32**(1): 65-77.

Evans, G. W. and T. D. Bowman (1992). "Chromium picolinate increases membrane fluidity and rate of insulin internalization." J Inorg Biochem **46**(4): 243-50.

Kumpulainen, J. T. (1992). "Chromium content of foods and diets." Biol Trace Elem Res **32**(1): 9-18.

Mertz, W. (1992). "Chromium. History and nutritional importance." Biol Trace Elem Res **32**(1): 3-8.

Morris, B. W., A. Blumsohn, et al. (1992). "The trace element chromium—a role in glucose homeostasis." Am J Clin Nutr **55**(5): 989-91.

Offenbacher, E. G. (1992). "Chromium in the elderly." Biol Trace Elem Res **32**(1): 123-31.

Uusitupa, M. I., L. Mykkanen, et al. (1992). "Chromium supplementation in impaired glucose tolerance of elderly: effects on blood glucose, plasma insulin, C-peptide and lipid levels(not helpful)." Br J Nutr **68**(1): 209-16.

Yoshimoto, S., K. Sakamoto, et al. (1992). "Effect of chromium administration on glucose tolerance in stroke-prone spontaneously hypertensive rats with streptozotocin-induced diabetes." Metabolism **41**(6): 636-42.

Abraham, A. S., B. A. Brooks, et al. (1991). "Chromium and cholesterol-induced atherosclerosis in rabbits." Ann Nutr Metab **35**(4): 203-7.

Anderson, R. A., M. M. Polansky, et al. (1991). "Supplemental-chromium effects on glucose, insulin, glucagon, and urinary chromium losses in subjects consuming controlled low-chromium diets." Am J Clin Nutr **54**(5): 909-16.

Lees, P. S. (1991). "Chromium and disease: review of epidemiologic studies with particular reference to etiologic information provided by measures of exposure." Environ Health Perspect **92**(1): 93-104.

Mahdi, G. S. and D. J. Naismith (1991). "Role of chromium in barley in modulating the symptoms of diabetes." Ann Nutr Metab **35**(2): 65-70.

Roeback, J. J., K. M. Hla, et al. (1991). "Effects of chromium supplementation on serum high-density lipoprotein cholesterol levels in men taking beta-blockers. A randomized, controlled trial [see comments]." Ann Intern Med **115**(12): 917-24.

Press, R. I., J. Geller, et al. (1990). "The effect of chromium picolinate on serum cholesterol and apolipoprotein fractions in human subjects [see comments]." West J Med **152**(1): 41-5.

Urberg, M., J. Benyi, et al. (1988). "Hypocholesterolemic effects of nicotinic acid and chromium supplementation." J Fam Pract **27**(6): 603-6.

Kozlovsky, A. S., P. B. Moser, et al. (1986). "Effects of diets high in simple sugars on urinary chromium losses." Metabolism **35**(6): 515-8.

Simonoff, M. (1984). "Chromium deficiency and cardiovascular risk." Cardiovasc Res **18**(10): 591-6.

Podell, R. N. (1983). "Chromium supplementation. Can it improve glucose and cholesterol metabolism?" Postgrad Med **74**(1): 135-8.

Check, W. A. (1982). "And if you add chromium, that's even better [news]." Jama **247**(22): 3046-7.

Clot-busters (Thrombolysis)

Davies, S. W., K. Ranjadayalan, et al. (1993). "Free radical activity and left ventricular function after thrombolysis for acute infarction." Br Heart J **69**(2): 114-20.

Grines, C. L., K. F. Browne, et al. (1993). "A comparison of immediate angioplasty with thrombolytic therapy for acute myocardial infarction. The Primary Angioplasty in Myocardial Infarction Study Group [see comments]." N Engl J Med **328**(10): 673-9.

Prager, N. A., S. R. Torr-Brown, et al. (1993). "Maintenance of patency after thrombolysis in stenotic coronary arteries requires combined inhibition of thrombin and platelets." J Am Coll Cardiol **22**(1): 296-301.

Benedict, C. R., S. Mueller, et al. (1992). "Thrombolytic therapy: a state of the art review." Hosp Pract **27**(6): 61-72.

Clotting

Badimon, J. J., V. Fuster, et al. (1993). "Coronary atherosclerosis. A multifactorial disease." Circulation **87**(3 Suppl): II3-16.

Barbash, G. I., H. D. White, et al. (1993). "Significance of smoking in patients receiving thrombolytic therapy for acute myocardial infarction. Experience gleaned from the International Tissue Plasminogen Activator/Streptokinase Mortality Trial [see comments]." Circulation **87**(1): 53-8.

Budd, J. S., K. Allen, et al. (1993). "The effectiveness of low dose slow release aspirin as an antiplatelet agent." J R Soc Med **86**(5): 261-3.

Colwell, J. A. (1993). "Vascular thrombosis in type II diabetes mellitus [editorial]." Diabetes **42**(1): 8-11.

Folsom, A. R., H. T. Qamhieh, et al. (1993). "Impact of weight loss on plasminogen activator inhibitor (PAI-1), factor VII, and other hemostatic factors in moderately overweight adults." Arterioscler Thromb **13**(2): 162-9.

Hajjar, K. A. (1993). "Homocysteine-induced modulation of tissue plasminogen activator binding to its endothelial cell membrane receptor." J Clin Invest **91**(6): 2873-9.

Harker, L. A., A. B. Kelly, et al. (1993). "Interruption of vascular thrombus formation and vascular lesion formation by dietary n-3 fatty acids in fish oil in nonhuman primates." Circulation **87**(3): 1017-29.

Huang, Z. S., C. M. Teng, et al. (1993). "Combined use of aspirin and heparin inhibits in vivo acute carotid thrombosis." Stroke **24**(6): 829-36.

Legnani, C., M. Frascaro, et al. (1993). "Effects of a dried garlic preparation on fibrinolysis and platelet aggregation in healthy subjects." Arzneimittelforschung **43**(2): 119-22.

Mohri, H. and T. Ohkubo (1993). "Single-dose effect of enteric-coated aspirin on platelet function and thromboxane generation in middle-aged men." Ann Pharmacother **27**(4): 405-10.

Nadler, J. L., T. Buchanan, et al. (1993). "Magnesium deficiency produces insulin resistance and increased thromboxane synthesis." Hypertension **21**: 1024-1029.

Schonwetter, D. J., J. M. Gerrard, et al. (1993). "Type A behavior and alcohol consumption: effects on resting and post-exercise bleeding time thromboxane and prostacyclin metabolites." Prostaglandins Leukot Essent Fatty Acids **48**(2): 143-8.

Schonwetter, D. J., J. M. Gerrard, et al. (1993). "Type A behavior and alcohol consumption: effects on resting and post-exercise bleeding time thromboxane and prostacyclin metabolites." Prostaglandins Leukot Essent Fatty Acids **48**(2): 143-8.

Steiner, M. (1993). "Vitamin E: more than an antioxidant." Clin Cardiol **16**(4 Suppl 1): I16-8.

Ware, J. A. and D. D. Heistad (1993). "Seminars in medicine of the Beth Israel Hospital, Boston. Platelet-endothelium interactions." N Engl J Med **328**(9): 628-35.

Andersen, P. (1992). "Hypercoagulability and reduced fibrinolysis in hyperlipidemia: relationship to the metabolic cardiovascular syndrome." J Cardiovasc Pharmacol **20**(1): S29-31.

Badimon, L., J. J. Badimon, et al. (1992). "Endothelium and atherosclerosis." J Hypertens Suppl **10**(2): S43-50.

Badimon, L., J. H. Chesebro, et al. (1992). "Thrombus formation on ruptured atherosclerotic plaques and rethrombosis on evolving thrombi." Circulation **86**(6 Suppl): III74-85.

Caine, Y. G., K. A. Bauer, et al. (1992). "Coagulation activation following estrogen administration to postmenopausal women." Thromb Haemost **68**(4): 392-5.

Cairns, J. A., J. Hirsh, et al. (1992). "Antithrombotic agents in coronary artery disease." Chest **102**(4 Suppl): 456S-481S.

Chesebro, J. H. and V. Fuster (1992). "Thrombosis in unstable angina [editorial; comment]." N Engl J Med **327**(3): 192-4.

Chesebro, J. H., M. W. Webster, et al. (1992). "Antithrombotic therapy and progression of coronary artery disease. Antiplatelet versus antithrombins." Circulation **86**(6 Suppl): III100-10.

Connelly, J. B., J. A. Cooper, et al. (1992). "Strenuous exercise, plasma fibrinogen, and factor VII activity." Br Heart J **67**(5): 351-4.

Dalen, J. E. and J. Hirsh (1992). "Antithrombotic therapy. Introduction." Chest **102**(4 Suppl): 303S-304S.

Davi, G., M. Averna, et al. (1992). "Increased thromboxane biosynthesis in type IIa hypercholesterolemia." Circulation **85**(5): 1792-8.

Dotevall, A., C. Rangemark, et al. (1992). "Cigarette smoking increases thromboxane A2 formation without affecting platelet survival in young healthy females." Thromb Haemost **68**(5): 583-8.

Fujii, S. and B. E. Sobel (1992). "Direct effects of gemfibrozil on the fibrinolytic system. Diminution of synthesis of plasminogen activator inhibitor type 1." Circulation **85**(5): 1888-93.

Gliksman, M. and A. Wilson (1992). "Are hemostatic factors responsible for the paradoxical risk factors for coronary heart disease and stroke?" Stroke **23**(4): 607-10.

Grignani, G., L. Pacchiarini, et al. (1992). "Effect of mental stress on platelet function in normal subjects and in patients with coronary artery disease." Haemostasis **22**(3): 138-46.

Grines, C. L. (1992). "Thrombolytic, antiplatelet, and antithrombotic agents." Am J Cardiol **70**(21): 18I-26I.

Harker, L. A. (1992). "What are the effects of dietary n-3 fatty acids on vascular thrombus and lesion formation in nonhuman primates?" Am J Clin Nutr **56**(4 Suppl): 817S-818S.

Harpel, P. C., V. T. Chang, et al. (1992). "Homocysteine and other sulfhydryl compounds enhance the binding of lipoprotein(a) to fibrin: a potential biochemical link between thrombosis, atherogenesis, and sulfhydryl compound metabolism." Proc Natl Acad Sci U S A **89**(21): 10193-7.

Kannel, W. B., et al (1992). "Update on fibrinogen as a cardiovascular risk factor." Ann Epidem **2**: 457-466.

Kario, K., T. Matsuo, et al. (1992). "Cigarette smoking increases the mean platelet volume in elderly patients with risk factors for atherosclerosis." Clin Lab Haematol **14**(4): 281-7.

Kelleher, C. C. (1992). "Plasma fibrinogen and factor VII as risk factors for cardiovascular disease." Eur J Epidemiol **8**(1): 79-82.

Kovacs, I. B., C. P. Ratnatunga, et al. (1992). "Significance of plasma fibrinogen in coronary arterial disease: marker or causative risk factor for arterial thrombosis?" Int J Cardiol **35**(1): 57-64.

Lam, J. Y., J. J. Badimon, et al. (1992). "Cod liver oil alters platelet-arterial wall response to injury in pigs." Circ Res **71**(4): 769-75.

Lawson, L. D., D. K. Ransom, et al. (1992). "Inhibition of whole blood platelet-aggregation by compounds in garlic clove extracts and commercial garlic products." Thromb Res **65**(2): 141-56.

Loscalzo, J. (1992). "Antiplatelet and antithrombotic effects of organic nitrates." Am J Cardiol **70**(8): 18B-22B.

Loscalzo, J. (1992). "The relation between atherosclerosis and thrombosis." Circulation **86**(6 Suppl): III95-9.

Lowe, G. D. (1992). "Blood viscosity and cardiovascular disease." Thromb Haemost **67**(5): 494-8.

Lowe, G. D. (1992). "Blood viscosity, lipoproteins, and cardiovascular risk [editorial; comment]." Circulation **85**(6): 2329-31.

Meydani, M. (1992). "Modulation of the platelet thromboxane A2 and aortic prostacyclin synthesis by dietary selenium and vitamin E." Biol Trace Elem Res **33**(1): 79-86.

Miller, G. J. (1992). "Hemostasis and cardiovascular risk. The British and European experience." Arch Pathol Lab Med **116**(12): 1318-21.

Mitropoulos, K. A., G. J. Miller, et al. (1992). "Lipolysis of triglyceride-rich lipoproteins activates coagulant factor XII: a study in familial lipoprotein-lipase deficiency." Atherosclerosis **95**(2-3): 119-25.

Mutanen, M., R. Freese, et al. (1992). "Rapeseed oil and sunflower oil diets enhance platelet in vitro aggregation and thromboxane production in healthy men when compared with milk fat or habitual diets." Thromb Haemost **67**(3): 352-6.

Prescott, S. M. (1992). "What are the effects of dietary fatty acid modification on platelet eicosanoid metabolism, platelet-activating factor, and platelet function? How might these metabolic alterations influence thrombosis?" Am J Clin Nutr **56**(4 Suppl): 801S-802S.

Rangemark, C., G. Benthin, et al. (1992). "Tobacco use and urinary excretion of thromboxane A2 and prostacyclin metabolites in women stratified by age." Circulation **86**(5): 1495-500.

Sakata, K., T. Hoshino, et al. (1992). "Circadian fluctuations of tissue plasminogen activator antigen and plasminogen activator inhibitor-1 antigens in vasospastic angina." Am Heart J **124**(4): 854-60.

Steiner, M. (1992). "Alpha-tocopherol: a potent inhibitor of platelet adhesion." J Nutr Sci Vitaminol **1**(5): 191-5.

Tracy, R. P. and E. G. Bovill (1992). "Thrombosis and cardiovascular risk in the elderly." Arch Pathol Lab Med **116**(12): 1307-12.

Wosornu, D., W. Allardyce, et al. (1992). "Influence of power and aerobic exercise training on haemostatic factors after coronary artery surgery." Br Heart J **68**(2): 181-6.

Badimon, L., J. J. Badimon, et al. (1991). "Vessel wall-related risk factors in acute vascular events." Drugs **42**(1): 1-9.

Becker, R. C. (1991). "Seminars in thrombosis, thrombolysis and vascular biology. 3. Platelet activity in cardiovascular disease." Cardiology **79**(1): 49-63.

Beretz, A. and J. P. Cazenave (1991). "Old and new natural products as the source of modern antithrombotic drugs." Planta Med **57**(7): S68-72.

Chesebro, J. H. and V. Fuster (1991). "Dynamic thrombosis and thrombolysis. Role of antithrombins [editorial; comment]." Circulation **83**(5): 1815-7.

Chesebro, J. H., P. Zoldhelyi, et al. (1991). "Role of thrombin in arterial thrombosis: implications for therapy." Thromb Haemost **66**(1): 1-5.

Chesebro, J. H., P. Zoldhelyi, et al. (1991). "Pathogenesis of thrombosis in unstable angina." Am J Cardiol **68**(7): 2B-10B.

Chesebro, J. H., P. Zoldhelyi, et al. (1991). "Plaque disruption and thrombosis in unstable angina pectoris." Am J Cardiol **68**(12): 9C-15C.

Ciavatti, M. and S. Renaud (1991). "Oxidative status and oral contraceptive. Its relevance to platelet abnormalities and cardiovascular risk." Free Radic Biol Med **10**(5): 325-38.

Cobiac, L., P. M. Clifton, et al. (1991). "Lipid, lipoprotein, and hemostatic effects of fish vs fish-oil n-3 fatty acids in mildly hyperlipidemic males." Am J Clin Nutr **53**(5): 1210-6.

Dahlen, G. H. (1991). "Lipoprotein(a), atherosclerosis and thrombosis." Prog Lipid Res **30**(2-3): 189-94.

Folsom, A. R., K. K. Wu, et al. (1991). "Population correlates of plasma fibrinogen and factor VII, putative cardiovascular risk factors." Atherosclerosis **91**(3): 191-205.

Force, T., R. Milani, et al. (1991). "Aspirin-induced decline in prostacyclin production in patients with coronary artery disease is due to decreased endoperoxide shift. Analysis of the effects of a combination of aspirin and n-3 fatty acids on the eicosanoid profile [see comments]." Circulation **84**(6): 2286-93.

Fuster, V., J. H. Ip, et al. (1991). "Importance of experimental models for the development of clinical trials on thromboatherosclerosis." Circulation **83**(6 Suppl): IV15-25.

Gadkari, J. V. and V. D. Joshi (1991). "Effect of ingestion of raw garlic on serum cholesterol level, clotting time and fibrinolytic activity in normal subjects." J Postgrad Med **37**(3): 128-31.

Heinrich, J., M. Sandkamp, et al. (1991). "Relationship of lipoprotein(a) to variables of coagulation and fibrinolysis in a healthy population." Clin Chem **37**(11): 1950-4.

Jansson, J. H., T. K. Nilsson, et al. (1991). "Tissue plasminogen activator and other risk factors as predictors of cardiovascular events in patients with severe angina pectoris." Eur Heart J **12**(2): 157-61.

Kiesewetter, H., F. Jung, et al. (1991). "Effect of garlic on thrombocyte aggregation, microcirculation, and other risk factors." Int J Clin Pharmacol Ther Toxicol **29**(4): 151-5.

Lenz, P. H., T. Watkins, et al. (1991). "Effect of dietary menhaden, Canola and partially hydrogenated soy oil supplemented with vitamin E upon plasma lipids and platelet aggregation." Thromb Res **61**(3): 213-24.

Lowe, G. D., D. A. Wood, et al. (1991). "Relationships of plasma viscosity, coagulation and fibrinolysis to coronary risk factors and angina." Thromb Haemost **65**(4): 339-43.

Miller, G. J., J. C. Martin, et al. (1991). "Plasma factor VII is activated by postprandial triglyceridaemia, irrespective of dietary fat composition." Atherosclerosis **86**(2-3): 163-71.

Nelson, G. J., P. C. Schmidt, et al. (1991). "The effect of a salmon diet on blood clotting, platelet aggregation and fatty acids in normal adult men." Lipids **26**(2): 87-96.

Neumann, F. J., H. A. Katus, et al. (1991). "Increased plasma viscosity and erythrocyte aggregation: indicators of an unfavourable clinical outcome in patients with unstable angina pectoris." Br Heart J **66**(6): 425-30.

Numminen, H., M. Hillbom, et al. (1991). "Effects of exercise and ethanol ingestion on platelet thromboxane release in healthy men." Metabolism **40**(7): 695-701.

Ridker, P. M. and C. H. Hennekens (1991). "Hemostatic risk factors for coronary heart disease [editorial; comment]." Circulation **83**(3): 1098-100.

Ridker, P. M., J. E. Manson, et al. (1991). "Clinical characteristics of nonfatal myocardial infarction among individuals on prophylactic low-dose aspirin therapy." Circulation **84**(2): 708-11.

Ridker, P. M., J. E. Manson, et al. (1991). "The effect of chronic platelet inhibition with low-dose aspirin on atherosclerotic progression and acute thrombosis: clinical evidence from the Physicians' Health Study." Am Heart J **122**(6): 1588-92.

Ridker, P. M., J. E. Manson, et al. (1991). "Low-dose aspirin therapy for chronic stable angina. A randomized, placebo-controlled clinical trial." Ann Intern Med **114**(10): 835-9.

Ridker, P. M., S. N. Willich, et al. (1991). "Aspirin, platelet aggregation, and the circadian variation of acute thrombotic events." Chronobiol Int **8**(5): 327-35.

Rouy, D., P. Grailhe, et al. (1991). "Lipoprotein(a) impairs generation of plasmin by fibrin-bound tissue-type plasminogen activator. In vitro studies in a plasma milieu." Arterioscler Thromb **11**(3): 629-38.

Salonen, J. T., R. Salonen, et al. (1991). "Effects of antioxidant supplementation on platelet function: a randomized pair-matched, placebo-controlled, double-blind trial in men with low antioxidant status [see comments]." Am J Clin Nutr **53**(5): 1222-9.

Sandset, P. M., H. Lund, et al. (1991). "Treatment with hydroxymethylglutaryl-coenzyme A reductase inhibitors in hypercholesterolemia induces changes in the components of the extrinsic coagulation system." Arterioscler Thromb **11**(1): 138-45.

Thaulow, E., J. Erikssen, et al. (1991). "Blood platelet count and function are related to total and cardiovascular death in apparently healthy men [see comments]." Circulation **84**(2): 613-7.

Vasilieva, E. J., A. V. Shpector, et al. (1991). "Platelet function and plasma lipid levels in patients with stable and unstable angina pectoris." Am J Cardiol **68**(9): 959-61.

Wander, R. C. and B. D. Patton (1991). "Comparison of three species of fish consumed as part of a Western diet: effects on platelet fatty acids and function, hemostasis, and production of thromboxane." Am J Clin Nutr **54**(2): 326-33.

Broadhurst, P., C. Kelleher, et al. (1990). "Fibrinogen, factor VII clotting activity and coronary artery disease severity." Atherosclerosis **85**(2-3): 169-73.

Fuster, V., B. Stein, et al. (1990). "Atherosclerotic plaque rupture and thrombosis. Evolving concepts." Circulation **82**(3 Suppl): II47-59.

Ridker, P. M., J. E. Manson, et al. (1990). "Circadian variation of acute myocardial infarction and the effect of low-dose aspirin in a randomized trial of physicians." Circulation **82**(3): 897-902.

Violi, F., D. Pratico, et al. (1990). "Inhibition of cyclooxygenase-independent platelet aggregation by low vitamin E concentration." Atherosclerosis **82**(3): 247-52.

Gisinger, C., J. Jeremy, et al. (1988). "Effect of vitamin E supplementation on platelet thromboxane A2 production in type I diabetic patients. Double-blind crossover trial." Diabetes **37**(9): 1260-4.

CoQ10

Ali, K., M. Morimoto, et al. (1993). "Improvement of cardiac function impaired by repeated ischemic arrests in isolated rat hearts." Ann Thorac Surg **55**(4): 902-7.

Folkers, K., R. Brown, et al. (1993). "Survival of cancer patients on therapy with coenzyme Q10." Biochem Biophys Res Commun **192**(1): 241-5.

Folkers, K., M. Morita, et al. (1993). "The activities of coenzyme Q10 and vitamin B6 for immune responses." Biochem Biophys Res Commun **193**(1): 88-92.

Ghirlanda, G., A. Oradei, et al. (1993). "Evidence of plasma CoQ10-lowering effect by HMG-CoA reductase inhibitors: a double-blind, placebo-controlled study." J Clin Pharmacol **33**(3): 226-9.

Ingold, K. U., V. W. Bowry, et al. (1993). "Autoxidation of lipids and antioxidation by alpha-tocopherol and ubiquinol in homogeneous solution and in aqueous dispersions of lipids: unrecognized consequences of lipid particle size as exemplified by oxidation of human low density lipoprotein." Proc Natl Acad Sci U S A **90**(1): 45-9.

Vadhanavikit, S. and H. E. Ganther (1993). "Decreased ubiquinone levels in tissues of rats deficient in selenium." Biochem Biophys Res Commun **190**(3): 921-6.

Beyer, R. E. (1992). "An analysis of the role of coenzyme Q in free radical generation and as an antioxidant." Biochem Cell Biol **70**(6): 390-403.

Digiesi, V., F. Cantini, et al. (1992). "Mechanisum of action of coenzyme Q10 in essential hypertension." Curr Ther Res **51**(5): 668-672.

Ernster, L., P. Forsmark, et al. (1992). "The mode of action of lipid-soluble antioxidants in biological membranes. Relationship between the effects of ubiquinol and vitamin E as inhibitors of lipid peroxidation in submitochondrial particles." J Nutr Sci Vitaminol **1**(51): 548-51.

Ernster, L., P. Forsmark, et al. (1992). "The mode of action of lipid-soluble antioxidants in biological membranes: relationship between the effects of ubiquinol and vitamin E as inhibitors of lipid peroxidation in submitochondrial particles." Biofactors **3**(4): 241-8.

Folkers, K., P. Langsjoen, et al. (1992). "Therapy with coenzyme Q10 of patients in heart failure who are eligible or ineligible for a transplant." Biochem Biophys Res Commun **182**(1): 247-53.

Giral, P. and E. Bruckert (1992). "Ratio of low-density lipoprotein cholesterol to ubiquinone as a coronary risk factor [letter; comment]." N Engl J Med **326**(6): 416-7.

Karlsson, J., B. Diamant, et al. (1992). "Plasma ubiquinone, alpha-tocopherol and cholesterol in man." Int J Vitam Nutr Res **62**(2): 160-4.

Kawasaki, T. (1992). "Antioxidant function of coenzyme Q." J Nutr Sci Vitaminol **1**(5): 552-5.

Matsushima, T., T. Sueda, et al. (1992). "Protection by coenzyme Q10 of canine myocardial reperfusion injury after preservation." J Thorac Cardiovasc Surg **103**(5): 945-51.

Merati, G., P. Pasquali, et al. (1992). "Antioxidant activity of ubiquinone-3 in human low density lipoprotein." Free Radic Res Commun **16**(1): 11-7.

Mohr, D., V. W. Bowry, et al. (1992). "Dietary supplementation with coenzyme Q10 results in increased levels of ubiquinol-10 within circulating lipoproteins and increased resistance of human low-density lipoprotein to the initiation of lipid peroxidation." Biochim Biophys Acta **1126**(3): 247-54.

Permanetter, B., W. Rossy, et al. (1992). "Ubiquinone (coenzyme Q10) in the long-term treatment of idiopathic dilated cardiomyopathy." Eur Heart J **13**(11): 1528-33.

Sun, I. L., E. E. Sun, et al. (1992). "Requirement for coenzyme Q in plasma membrane electron transport." Proc Natl Acad Sci U S A **89**(23): 11126-30.

Yokoyama, K., M. Itoman, et al. (1992). "Protective effects of coenzyme Q10 on ischemia-induced reperfusion injury in ischemic limb models." Plast Reconstr Surg **90**(5): 890-8.

Cabrini, L., C. Stefanelli, et al. (1991). "Ubiquinol prevents alpha-tocopherol consumption during liposome peroxidation." Biochem Int **23**(4): 743-9.

Elmberger, P. G., A. Kalen, et al. (1991). "Effects of pravastatin and cholestyramine on products of the mevalonate pathway in familial hypercholesterolemia." J Lipid Res **32**(6): 935-40.

Forsmark, P., F. Aberg, et al. (1991). "Inhibition of lipid peroxidation by ubiquinol in submitochondrial particles in the absence of vitamin E." Febs Lett **285**(1): 39-43.

Hanaki, Y., S. Sugiyama, et al. (1991). "Ratio of low-density lipoprotein cholesterol to ubiquinone as a coronary risk factor [letter] [see comments]." N Engl J Med **325**(11): 814-5.

Johansen, K., H. Theorell, et al. (1991). "Coenzyme Q10, alpha-tocopherol and free cholesterol in HDL and LDL fractions." Ann Med **23**(6): 649-56.

Okamoto, H., H. Kawaguchi, et al. (1991). "Effect of coenzyme Q10 on structural alterations in the renal membrane of stroke-prone spontaneously hypertensive rats." Biochem Med Metab Biol **45**(2): 216-26.

Shimomura, Y., M. Suzuki, et al. (1991). "Protective effect of coenzyme Q10 on exercise-induced muscular injury." Biochem Biophys Res Commun **176**(1): 349-55.

Stocker, R., V. W. Bowry, et al. (1991). "Ubiquinol-10 protects human low density lipoprotein more efficiently against lipid peroxidation than does alpha-tocopherol." Proc Natl Acad Sci U S A **88**(5): 1646-50.

Sunamori, M., H. Tanaka, et al. (1991). "Clinical experience of coenzyme Q10 to enhance intraoperative myocardial protection in coronary artery revascularization." Cardiovasc Drugs Ther **5**(1): 297-300.

Wang, Y. L., Y. S. Li, et al. (1991). "Effect of ubiquinone on ischemic arrhythmia in conscious rats." Chung Kuo Yao Li Hsueh Pao **12**(3): 202-6.

Zamora, R., F. J. Hidalgo, et al. (1991). "Comparative antioxidant effectiveness of dietary beta-carotene, vitamin E, selenium and coenzyme Q10 in rat erythrocytes and plasma." J Nutr **121**(1): 50-6.

Folkers, K., P. Langsjoen, et al. (1990). "Lovastatin decreases coenzyme Q levels in humans." Proc Natl Acad Sci U S A **87**(22): 8931-4.

Frei, B., M. C. Kim, et al. (1990). "Ubiquinol-10 is an effective lipid-soluble antioxidant at physiological concentrations." Proc Natl Acad Sci U S A **87**(12): 4879-83.

Langsjoen, P. H., P. H. Langsjoen, et al. (1990). "Long-term efficacy and safety of coenzyme Q10 therapy for idiopathic dilated cardiomyopathy." Am J Cardiol **65**(7): 521-3.

Leibovitz, B., M. L. Hu, et al. (1990). "Dietary supplements of vitamin E, beta-carotene, coenzyme Q10 and selenium protect tissues against lipid peroxidation in rat tissue slices." J Nutr **120**(1): 97-104.

Greenberg, S. M. and W. H. Frishman (1988). "Coenzyme Q10: a new drug for myocardial ischemia?" Med Clin North Am **72**(1): 243-58.

Kamikawa, T., A. Kobayashi, et al. (1985). "Effects of coenzyme Q10 on exercise tolerance in chronic stable angina pectoris." Am J Cardiol **56**(4): 247-51.

Coffee

Hofer, I. and K. Battig (1993). "Coffee consumption, blood pressure tonus and reactivity to physical challenge in 338 women." Pharmacol Biochem Behav **44**(3): 573-6.

Pirich, C., J. O'Grady, et al. (1993). "Coffee, lipoproteins and cardiovascular disease." Wien Klin Wochenschr **105**(1): 3-6.

(1992). "Regular or decaf? Coffee consumption and serum lipoproteins." Nutr Rev **50**(6): 175-8.

Casiglia, E., C. D. Paleari, et al. (1992). "Haemodynamic effects of coffee and purified caffeine in normal volunteers: a placebo-controlled clinical study." J Hum Hypertens **6**(2): 95-9.

Fried, R. E., D. M. Levine, et al. (1992). "The effect of filtered-coffee consumption on plasma lipid levels. Results of a randomized clinical trial." Jama **267**(6): 811-5.

Green, M. S. and G. Harari (1992). "Association of serum lipoproteins and health-related habits with coffee and tea consumption in free-living subjects examined in the Israeli CORDIS Study." Prev Med **21**(4): 532-45.

Hostmark, A. T., J. Berg, et al. (1992). "Coronary risk factors in middle-aged men as related to smoking, coffee intake and physical activity." Scand J Soc Med **20**(4): 196-203.

Myers, M. G. and A. Basinski (1992). "Coffee and coronary heart disease." Arch Intern Med **152**(9): 1767-72.

Ahola, I., M. Jauhiainen, et al. (1991). "The hypercholesterolaemic factor in boiled coffee is retained by a paper filter." J Intern Med **230**(4): 293-7.

Bak, A. A. and D. E. Grobbee (1991). "Caffeine, blood pressure, and serum lipids." Am J Clin Nutr **53**(4): 971-5.

Casiglia, E., S. Bongiovi, et al. (1991). "Haemodynamic effects of coffee and caffeine in normal volunteers: a placebo-controlled clinical study." J Intern Med **229**(6): 501-4.

Kohlmeier, L., G. Mensink, et al. (1991). "The relationship between coffee consumption and lipid levels in young and older people in the Heidelberg-Michelstadt-Berlin study." Eur Heart J **12**(8): 869-74.

Lindahl, B., I. Johansson, et al. (1991). "Coffee drinking and blood cholesterol—effects of brewing method, food intake and life style." J Intern Med **230**(4): 299-305.

Mac Donald, T. M., K. Sharpe, et al. (1991). "Caffeine restriction: effect on mild hypertension." Bmj **303**(6812): 1235-8.

Rosengren, A. and L. Wilhelmsen (1991). "Coffee, coronary heart disease and mortality in middle-aged Swedish men: findings from the Primary Prevention Study." J Intern Med **230**(1): 67-71.

Salvaggio, A., M. Periti, et al. (1991). "Coffee and cholesterol, an Italian study." Am J Epidemiol **134**(2): 149-56.

Sedor, F. A., K. A. Schneider, et al. (1991). "Effect of coffee on cholesterol and apolipoproteins, corroborated by caffeine levels." Am J Prev Med **7**(6): 391-6.

Superko, H. R., W. Bortz Jr., et al. (1991). "Caffeinated and decaffeinated coffee effects on plasma lipoprotein cholesterol, apolipoproteins, and lipase activity: a controlled, randomized trial." Am J Clin Nutr **54**(3): 599-605.

Thelle, D. S. (1991). "Coffee, cholesterol, and coronary heart disease [editorial]." Bmj **302**(6780): 804.

van Dusseldorp, M., M. B. Katan, et al. (1991). "Cholesterol-raising factor from boiled coffee does not pass a paper filter." Arterioscler Thromb **11**(3): 586-93.

van Dusseldorp, M., P. Smits, et al. (1991). "Boiled coffee and blood pressure. A 14-week controlled trial." Hypertension **18**(5): 607-13.

Congestive Heart Failure/Cardiomyopathy

Roberts, W. C. (1993). "The best anti-heart failure agent will be a lipid-lowering agent [editorial]." Am J Cardiol **71**(7): 628.

Azuma, J., A. Sawamura, et al. (1992). "Usefulness of taurine in chronic congestive heart failure and its prospective application." Jpn Circ J **56**(1): 95-9.

Folkers, K., P. Langsjoen, et al. (1992). "Therapy with coenzyme Q10 of patients in heart failure who are eligible or ineligible for a transplant." Biochem Biophys Res Commun **182**(1): 247-53.

Kobayashi, A., Y. Masumura, et al. (1992). "L-carnitine treatment for congestive heart failure—experimental and clinical study." Jpn Circ J **56**(1): 86-94.

Pasini, E., L. Comini, et al. (1992). "Effect of propionyl-L-carnitine on experimental induced cardiomyopathy in rats." Am J Cardiovasc Pathol **4**(3): 216-22.

Permanetter, B., W. Rossy, et al. (1992). "Ubiquinone (coenzyme Q10) in the long-term treatment of idiopathic dilated cardiomyopathy." Eur Heart J **13**(11): 1528-33.

Pucciarelli, G., M. Mastursi, et al. (1992). "[The clinical and hemodynamic effects of propionyl-L-carnitine in the treatment of congestive heart failure]." Clin Ter **141**(11): 379-84.

Teo, K. K., A. P. Ignaszewski, et al. (1992). "Contemporary medical management of left ventricular dysfunction and congestive heart failure." Can J Cardiol **8**(6): 611-9.

Weglicki, W. B., S. Bloom, et al. (1992). "Antioxidants and the cardiomyopathy of Mg-deficiency." Am J Cardiovasc Pathol **4**(3): 210-5.

Belch, J. J., A. B. Bridges, et al. (1991). "Oxygen free radicals and congestive heart failure." Br Heart J **65**(5): 245-8.

Ganguly, P. K. (1991). "Antioxidant therapy in congestive heart failure: is there any advantage? [editorial] [see comments]." J Intern Med **229**(3): 205-8.

Langsjoen, P. H., P. H. Langsjoen, et al. (1990). "Long-term efficacy and safety of coenzyme Q10 therapy for idiopathic dilated cardiomyopathy." Am J Cardiol **65**(7): 521-3.

Regitz, V., A. L. Shug, et al. (1990). "Defective myocardial carnitine metabolism in congestive heart failure secondary to dilated cardiomyopathy and to coronary, hypertensive and valvular heart diseases." Am J Cardiol **65**(11): 755-60.

Coronary Bypass Surgery, Angioplasty and Restenosis

Fremes, S. E., C. Levinton, et al. (1993). "Optimal antithrombotic therapy following aorto-coronary bypass: a meta-analysis." Eur J Cardiothorac Surg **7**(4): 169-80.

Grines, C. L., K. F. Browne, et al. (1993). "A comparison of immediate angioplasty with thrombolytic therapy for acute myocardial infarction. The Primary Angioplasty in Myocardial Infarction Study Group [see comments]." N Engl J Med **328**(10): 673-9.

Mezzetti, A., D. Lapenna, et al. (1993). "Myocardial antioxidant defenses during cardiopulmonary bypass." J Card Surg **8**(2): 167-71.

Davis, K. B., E. L. Alderman, et al. (1992). "Early mortality of acute myocardial infarction in patients with and without prior coronary revascularization surgery. A Coronary Artery Surgery Study Registry Study." Circulation **85**(6): 2100-9.

De Maio, S. J., S. 3. King, et al. (1992). "Vitamin E supplementation, plasma lipids and incidence of restenosis after percutaneous transluminal coronary angioplasty (PTCA)." J Am Coll Nutr **11**(1): 68-73.

DeMaio, S. J., S. B. 3. King, et al. (1992). "Vitamin E supplementation, plasma lipids and incidence of restenosis after percutaneous transluminal coronary angioplasty (PTCA)." J Am Coll Nutr **11**(1): 68-73.

England, M. R., G. Gordon, et al. (1992). "Magnesium administration and dysrhythmias after cardiac surgery. A placebo-controlled, double-blind, randomized trial." Jama **268**(17): 2395-402.

Fasol, R., M. Schindler, et al. (1992). "The influence of obesity on perioperative morbidity: retrospective study of 502 aortocoronary bypass operations." Thorac Cardiovasc Surg **40**(3): 126-9.

Hearn, J. A., B. C. Donohue, et al. (1992). "Usefulness of serum lipoprotein (a) as a predictor of restenosis after percutaneous transluminal coronary angioplasty." Am J Cardiol **69**(8): 736-9.

Israel, D. H. and R. Gorlin (1992). "Fish oils in the prevention of atherosclerosis." J Am Coll Cardiol **19**(1): 174-85.

Johnson, W. D., K. L. Kayser, et al. (1992). "Aspirin use and survival after coronary bypass surgery." Am Heart J **123**(3): 603-8.

Kaul, U., S. Sanghvi, et al. (1992). "Fish oil supplements for prevention of restenosis after coronary angioplasty." Int J Cardiol **35**(1): 87-93.

Libby, P., D. Schwartz, et al. (1992). "A cascade model for restenosis. A special case of atherosclerosis progression." Circulation **86**(6 Suppl): III47-52.

O'Connor, G. T., D. J. Malenka, et al. (1992). "A meta-analysis of randomized trials of fish oil in prevention of restenosis following coronary angioplasty." Am J Prev Med **8**(3): 186-92.

Shah, P. K. and J. Amin (1992). "Low high density lipoprotein level is associated with increased restenosis rate after coronary angioplasty [see comments]." Circulation **85**(4): 1279-85.

Terres, W., C. W. Hamm, et al. (1992). "Residual platelet function under acetylsalicylic acid and the risk of restenosis after coronary angioplasty." J Cardiovasc Pharmacol **19**(2): 190-3.

Wosornu, D., W. Allardyce, et al. (1992). "Influence of power and aerobic exercise training on haemostatic factors after coronary artery surgery." Br Heart J **68**(2): 181-6.

Gellman, J., M. D. Ezekowitz, et al. (1991). "Effect of lovastatin on intimal hyperplasia after balloon angioplasty: a study in an atherosclerotic hypercholesterolemic rabbit." J Am Coll Cardiol **17**(1): 251-9.

Qiao, J. H., A. E. Walts, et al. (1991). "The severity of atherosclerosis at sites of plaque rupture with occlusive thrombosis in saphenous vein coronary artery bypass grafts." Am Heart J **122**(4 Pt 1): 955-8.

Reis, G. J., R. E. Kuntz, et al. (1991). "Effects of serum lipid levels on restenosis after coronary angioplasty." Am J Cardiol **68**(15): 1431-5.

Taylor, R. R., F. A. Gibbons, et al. (1991). "Effects of low-dose aspirin on restenosis after coronary angioplasty." Am J Cardiol **68**(9): 874-8.

Milner, M. R., R. A. Gallino, et al. (1989). "Usefulness of fish oil supplements in preventing clinical evidence of restenosis after percutaneous transluminal coronary angioplasty [see comments]." Am J Cardiol **64**(5): 294-9.

Reis, G. J., T. M. Boucher, et al. (1989). "Randomised trial of fish oil for prevention of restenosis after coronary angioplasty [see comments]." Lancet **2**(8656): 177-81.

Dehmer, G. J., J. J. Popma, et al. (1988). "Reduction in the rate of early restenosis after coronary angioplasty by a diet supplemented with n-3 fatty acids." N Engl J Med **319**(12): 733-40.

Coronary Heart Disease

(1993). "NIH Consensus conference. Triglyceride, high-density lipoprotein, and coronary heart disease. NIH Consensus Development Panel on Triglyceride, High-Density Lipoprotein, and Coronary Heart Disease." Jama **269**(4): 505-10.

Badimon, J. J., V. Fuster, et al. (1993). "Coronary atherosclerosis. A multifactorial disease." Circulation **87**(3 Suppl): II3-16.

Becker, R. C. (1993). "Antiplatelet therapy in coronary heart disease. Emerging strategies for the treatment and prevention of acute myocardial infarction." Arch Pathol Lab Med **117**(1): 89-96.

Duthie, G. G., J. R. Arthur, et al. (1993). "Cigarette smoking, antioxidants, lipid peroxidation, and coronary heart disease." Ann N Y Acad Sci **686**(1): 120-9.

Gey, K. F., H. B. Stahelin, et al. (1993). "Poor plasma status of carotene and vitamin C is associated with higher mortality from ischemic heart disease and stroke: Basel Prospective Study." Clin Investig **71**(1): 3-6.

(1992). "Triglyceride, high density lipoprotein, and coronary heart disease." Consens Statement **10**(2): 1-28.

Bainton, D., N. E. Miller, et al. (1992). "Plasma triglyceride and high density lipoprotein cholesterol as predictors of ischaemic heart disease in British men. The Caerphilly and Speedwell Collaborative Heart Disease Studies." Br Heart J **68**(1): 60-6.

Bairati, I., L. Roy, et al. (1992). "Effects of a fish oil supplement on blood pressure and serum lipids in patients treated for coronary artery disease." Can J Cardiol **8**(1): 41-6.

Benotti, P. N., B. Bistrain, et al. (1992). "Heart disease and hypertension in severe obesity: the benefits of weight reduction." Am J Clin Nutr **55**(2 Suppl): 586S-590S.

Coleman, M. P., T. J. Key, et al. (1992). "A prospective study of obesity, lipids, apolipoproteins and ischaemic heart disease in women." Atherosclerosis **92**(2-3): 177-85.

Douglas, P. S., T. B. Clarkson, et al. (1992). "Exercise and atherosclerotic heart disease in women." Med Sci Sports Exerc **24**(6 Suppl): S266-76.

Eichholzer, M., H. B. Stahelin, et al. (1992). "Inverse correlation between essential antioxidants in plasma and subsequent risk to develop cancer, ischemic heart disease and stroke respectively: 12-year follow-up of the Prospective Basel Study." Exs **62**(1): 398-410.

Eysenck, H. J. (1992). "Psychosocial factors, cancer, and ischaemic heart disease." Bmj **305**(6851): 457-9.

Franklin, B. A., S. Gordon, et al. (1992). "Amount of exercise necessary for the patient with coronary artery disease." Am J Cardiol **69**(17): 1426-32.

Glantz, S. A. and W. W. Parmley (1992). "Passive smoking causes heart disease and lung cancer." J Clin Epidemiol **45**(8): 815-9.

Gliksman, M. and A. Wilson (1992). "Are hemostatic factors responsible for the paradoxical risk factors for coronary heart disease and stroke?" Stroke **23**(4): 607-10.

Hong, M. K., P. A. Romm, et al. (1992). "Effects of estrogen replacement therapy on serum lipid values and angiographically defined coronary artery disease in postmenopausal women." Am J Cardiol **69**(3): 176-8.

Karnegis, J. N., J. P. Matts, et al. (1992). "Correlation of coronary with peripheral arterial stenosis. The POSCH Group." Atherosclerosis **92**(1): 25-30.

Kwiterovich, P., Jr., J. Coresh, et al. (1992). "Comparison of the plasma levels of apolipoproteins B and A-1, and other risk factors in men and women with premature coronary artery disease." Am J Cardiol **69**(12): 1015-21.

Curb, J. D. and E. B. Marcus (1991). "Body fat, coronary heart disease, and stroke in Japanese men." Am J Clin Nutr **53**(6 Suppl): 1612S-1615S.

Gey, K. F., P. Puska, et al. (1991). "Inverse correlation between plasma vitamin E and mortality from ischemic heart disease in cross-cultural epidemiology." Am J Clin Nutr **53**(1 Suppl): 326S-334S.

d-limonene

Crowell, P. L., W. S. Kennan, et al. (1992). "Chemoprevention of mammary carcinogenesis by hydroxylated derivatives of d-limonene." Carcinogenesis **13**(7): 1261-4.

Haag, J. D., M. J. Lindstrom, et al. (1992). "Limonene-induced regression of mammary carcinomas." Cancer Res **52**(14): 4021-6.

Igimi, H., D. Watanabe, et al. (1992). "A useful cholesterol solvent for medical dissolution of gallstones." Gastroenterol Jpn **27**(4): 536-45.

Karlberg, A. T., K. Magnusson, et al. (1992). "Air oxidation of d-limonene (the citrus solvent) creates potent allergens." Contact Dermatitis **26**(5): 332-40.

Falk, A., T. Fischer, et al. (1991). "Purpuric rash caused by dermal exposure to d-limonene." Contact Dermatitis **25**(3): 198-9.

Igimi, H., R. Tamura, et al. (1991). "Medical dissolution of gallstones. Clinical experience of d-limonene as a simple, safe, and effective solvent." Dig Dis Sci **36**(2): 200-8.

Karlberg, A. T., A. Boman, et al. (1991). "Animal experiments on the allergenicity of d-limonene—the citrus solvent." Ann Occup Hyg **35**(4): 419-26.

Saito, K., S. Uwagawa, et al. (1991). "Behavior of alpha 2u-globulin accumulating in kidneys of male rats treated with d-limonene: kidney-type alpha 2u-globulin in the urine as a marker of d-limonene nephropathy." Toxicology **70**(2): 173-83.

Vergunst, H., O. T. Terpstra, et al. (1991). "In vitro comparison of different gall stone dissolution solvents." Gut **32**(2): 211-4.

Cardullo, A. C., A. M. Ruszkowski, et al. (1989). "Allergic contact dermatitis resulting from sensitivity to citrus peel, geraniol, and citral." J Am Acad Dermatol **21**(2 Pt 2): 395-7.

Gureshi, A., W. Mangels, et al. (1988). "Inhibition of hepatic mevalonate biosynthesis by the monoterpene, d-limonene." J Agricult Food Chem **36**: 1220-1224.

DHEA

Eich, D. M., J. E. Nestler, et al. (1993). "Inhibition of accelerated coronary atherosclerosis with dehydroepiandrosterone in the heterotopic rabbit model of cardiac transplantation." Circulation **87**(1): 261-9.

Gordon, G. B., K. J. Helzlsouer, et al. (1993). "Serum levels of dehydroepiandrosterone and dehydroepiandrosterone sulfate and the risk of developing gastric cancer." Cancer Epidemiol Biomarkers Prev **2**(1): 33-5.

McIntosh, M. K., A. H. Goldfarb, et al. (1993). "Vitamin E alters hepatic antioxidant enzymes in rats treated with dehydroepiandrosterone (DHEA)." J Nutr **123**(2): 216-24.

Glaser, J. L., J. L. Brind, et al. (1992). "Elevated serum dehydroepiandrosterone sulfate levels in practitioners of the Transcendental Meditation (TM) and TM-Sidhi programs." J Behav Med **15**(4): 327-41.

Ishihara, F., K. Hiramatsu, et al. (1992). "Role of adrenal androgens in the development of arteriosclerosis as judged by pulse wave velocity and calcification of the aorta." Cardiology **80**(5-6): 332-8.

La Croix, A. Z., K. Yano, et al. (1992). "Dehydroepiandrosterone sulfate, incidence of myocardial infarction, and extent of atherosclerosis in men [see comments]." Circulation **86**(5): 1529-35.

Nestler, J. E., J. N. Clore, et al. (1992). "Dehydroepiandrosterone: the "missing link" between hyperinsulinemia and atherosclerosis?" Faseb J **6**(12): 3073-5.

Ruiz Salmeron, R. J., J. L. del Arbol, et al. (1992). "[Dehydroepiandrosterone sulfate and lipids in acute myocardial infarct]." Rev Clin Esp **190**(8): 398-402.

Salvini, S., M. J. Stampfer, et al. (1992). "Effects of age, smoking and vitamins on plasma DHEAS levels: a cross-sectional study in men." J Clin Endocrinol Metab **74**(1): 139-43.

Herrington, D. M., G. B. Gordon, et al. (1990). "Plasma dehydroepiandrosterone and dehydroepiandrosterone sulfate in patients undergoing diagnostic coronary angiography [corrected and republished with original paging, article originally printed in J Am Coll Cardiol 1990 Oct; 16(4):862-70]." J Am Coll Cardiol **16**(6): 862-70.

Rudman, D., K. R. Shetty, et al. (1990). "Plasma dehydroepiandrosterone sulfate in nursing home men." J Am Geriatr Soc **38**(4): 421-7.

Diabetes

Colwell, J. A. (1993). "Vascular thrombosis in type II diabetes mellitus [editorial]." Diabetes **42**(1): 8-11.

Glassman, A. B. (1993). "Platelet abnormalities in diabetes mellitus." Ann Clin Lab Sci **23**(1): 47-50.

Haffner, S. M., P. A. Morales, et al. (1993). "Cardiovascular risk factors in non-insulin-dependent diabetic subjects with microalbuminuria." Arterioscler Thromb **13**(2): 205-10.

Jiang, X., S. R. Srinivasan, et al. (1993). "Association of fasting insulin with blood pressure in young individuals. The Bogalusa Heart Study [see comments]." Arch Intern Med **153**(3): 323-8.

Kahler, W., B. Kuklinski, et al. (1993). "[Diabetes mellitus—a free radical-associated disease. Results of adjuvant antioxidant supplementation]." Z Gesamte Inn Med **48**(5): 223-32.

Mac Rury, S. M., S. E. Lennie, et al. (1993). "Increased red cell aggregation in diabetes mellitus: association with cardiovascular risk factors." Diabet Med **10**(1): 21-6.

Paolisso, G., A. D'Amore, et al. (1993). "Pharmacologic doses of vitamin E improve insulin action in healthy subjects and non-insulin-dependent diabetic patients." Am J Clin Nutr **57**(5): 650-6.

Rimm, E. B., J. E. Manson, et al. (1993). "Cigarette smoking and the risk of diabetes in women." Am J Public Health **83**(2): 211-4.

Schneider, D. J., T. K. Nordt, et al. (1993). "Attenuated fibrinolysis and accelerated atherogenesis in type II diabetic patients." Diabetes **42**(1): 1-7.

Stamler, J., O. Vaccaro, et al. (1993). "Diabetes, other risk factors, and 12-yr cardiovascular mortality for men screened in the Multiple Risk Factor Intervention Trial." Diabetes Care **16**(2): 434-44.

(1992). "Aspirin effects on mortality and morbidity in patients with diabetes mellitus. Early Treatment Diabetic Retinopathy Study report 14. ETDRS Investigators." Jama **268**(10): 1292-300.

(1992). "Dietary recommendations for people with diabetes: an update for the 1990s. Nutrition Subcommittee of the British Diabetic Association's Professional Advisory Committee." Diabet Med **9**(2): 189-202.

(1992). "Magnesium supplementation in the treatment of diabetes. American Diabetes Association." Diabetes Care **15**(8): 1065-7.

Anderson, J. W. (1992). "Dietary fiber and diabetes: what else do we need to know? [editorial]." Diabetes Res Clin Pract **17**(2): 71-3.

Anderson, R. A. (1992). "Chromium, glucose tolerance, and diabetes." Biol Trace Elem Res **32**(1): 19-24.

Arauz-Pacheco, C. and P. Raskin (1992). "Management of hypertension in diabetes." Endocrinol Metab Clin North Am **21**(2): 371-94.

Babiy, A. V., J. M. Gebicki, et al. (1992). "Increased oxidizability of plasma lipoproteins in diabetic patients can be decreased by probucol therapy and is not due to glycation." Biochem Pharmacol **43**(5): 995-1000.

Bagdade, J. D. and F. L. Dunn (1992). "Effects of insulin treatment on lipoprotein composition and function in patients with IDDM." Diabetes **41**(1): 107-10.

Baker, D. E. and R. K. Campbell (1992). "Vitamin and mineral supplementation in patients with diabetes mellitus." Diabetes Educ **18**(5): 420-7.

Bantle, J. P., J. E. Swanson, et al. (1992). "Metabolic effects of dietary fructose in diabetic subjects." Diabetes Care **15**(11): 1468-76.

Barnard, R. J., E. J. Ugianskis, et al. (1992). "Role of diet and exercise in the management of hyperinsulinemia and associated atherosclerotic risk factors." Am J Cardiol **69**(5): 440-4.

Barrett-Connor, E. (1992). "Lower endogenous androgen levels and dyslipidemia in men with non-insulin-dependent diabetes mellitus [see comments]." Ann Intern Med **117**(10): 807-11.

Bell, D. S. (1992). "Exercise for patients with diabetes. Benefits, risks, precautions." Postgrad Med **92**(1): 183-4.

Berliner, J. A., M. Territo, et al. (1992). "Minimally modified lipoproteins in diabetes." Diabetes **41**(1): 74-6.

Bjorntorp, P. A. (1992). "Efficacy of training in obese diabetic patients." Diabetes Care **15**(11): 1783-6.

Blake, G. H. (1992). "Control of type II diabetes. Reaping the rewards of exercise and weight loss." Postgrad Med **92**(6): 129-32.

Brownlee, M. (1992). "Glycosylation of proteins and microangiopathy [see comments]." Hosp Pract **27**(1): 46-50.

Brunzell, J. D. (1992). "Lipoprotein abnormalities in diabetes mellitus." Hosp Pract **27**(1): 55-8.

Burchfiel, C. M., S. M. Shetterly, et al. (1992). "The roles of insulin, obesity, and fat distribution in the elevation of cardiovascular risk factors in impaired glucose tolerance. The San Luis Valley Diabetes Study." Am J Epidemiol **136**(9): 1101-9.

Ceriello, A., A. Quatraro, et al. (1992). "New insights on non-enzymatic glycosylation may lead to therapeutic approaches for the prevention of diabetic complications." Diabet Med **9**(3): 297-9.

Chalmers, T. C. (1992). "Oral hypoglycemic agents? Negative [comment]." Hosp Pract **27**(1): 32-4.

Chisolm, G. M., K. C. Irwin, et al. (1992). "Lipoprotein oxidation and lipoprotein-induced cell injury in diabetes." Diabetes **41**(1): 61-6.

Colditz, G. A., J. E. Manson, et al. (1992). "Diet and risk of clinical diabetes in women." Am J Clin Nutr **55**(5): 1018-23.

Colwell, J. A. (1992). "Antiplatelet drugs and prevention of macrovascular disease in diabetes mellitus." Metabolism **41**(5 Suppl 1): 7-10.

Davie, S. J., B. J. Gould, et al. (1992). "Effect of vitamin C on glycosylation of proteins." Diabetes **41**(2): 167-73.

De Fronzo, R. A., R. C. Bonadonna, et al. (1992). "Pathogenesis of NIDDM. A balanced overview." Diabetes Care **15**(3): 318-68.

De Leeuw, I. (1992). "Atherogenic profiles in insulin-dependent diabetic patients and their treatment." Eur J Epidemiol **8**(1): 125-8.

Dunn, F. L. (1992). "Management of hyperlipidemia in diabetes mellitus." Endocrinol Metab Clin North Am **21**(2): 395-414.

Dunn, F. L. (1992). "Plasma lipid and lipoprotein disorders in IDDM." Diabetes **41**(1): 102-6.

Durrington, P. N. (1992). "Is insulin atherogenic?" Diabet Med **9**(7): 597-600.

Everhart, J. E., D. J. Pettitt, et al. (1992). "Duration of obesity increases the incidence of NIDDM." Diabetes **41**(2): 235-40.

Feskens, E. J. and D. Kromhout (1992). "Glucose tolerance and the risk of cardiovascular disease: the Zutphen Study." J Clin Epidemiol **45**(11): 1327-34.

Garg, A., S. M. Grundy, et al. (1992). "Comparison of effects of high and low carbohydrate diets on plasma lipoproteins and insulin sensitivity in patients with mild NIDDM." Diabetes **41**(10): 1278-85.

Garland, H. O. (1992). "New experimental data on the relationship between diabetes mellitus and magnesium." Magnes Res **5**(3): 193-202.

Grafton, G. and M. A. Baxter (1992). "The role of magnesium in diabetes mellitus. A possible mechanism for the development of diabetic complications." J Diabetes Complications **6**(2): 143-9.

Grafton, G., C. M. Bunce, et al. (1992). "Effect of Mg2+ on Na(+)-dependent inositol transport. Role for Mg2+ in etiology of diabetic complications." Diabetes **41**(1): 35-9.

Greco, A. V., G. Mingrone, et al. (1992). "Effect of propionyl-L-carnitine in the treatment of diabetic angiopathy: controlled double blind trial versus placebo." Drugs Exp Clin Res **18**(2): 69-80.

Haffner, S. M., S. E. Moss, et al. (1992). "Lack of association between lipoprotein (a) concentrations and coronary heart disease mortality in diabetes: the Wisconsin Epidemiologic Study of Diabetic Retinopathy." Metabolism **41**(2): 194-7.

Haffner, S. M., K. R. Tuttle, et al. (1992). "Lack of change of lipoprotein (a) concentration with improved glycemic control in subjects with type II diabetes." Metabolism **41**(2): 116-20.

Hebert, P. R., J. E. Manson, et al. (1992). "Pharmacologic therapy of mild to moderate hypertension: possible generalizability to diabetics." J Am Soc Nephrol **3**(4 Suppl): S135-9.

Hunt, J. V., M. A. Bottoms, et al. (1992). "Ascorbic acid oxidation: a potential cause of the elevated severity of atherosclerosis in diabetes mellitus?" Febs Lett **311**(2): 161-4.

Karam, J. H. (1992). "Type II diabetes and syndrome X. Pathogenesis and glycemic management." Endocrinol Metab Clin North Am **21**(2): 329-50.

Manna, R., A. Migliore, et al. (1992). "Nicotinamide treatment in subjects at high risk of developing IDDM improves insulin secretion." Br J Clin Pract **46**(3): 177-9.

Manson, J. E., D. M. Nathan, et al. (1992). "A prospective study of exercise and incidence of diabetes among US male physicians." Jama **268**(1): 63-7.

Morisaki, N., M. Kawano, et al. (1992). "Role of obesity in development of ischemic heart disease in elderly diabetic patients." Gerontology **38**(3): 167-73.

Morris, B. W., A. Blumsohn, et al. (1992). "The trace element chromium—a role in glucose homeostasis." Am J Clin Nutr **55**(5): 989-91.

Murthy, V. K., J. C. Shipp, et al. (1992). "Delayed onset and decreased incidence of diabetes in BB rats fed free radical scavengers." Diabetes Res Clin Pract **18**(1): 11-6.

Nadler, J. L., S. Malayan, et al. (1992). "Intracellular free magnesium deficiency plays a key role in increased platelet reactivity in type II diabetes mellitus." Diabetes Care **15**(7): 835-41.

Paolisso, G., S. Sgambato, et al. (1992). "Daily magnesium supplements improve glucose handling in elderly subjects." Am J Clin Nutr **55**(6): 1161-7.

Parillo, M., A. A. Rivellese, et al. (1992). "A high-monounsaturated-fat/low-carbohydrate diet improves peripheral insulin sensitivity in non-insulin-dependent diabetic patients." Metabolism **41**(12): 1373-8.

Paulson, D. J., A. L. Shug, et al. (1992). "Protection of the ischemic diabetic heart by L-propionylcarnitine therapy." Mol Cell Biochem **116**(1-2): 131-7.

Rude, R. K. (1992). "Magnesium deficiency and diabetes mellitus. Causes and effects." Postgrad Med **92**(5): 217-9.

Schnack, C., I. Bauer, et al. (1992). "Hypomagnesaemia in type 2 (non-insulin-dependent) diabetes mellitus is not corrected by improvement of long-term metabolic control." Diabetologia **35**(1): 77-9.

Sheela, C. G. and K. T. Augusti (1992). "Antidiabetic effects of S-allyl cysteine sulphoxide isolated from garlic Allium sativum Linn." Indian J Exp Biol **30**(6): 523-6.

Sivenius, J., M. Laakso, et al. (1992). "European stroke prevention study: effectiveness of antiplatelet therapy in diabetic patients in secondary prevention of stroke." Stroke **23**(6): 851-4.

Uusitupa, M. I., L. Mykkanen, et al. (1992). "Chromium supplementation in impaired glucose tolerance of elderly: effects on blood glucose, plasma insulin, C-peptide and lipid levels(not helpful)." Br J Nutr **68**(1): 209-16.

Vinik, A. I. and R. R. Wing (1992). "The good, the bad, and the ugly in diabetic diets." Endocrinol Metab Clin North Am **21**(2): 237-79.

Vuorinen-Markkola, H., M. Sinisalo, et al. (1992). "Guar gum in insulin-dependent diabetes: effects on glycemic control and serum lipoproteins." Am J Clin Nutr **56**(6): 1056-60.

Wu, H. P., T. Y. Tai, et al. (1992). "Effect of tocopherol on platelet aggregation in non-insulin-dependent diabetes mellitus: ex vivo and in vitro studies." Taiwan I Hsueh Hui Tsa Chih **91**(3): 270-5.

Anderson, R. A., M. M. Polansky, et al. (1991). "Supplemental-chromium effects on glucose, insulin, glucagon, and urinary chromium losses in subjects consuming controlled low-chromium diets." Am J Clin Nutr **54**(5): 909-16.

Behrens, W. A. and R. Madere (1991). "Vitamin C and vitamin E status in the spontaneously diabetic BB rat before the onset of diabetes." Metabolism **40**(1): 72-6.

Bonanome, A., A. Visona, et al. (1991). "Carbohydrate and lipid metabolism in patients with non-insulin-dependent diabetes mellitus: effects of a low-fat, high-carbohydrate diet vs a diet high in monounsaturated fatty acids." Am J Clin Nutr **54**(3): 586-90.

Ceriello, A., D. Giugliano, et al. (1991). "Vitamin E reduction of protein glycosylation in diabetes. New prospect for prevention of diabetic complications?" Diabetes Care **14**(1): 68-72.

Ceriello, A., D. Giugliano, et al. (1991). "Anti-oxidants show an anti-hypertensive effect in diabetic and hypertensive subjects." Clin Sci **81**(6): 739-42.

Feskens, E. J., C. H. Bowles, et al. (1991). "Inverse association between fish intake and risk of glucose intolerance in normoglycemic elderly men and women." Diabetes Care **14**(11): 935-41.

Grundy, S. M. (1991). "Dietary therapy in diabetes mellitus. Is there a single best diet?" Diabetes Care **14**(9): 796-801.

Anderson, J. W., B. M. Smith, et al. (1990). "High-fiber diet for diabetes. Safe and effective treatment." Postgrad Med **88**(2): 157-61.

Gisinger, C., J. Jeremy, et al. (1988). "Effect of vitamin E supplementation on platelet thromboxane A2 production in type I diabetic patients. Double-blind crossover trial." Diabetes **37**(9): 1260-4.

Dairy Products

Gatti, E., D. Noe, et al. (1992). "Differential effect of unsaturated oils and butter on blood glucose and insulin response to carbohydrate in normal volunteers." Eur J Clin Nutr **46**(3): 161-6.

Jacques, H., D. Laurin, et al. (1992). "Influence of diets containing cow's milk or soy protein beverage on plasma lipids in children with familial hypercholesterolemia." J Am Coll Nutr **11**(1): 69S-73S.

Trevisan, M., V. Krogh, et al. (1990). "Consumption of olive oil, butter, and vegetable oils and coronary heart disease risk factors. The Research Group ATS-RF2 of the Italian National Research Council [published erratum appears in JAMA 1990 Apr;263(13):1768]." Jama **263**(5): 688-92.

Diet and Cholesterol

Hopkins, P. N. (1992). "Effects of dietary cholesterol on serum cholesterol: a meta-analysis and review." Am J Clin Nutr **55**(6): 1060-70.

Mott, G. E., E. M. Jackson, et al. (1992). "Dietary cholesterol and type of fat differentially affect cholesterol metabolism and atherosclerosis in baboons." J Nutr **122**(7): 1397-406.

Gotto, A. M. (1991). "Cholesterol intake and serum cholesterol level [editorial; comment]." N Engl J Med **324**(13): 912-3.

McMurry, M. P., M. T. Cerqueira, et al. (1991). "Changes in lipid and lipoprotein levels and body weight in Tarahumara Indians after consumption of an affluent diet [see comments]." N Engl J Med **325**(24): 1704-8.

Johnson, C. and P. Greenland (1990). "Effects of exercise, dietary cholesterol, and dietary fat on blood lipids." Arch Intern Med **150**(1): 137-41.

Edington, J., M. Geekie, et al. (1987). "Effect of dietary cholesterol on plasma cholesterol concentration in subjects following reduced fat, high fibre diet." Br Med J **294**(6568): 333-6.

Beynen, A. C. and M. B. Katan (1985). "Reproducibility of the variations between humans in the response of serum cholesterol to cessation of egg consumption." Atherosclerosis **57**(1): 19-31.

Diet and Coronary Heart Disease

Kant, A. K., A. Schatzkin, et al. (1993). "Dietary diversity and subsequent mortality in the First National Health and Nutrition Examination Survey Epidemiologic Follow-up Study." Am J Clin Nutr **57**(3): 434-40.

Bolton-Smith, C., M. Woodward, et al. (1992). "The Scottish Heart Health Study. Dietary intake by food frequency questionnaire and odds ratios for coronary heart disease risk. II. The antioxidant vitamins and fibre." Eur J Clin Nutr **46**(2): 85-93.

Bolton-Smith, C., M. Woodward, et al. (1992). "The Scottish Heart Health Study. Dietary intake by food frequency questionnaire and odds ratios for coronary heart disease risk. I. The macronutrients." Eur J Clin Nutr **46**(2): 75-84.

Burr, M. L. (1992). "Particular diets and cardiovascular risk." Bibl Nutr Dieta **49**: 102-10.

Farinaro, E., S. Panico, et al. (1992). "[Diet and cardiovascular risk among women in Italy]." Ann Ist Super Sanita **28**(3): 349-53.

Foley, M., M. Ball, et al. (1992). "Should mono- or poly-unsaturated fats replace saturated fat in the diet?" Eur J Clin Nutr **46**(6): 429-36.

Leaf, A. and H. A. Hallaq (1992). "The role of nutrition in the functioning of the cardiovascular system." Nutr Rev **50**(12): 402-6.

Shrapnel, W. S., G. D. Calvert, et al. (1992). "Diet and coronary heart disease. The National Heart Foundation of Australia (one of the best review articles I have read)." Med J Aust **156**(1): 16.

Singh, R. B. and M. A. Niaz (1992). "Diets that protect against coronary heart disease [letter]." Bmj **305**(6851): 473.

Singh, R. B., A. R. Sircar, et al. (1992). "Dietary modulators of lipid metabolism in the Indian diet-heart study (I.D.H.S.)." Int J Vitam Nutr Res **62**(1): 73-82.

Bolton-Smith, C., M. Woodward, et al. (1991). "Dietary and non-dietary predictors of serum total and HDL-cholesterol in men and women: results from the Scottish Heart Health Study." Int J Epidemiol **20**(1): 95-104.

Gurr, M. I. (1991). "Diet, nutrition and the prevention of chronic diseases (WHO, 1990) [letter]." Eur J Clin Nutr **45**(12): 619-23.

Kafatos, A., I. Kouroumalis, et al. (1991). "Coronary-heart-disease risk-factor status of the Cretan urban population in the 1980s." Am J Clin Nutr **54**(3): 591-8.

Porrini, M., P. Simonetti, et al. (1991). "Relation between diet composition and coronary heart disease risk factors." J Epidemiol Community Health **45**(2): 148-51.

Posner, B. M., J. L. Cobb, et al. (1991). "Dietary lipid predictors of coronary heart disease in men. The Framingham Study." Arch Intern Med **151**(6): 1181-7.

Sacks, F. M. and W. W. Willett (1991). "More on chewing the fat. The good fat and the good cholesterol [editorial; comment]." N Engl J Med **325**(24): 1740-2.

Singh, R. B., S. S. Rastogi, et al. (1991). "Dietary strategies for risk-factor modification to prevent cardiovascular diseases." Nutrition **7**(3): 210-4.

Ulbricht, T. L. and D. A. Southgate (1991). "Coronary heart disease: seven dietary factors [see comments]." Lancet **338**(8773): 985-92.

Willett, W. and F. M. Sacks (1991). "Chewing the fat—how much and what kind? [editorial; comment] [see comments]." N Engl J Med **324**(2): 121-3.

Trevisan, M., V. Krogh, et al. (1990). "Consumption of olive oil, butter, and vegetable oils and coronary heart disease risk factors. The Research Group ATS-RF2 of the Italian National Research Council [published erratum appears in JAMA 1990 Apr;263(13):1768]." Jama **263**(5): 688-92.

Gotto, A., Jr. (1989). "Diet and cholesterol guidelines and coronary heart disease." J Am Coll Cardiol **13**(2): 503-7.

Kromhout, D., A. Keys, et al. (1989). "Food consumption patterns in the 1960s in seven countries." Am J Clin Nutr **49**(5): 889-94.

Connor, S. L., J. R. Gustafson, et al. (1986). "The cholesterol/saturated-fat index: an indication of the hypercholesterolaemic and atherogenic potential of food." Lancet **1**(8492): 1229-32.

Kromhout, D., E. B. Bosschieter, et al. (1985). "The inverse relation between fish consumption and 20-year mortality from coronary heart disease." N Engl J Med **312**(19): 1205-9.

Diet and Fat

Corboy, J., W. H. Sutherland, et al. (1993). "Fatty acid composition and the oxidation of low-density lipoproteins." Biochem Med Metab Biol **49**(1): 25-35.

Harlan, L. C., R. J. Coates, et al. (1993). "Estrogen receptor status and dietary intakes in breast cancer patients." Epidemiology **4**(1): 25-31.

Sheehy, P. J., P. A. Morrissey, et al. (1993). "Influence of heated vegetable oils and alpha-tocopheryl acetate supplementation on alpha-tocopherol, fatty acids and lipid peroxidation in chicken muscle." Br Poult Sci **34**(2): 367-81.

Barr, S. L., R. Ramakrishnan, et al. (1992). "Reducing total dietary fat without reducing saturated fatty acids does not significantly lower total plasma cholesterol concentrations in normal males." Am J Clin Nutr **55**(3): 675-81.

Cabre, E., J. L. Periago, et al. (1992). "Factors related to the plasma fatty acid profile in healthy subjects, with special reference to antioxidant micronutrient status: a multivariate analysis." Am J Clin Nutr **55**(4): 831-7.

Charnock, J. S., P. L. McLennan, et al. (1992). "Dietary modulation of lipid metabolism and mechanical performance of the heart." Mol Cell Biochem **116**(1-2): 19-25.

Drewnowski, A., C. Kurth, et al. (1992). "Food preferences in human obesity: carbohydrates versus fats." Appetite **18**(3): 207-21.

Foley, M., M. Ball, et al. (1992). "Should mono- or poly-unsaturated fats replace saturated fat in the diet?" Eur J Clin Nutr **46**(6): 429-36.

Gustafsson, I. B., B. Vessby, et al. (1992). "Effects of lipid-lowering diets enriched with monounsaturated and polyunsaturated fatty acids on serum lipoprotein composition in patients with hyperlipoproteinaemia." Atherosclerosis **96**(2-3): 109-18.

Hayes, K. C. and P. Khosla (1992). "Dietary fatty acid thresholds and cholesterolemia." Faseb J **6**(8): 2600-7.

Horrobin, D. F. (1992). "Nutritional and medical importance of gamma-linolenic acid." Prog Lipid Res **31**(2): 163-94.

Howe, G. R. (1992). "High-fat diets and breast cancer risk. The epidemiologic evidence [editorial; comment]." Jama **268**(15): 2080-1.

Khosla, P. and K. C. Hayes (1992). "Comparison between the effects of dietary saturated (16:0), monounsaturated (18:1), and polyunsaturated (18:2) fatty acids on plasma lipoprotein metabolism in cebus and rhesus monkeys fed cholesterol-free diets." Am J Clin Nutr **55**(1): 51-62.

Krebs-Smith, S. M., F. J. Cronin, et al. (1992). "Food sources of energy, macronutrients, cholesterol, and fiber in diets of women." J Am Diet Assoc **92**(2): 168-74.

Kromhout, D. (1992). "Dietary fats: long-term implications for health." Nutr Rev **50**(4 (Pt 2): 49-53.

McNamara, D. J. (1992). "Dietary fatty acids, lipoproteins, and cardiovascular disease." Adv Food Nutr Res **36**(1): 253-351.

Mensink, R. P. and M. B. Katan (1992). "Effect of dietary fatty acids on serum lipids and lipoproteins. A meta-analysis of 27 trials." Arterioscler Thromb **12**(8): 911-9.

Mott, G. E., E. M. Jackson, et al. (1992). "Dietary cholesterol and type of fat differentially affect cholesterol metabolism and atherosclerosis in baboons." J Nutr **122**(7): 1397-406.

Mutanen, M., R. Freese, et al. (1992). "Rapeseed oil and sunflower oil diets enhance platelet in vitro aggregation and thromboxane production in healthy men when compared with milk fat or habitual diets." Thromb Haemost **67**(3): 352-6.

Nestel, P. J., M. Noakes, et al. (1992). "Plasma cholesterol-lowering potential of edible-oil blends suitable for commercial use." Am J Clin Nutr **55**(1): 46-50.

Parks, J. S. and J. R. Crouse (1992). "Reduction of cholesterol absorption by dietary oleinate and fish oil in African green monkeys." J Lipid Res **33**(4): 559-68.

Reimer, L. (1992). "Role of dietary fat in obesity. Fat is fattening." J Fla Med Assoc **79**(6): 382-4.

Sirtori, C. R., E. Gatti, et al. (1992). "Olive oil, corn oil, and n-3 fatty acids differently affect lipids, lipoproteins, platelets, and superoxide formation in type II hypercholesterolemia." Am J Clin Nutr **56**(1): 113-22.

Willett, W. C., D. J. Hunter, et al. (1992). "Dietary fat and fiber in relation to risk of breast cancer. An 8-year follow-up [see comments]." Jama **268**(15): 2037-44.

Beswick, A. D., A. M. Fehily, et al. (1991). "Long-term diet modification and platelet activity." J Intern Med **229**(6): 511-5.

Burri, B. J., R. M. Dougherty, et al. (1991). "Platelet aggregation in humans is affected by replacement of dietary linoleic acid with oleic acid." Am J Clin Nutr **54**(2): 359-62.

Carroll, K. K. (1991). "Dietary fats and cancer." Am J Clin Nutr **53**(4 Suppl): 1064S-1067S.

Katsouyanni, K., Y. Skalkidis, et al. (1991). "Diet and peripheral arterial occlusive disease: the role of poly-, mono-, and saturated fatty acids." Am J Epidemiol **133**(1): 24-31.

Lenz, P. H., T. Watkins, et al. (1991). "Effect of dietary menhaden, Canola and partially hydrogenated soy oil supplemented with vitamin E upon plasma lipids and platelet aggregation." Thromb Res **61**(3): 213-24.

Rozewicka, L., W. B. Barcew, et al. (1991). "Protective effect of selenium and vitamin E against changes induced in heart vessels of rabbits fed chronically on a high-fat diet." Kitasato Arch Exp Med **64**(4): 183-92.

Salonen, J. T. (1991). "Dietary fats, antioxidants and blood pressure." Ann Med **23**(3): 295-8.

La Rosa, J. C., D. Hunninghake, et al. (1990). "The cholesterol facts. A summary of the evidence relating dietary fats, serum cholesterol, and coronary heart disease. A joint statement by the American Heart Association and the National Heart, Lung, and Blood Institute. The Task Force on Cholesterol Issues, American Heart Association." Circulation **81**(5): 1721-33.

Thorogood, M., L. Roe, et al. (1990). "Dietary intake and plasma lipid levels: lessons from a study of the diet of health conscious groups [see comments]." Bmj **300**(6735): 1297-301.

Willett, W. C., M. J. Stampfer, et al. (1990). "Relation of meat, fat, and fiber intake to the risk of colon cancer in a prospective study among women [see comments]." N Engl J Med **323**(24): 1664-72.

Diet/Exercise—Lifestyle

Barnard, R. J., E. J. Ugianskis, et al. (1992). "Role of diet and exercise in the management of hyperinsulinemia and associated atherosclerotic risk factors." Am J Cardiol **69**(5): 440-4.

Evans, W. J. (1992). "Exercise, nutrition and aging." J Nutr **122**(3 Suppl): 796-801.

Gould, K. L., D. Ornish, et al. (1992). "Improved stenosis geometry by quantitative coronary arteriography after vigorous risk factor modification." Am J Cardiol **69**(9): 845-53.

Ornish, D. (1992). "What if Americans ate less fat? [letter]." Jama **267**(3): 363-4.

Singh, R. B. and H. Mori (1992). "Risk factors for coronary heart disease: synthesis of a new hypothesis through adaptation." Med Hypotheses **39**(4): 334-41.

Singh, R. B., S. S. Rastogi, et al. (1992). "The diet and moderate exercise trial (DAMET): results after 24 weeks." Acta Cardiol **47**(6): 543-57.

Singh, R. B., V. K. Sharma, et al. (1992). "Nutritional modulators of lipoprotein metabolism in patients with risk factors for coronary heart disease: diet and moderate exercise trial." J Am Coll Nutr **11**(4): 391-8.

Singh, V. N. (1992). "A current perspective on nutrition and exercise." J Nutr **122**(3 Suppl): 760-5.

Barnard, R. J. (1991). "Effects of life-style modification on serum lipids [see comments]." Arch Intern Med **151**(7): 1389-94.

Ornish, D. (1991). "Can life-style changes reverse coronary atherosclerosis?" Hosp Pract **26**(5): 123-6.

Schuler, G., R. Hambrecht, et al. (1991). "[Modification of risk factors through physical training and low-fat diet]." Herz **16**(4): 237-42.

Ornish, D., S. E. Brown, et al. (1990). "Can lifestyle changes reverse coronary heart disease? The Lifestyle Heart Trial [see comments]." Lancet **336**(8708): 129-33.

Peterkin, B. B. (1990). "Dietary Guidelines for Americans, 1990 edition [published erratum appears in J Am Diet Assoc 1991 Mar; 91(3):292] [see comments]." J Am Diet Assoc **90**(12): 1725-7.

Diet Therapy

Cobb, M. M. and N. Risch (1993). "Low-density lipoprotein cholesterol responsiveness to diet in normolipidemic subjects." Metabolism **42**(1): 7-13.

(1992). "Dietary recommendations for people with diabetes: an update for the 1990s. Nutrition Subcommittee of the British Diabetic Association's Professional Advisory Committee." Diabet Med **9**(2): 189-202.

Barr, S. L., R. Ramakrishnan, et al. (1992). "Reducing total dietary fat without reducing saturated fatty acids does not significantly lower total plasma cholesterol concentrations in normal males." Am J Clin Nutr **55**(3): 675-81.

Edelstein, S. L., E. L. Barrett-Connor, et al. (1992). "Increased meal frequency associated with decreased cholesterol concentrations; Rancho Bernardo, CA, 1984-1987." Am J Clin Nutr **55**(3): 664-9.

Gabel, L. L., P. J. Fahey, et al. (1992). "Dietary prevention and treatment of disease." Am Fam Physician **46**(5 Suppl): 41S-48S.

Garry, P. J., W. C. Hunt, et al. (1992). "Longitudinal study of dietary intakes and plasma lipids in healthy elderly men and women." Am J Clin Nutr **55**(3): 682-8.

Gotto, A., Jr. (1992). "Therapeutic intervention for hypercholesterolemia." Clin Cardiol **15**(11): III22-4.

Grover, S. A., M. Abrahamowicz, et al. (1992). "The benefits of treating hyperlipidemia to prevent coronary heart disease. Estimating changes in life expectancy and morbidity." Jama **267**(6): 816-22.

Henkin, Y., D. W. Garber, et al. (1992). "Saturated fats, cholesterol, and dietary compliance [see comments]." Arch Intern Med **152**(6): 1167-74.

Silvis, N. (1992). "Nutritional recommendations for individuals with diabetes mellitus." S Afr Med J **81**(3): 162-6.

Singh, R. B., S. S. Rastogi, et al. (1992). "Effect of fat-modified and fruit- and vegetable-enriched diets on blood lipids in the Indian Diet Heart Study." Am J Cardiol **70**(9): 869-74.

Singh, R. B., S. S. Rastogi, et al. (1992). "An Indian experiment with nutritional modulation in acute myocardial infarction." Am J Cardiol **69**(9): 879-85.

Singh, R. B., S. S. Rastogi, et al. (1992). "Randomised controlled trial of cardioprotective diet in patients with recent acute myocardial infarction: results of one year follow up." Bmj **304**(6833): 1015-9.

Beebe, C. A., J. G. Pastors, et al. (1991). "Nutrition management for individuals with noninsulin-dependent diabetes mellitus in the 1990s: a review by the Diabetes Care and Education dietetic practice group." J Am Diet Assoc **91**(2): 196-202.

Brown, S. A., J. Morrisett, et al. (1991). "Influence of short term dietary cholesterol and fat on human plasma Lp[a] and LDL levels." J Lipid Res **32**(8): 1281-9.

Gaddi, A., A. Ciarrocchi, et al. (1991). "Dietary treatment for familial hypercholesterolemia—differential effects of dietary soy protein according to the apolipoprotein E phenotypes." Am J Clin Nutr **53**(5): 1191-6.

Grundy, S. M. (1991). "Dietary therapy in diabetes mellitus. Is there a single best diet?" Diabetes Care **14**(9): 796-801.

Stacpoole, P. W., K. von Bergmann, et al. (1991). "Nutritional regulation of cholesterol synthesis and apolipoprotein B kinetics: studies in patients with familial hypercholesterolemia and normal subjects treated with a high carbohydrate, low fat diet." J Lipid Res **32**(11): 1837-48.

Eggs

Elkin, R. G., M. Freed, et al. (1993). "Evaluation of two novel biochemicals on plasma and egg yolk lipid composition and laying hen performance." Poult Sci **72**(3): 513-20.

Garber, D. W., Y. Henkin, et al. (1992). "Plasma lipoproteins in hyperlipidemic subjects eating iodine-enriched eggs." J Am Coll Nutr **11**(3): 294-303.

Garwin, J. L., J. M. Morgan, et al. (1992). "Modified eggs are compatible with a diet that reduces serum cholesterol concentrations in humans." J Nutr **122**(11): 2153-60.

Hall, L. M. and J. C. McKay (1992). "Variation in egg yolk cholesterol concentration between and within breeds of the domestic fowl." Br Poult Sci **33**(5): 941-6.

Jiang, Z. and J. S. Sim (1992). "Effects of dietary n-3 fatty acid-enriched chicken eggs on plasma and tissue cholesterol and fatty acid composition of rats." Lipids **27**(4): 279-84.

Shafey, T. M., J. G. Dingle, et al. (1992). "Comparison between wheat, triticale, rye, soyabean oil and strain of laying bird on the production, and cholesterol and fatty acid contents of eggs." Br Poult Sci **33**(2): 339-46.

Vorster, H. H., A. J. Benade, et al. (1992). "Egg intake does not change plasma lipoprotein and coagulation profiles." Am J Clin Nutr **55**(2): 400-10.

Kern, F., Jr. (1991). "Normal plasma cholesterol in an 88-year-old man who eats 25 eggs a day. Mechanisms of adaptation [see comments]." N Engl J Med **324**(13): 896-9.

Leeson, S., L. J. Caston, et al. (1991). "Response of laying hens to supplemental niacin (no effect)." Poult Sci **70**(5): 1231-5.

Oh, S. Y., J. Ryue, et al. (1991). "Eggs enriched in omega-3 fatty acids and alterations in lipid concentrations in plasma and lipoproteins and in blood pressure." Am J Clin Nutr **54**(4): 689-95.

Yoshizawa, Y., T. Miki, et al. (1991). "Effects of vitamin E-enriched egg yolk on lipid peroxidation, hemolysis and serum lipid concentration in young and old rats." J Nutr Sci Vitaminol **37**(3): 213-27.

Beynen, A. C. and M. B. Katan (1985). "Reproducibility of the variations between humans in the response of serum cholesterol to cessation of egg consumption." Atherosclerosis **57**(1): 19-31.

Sacks, F. M., J. Salazar, et al. (1984). "Ingestion of egg raises plasma low density lipoproteins in free-living subjects." Lancet **1**(8378): 647-9.

Packard, C. J., L. McKinney, et al. (1983). "Cholesterol feeding increases low density lipoprotein synthesis." J Clin Invest **72**(1): 45-51.

Exercise

Boyden, T. W., R. W. Pamenter, et al. (1993). "Resistance exercise training is associated with decreases in serum low-density lipoprotein cholesterol levels in premenopausal women." Arch Intern Med **153**(1): 97-100.

Curfman, G. D. (1993). "The health benefits of exercise. A critical reappraisal [editorial; comment]." N Engl J Med **328**(8): 574-6.

Elwood, P. C., J. W. Yarnell, et al. (1993). "Exercise, fibrinogen, and other risk factors for ischaemic heart disease. Caerphilly Prospective Heart Disease Study." Br Heart J **69**(2): 183-7.

Featherstone, J. F., R. G. Holly, et al. (1993). "Physiologic responses to weight lifting in coronary artery disease." Am J Cardiol **71**(4): 287-92.

Kanter, M. M., L. A. Nolte, et al. (1993). "Effects of an antioxidant vitamin mixture on lipid peroxidation at rest and postexercise." J Appl Physiol **74**(2): 965-9.

Meydani, M., W. J. Evans, et al. (1993). "Protective effect of vitamin E on exercise-induced oxidative damage in young and older adults." Am J Physiol **264**(5 Pt 2): R992-8.

Nichols, J. F., D. K. Omizo, et al. (1993). "Efficacy of heavy-resistance training for active women over sixty: muscular strength, body composition, and program adherence." J Am Geriatr Soc **41**(3): 205-10.

Paffenbarger, R., Jr., S. N. Blair, et al. (1993). "Measurement of physical activity to assess health effects in free-living populations." Med Sci Sports Exerc **25**(1): 60-70.

Paffenbarger, R., Jr., R. T. Hyde, et al. (1993). "The association of changes in physical-activity level and other lifestyle characteristics with mortality among men [see comments]." N Engl J Med **328**(8): 538-45.

Sandvik, L., J. Erikssen, et al. (1993). "Physical fitness as a predictor of mortality among healthy, middle-aged Norwegian men [see comments]." N Engl J Med **328**(8): 533-7.

Taylor, P. A. and A. Ward (1993). "Women, high-density lipoprotein cholesterol, and exercise." Arch Intern Med **153**(10): 1178-84.

Taylor, P. A. and A. Ward (1993). "Women, High-density lipoprotein cholesterol, and exercise." Arch Intern Med **153**: 1178-1184.

Ades, P. A., D. Huang, et al. (1992). "Cardiac rehabilitation participation predicts lower rehospitalization costs." Am Heart J **123**(4 Pt 1): 916-21.

Ades, P. A., M. L. Waldmann, et al. (1992). "Referral patterns and exercise response in the rehabilitation of female coronary patients aged greater than or equal to 62 years." Am J Cardiol **69**(17): 1422-5.

Arroll, B. and R. Beaglehole (1992). "Does physical activity lower blood pressure: a critical review of the clinical trials." J Clin Epidemiol **45**(5): 439-47.

Astrand, P. O. (1992). "J.B. Wolffe Memorial Lecture. "Why exercise?"." Med Sci Sports Exerc **24**(2): 153-62.

Astrand, P. O. (1992). "Physical activity and fitness." Am J Clin Nutr **55**(6 Suppl): 1231S-1236S.

Ballor, D. L. and E. T. Poehlman (1992). "Resting metabolic rate and coronary-heart-disease risk factors in aerobically and resistance-trained women." Am J Clin Nutr **56**(6): 968-74.

Bell, D. S. (1992). "Exercise for patients with diabetes. Benefits, risks, precautions." Postgrad Med **92**(1): 183-4.

Bjorntorp, P. A. (1992). "Efficacy of training in obese diabetic patients." Diabetes Care **15**(11): 1783-6.

Blair, S. N., H. W. Kohl, et al. (1992). "How much physical activity is good for health?" Annu Rev Public Health **13**(1): 99-126.

Blake, G. H. (1992). "Control of type II diabetes. Reaping the rewards of exercise and weight loss." Postgrad Med **92**(6): 129-32.

Connelly, J. B., J. A. Cooper, et al. (1992). "Strenuous exercise, plasma fibrinogen, and factor VII activity." Br Heart J **67**(5): 351-4.

Douglas, P. S., T. B. Clarkson, et al. (1992). "Exercise and atherosclerotic heart disease in women." Med Sci Sports Exerc **24**(6 Suppl): S266-76.

Eaton, C. B. (1992). "Relation of physical activity and cardiovascular fitness to coronary heart disease, Part I: A meta-analysis of the independent relation of physical activity and coronary heart disease." J Am Board Fam Pract **5**(1): 31-42.

Evans, W. J. (1992). "Exercise, nutrition and aging." J Nutr **122**(3 Suppl): 796-801.

Fletcher, G. F., S. N. Blair, et al. (1992). "Statement on exercise. Benefits and recommendations for physical activity programs for all Americans. A statement for health professionals by the Committee on Exercise and Cardiac Rehabilitation of the Council on Clinical Cardiology, American Heart association." Circulation **86**(1): 340-4.

Franklin, B. A., S. Gordon, et al. (1992). "Amount of exercise necessary for the patient with coronary artery disease." Am J Cardiol **69**(17): 1426-32.

Grassi, G., G. Seravalle, et al. (1992). "Physical exercise in essential hypertension." Chest **101**(5 Suppl): 312S-314S.

Haennel, R. G., G. D. Snydmiller, et al. (1992). "Changes in blood pressure and cardiac output during maximal isokinetic exercise." Arch Phys Med Rehabil **73**(2): 150-5.

Haskell, W. L., A. S. Leon, et al. (1992). "Cardiovascular benefits and assessment of physical activity and physical fitness in adults." Med Sci Sports Exerc **24**(6 Suppl): S201-20.

Hostmark, A. T., J. Berg, et al. (1992). "Coronary risk factors in middle-aged men as related to smoking, coffee intake and physical activity." Scand J Soc Med **20**(4): 196-203.

Jette, M., K. Sidney, et al. (1992). "Relation between cardiorespiratory fitness and selected risk factors for coronary heart disease in a population of Canadian men and women." Can Med Assoc J **146**(8): 1353-60.

Kohl, H. 3., K. E. Powell, et al. (1992). "Physical activity, physical fitness, and sudden cardiac death." Epidemiol Rev **14**(1): 37-58.

Kokkinos, P., J. Holland, et al. (1992). "Exercise threshold for favorable HDL changes in middle-aged men. (abstract)." J Am Coll Cardiol **19**(3): 346A #825-6.

Kumar, C. T., V. K. Reddy, et al. (1992). "Dietary supplementation of vitamin E protects heart tissue from exercise-induced oxidant stress." Mol Cell Biochem **111**(1-2): 109-15.

Lakka, T. A. and J. T. Salonen (1992). "Physical activity and serum lipids: a cross-sectional population study in eastern Finnish men." Am J Epidemiol **136**(7): 806-18.

Lavie, C. J., R. V. Milani, et al. (1992). "Exercise and the heart. Good, benign, or evil?" Postgrad Med **91**(2): 130-4.

Leclerc, K. M. (1992). "The role of exercise in reducing coronary heart disease and associated risk factors." J Okla State Med Assoc **85**(6): 283-90.

Manson, J. E., D. M. Nathan, et al. (1992). "A prospective study of exercise and incidence of diabetes among US male physicians." Jama **268**(1): 63-7.

Meydani, M., W. Evans, et al. (1992). "Antioxidant response to exercise-induced oxidative stress and protection by vitamin E." Ann N Y Acad Sci **669**(1): 363-4.

Owens, J. F., K. A. Matthews, et al. (1992). "Can physical activity mitigate the effects of aging in middle-aged women?" Circulation **85**(4): 1265-70.

Poehlman, E. T. (1992). "Energy expenditure and requirements in aging humans." J Nutr **122**(11): 2057-65.

Poehlman, E. T., A. W. Gardner, et al. (1992). "Resting energy metabolism and cardiovascular disease risk in resistance-trained and aerobically trained males." Metabolism **41**(12): 1351-60.

Posner, J. D., K. M. Gorman, et al. (1992). "Low to moderate intensity endurance training in healthy older adults: physiological responses after four months." J Am Geriatr Soc **40**(1): 1-7.

Rejeski, W. J., A. Thompson, et al. (1992). "Acute exercise: buffering psychosocial stress responses in women." Health Psychol **11**(6): 355-62.

Reznick, A. Z., E. Witt, et al. (1992). "Vitamin E inhibits protein oxidation in skeletal muscle of resting and exercised rats." Biochem Biophys Res Commun **189**(2): 801-6.

Reznick, A. Z., E. H. Witt, et al. (1992). "The threshold of age in exercise and antioxidants action." Exs **62**(1): 423-7.

Ruderman, N. B. and S. H. Schneider (1992). "Diabetes, exercise, and atherosclerosis." Diabetes Care **15**(11): 1787-93.

Schuler, G., R. Hambrecht, et al. (1992). "Myocardial perfusion and regression of coronary artery disease in patients on a regimen of intensive physical exercise and low fat diet." J Am Coll Cardiol **19**(1): 34-42.

Schuler, G., R. Hambrecht, et al. (1992). "Regular physical exercise and low-fat diet. Effects on progression of coronary artery disease." Circulation **86**(1): 1-11.

Schwartz, R. S., K. C. Cain, et al. (1992). "Effect of intensive endurance training on lipoprotein profiles in young and older men." Metabolism **41**(6): 649-54.

Selam, J. L., P. Casassus, et al. (1992). "Exercise is not associated with better diabetes control in type 1 and type 2 diabetic subjects." Acta Diabetol **29**(1): 11-3.

Sopko, G., E. Obarzanek, et al. (1992). "Overview of the National Heart, Lung, and Blood Institute Workshop on physical activity and cardiovascular health." Med Sci Sports Exerc **24**(6 Suppl): S192-5.

Stetson, B., D. G. Schlundt, et al. (1992). "The effects of aerobic exercise on psychological adjustment: a randomized study of sedentary obese women attempting weight loss." Women Health **19**(4): 1-14.

Tanaka, H. and M. Shindo (1992). "The benefits of the low intensity training." Ann Physiol Anthropol **11**(3): 365-8.

Tanji, J. L. (1992). "Exercise and the hypertensive athlete." Clin Sports Med **11**(2): 291-302.

Todd, I. C. and D. Ballantyne (1992). "Effect of exercise training on the total ischaemic burden: an assessment by 24 hour ambulatory electrocardiographic monitoring." Br Heart J **68**(6): 560-6.

Veera Reddy, K., T. Charles Kumar, et al. (1992). "Exercise-induced oxidant stress in the lung tissue: role of dietary supplementation of vitamin E and selenium." Biochem Int **26**(5): 863-71.

Wannamethee, G. and A. G. Shaper (1992). "Physical activity and stroke in British middle aged men." Bmj **304**(6827): 597-601.

Westheim, A. and I. Os (1992). "Physical activity and the metabolic cardiovascular syndrome." J Cardiovasc Pharmacol **20**(1): S49-53.

Winther, K., W. Hillegass, et al. (1992). "Effects on platelet aggregation and fibrinolytic activity during upright posture and exercise in healthy men." Am J Cardiol **70**(11): 1051-5.

Witt, E. H., A. Z. Reznick, et al. (1992). "Exercise, oxidative damage and effects of antioxidant manipulation." J Nutr **122**(3 Suppl): 766-73.

Wosornu, D., W. Allardyce, et al. (1992). "Influence of power and aerobic exercise training on haemostatic factors after coronary artery surgery." Br Heart J **68**(2): 181-6.

Yeater, R. A. and I. H. Ullrich (1992). "Hypertension and exercise. Where do we stand?" Postgrad Med **91**(5): 429-36.

Bauman, A. and N. Owen (1991). "Habitual physical activity and cardiovascular risk factors." Med J Aust **154**(1): 22-8.

Blair, S. N., H. 3. Kohl, et al. (1991). "Physical fitness and all-cause mortality in hypertensive men." Ann Med **23**(3): 307-12.

Blumenthal, J. A., C. F. Emery, et al. (1991). "Effects of exercise training on cardiorespiratory function in men and women older than 60 years of age." Am J Cardiol **67**(7): 633-9.

Blumenthal, J. A., W. C. Siegel, et al. (1991). "Failure of exercise to reduce blood pressure in patients with mild hypertension. Results of a randomized controlled trial [see comments]." Jama **266**(15): 2098-104.

Camacho, T. C., R. E. Roberts, et al. (1991). "Physical activity and depression: evidence from the Alameda County Study." Am J Epidemiol **134**(2): 220-31.

Caspersen, C. J., B. P. Bloemberg, et al. (1991). "The prevalence of selected physical activities and their relation with coronary heart disease risk factors in elderly men: the Zutphen Study, 1985." Am J Epidemiol **133**(11): 1078-92.

Chandrashekhar, Y. and I. S. Anand (1991). "Exercise as a coronary protective factor." Am Heart J **122**(6): 1723-39.

Cohen, J. C., J. Stray-Gundersen, et al. (1991). "Dissociation between postprandial lipemia and high density lipoprotein cholesterol concentrations in endurance-trained men." Arterioscler Thromb **11**(4): 838-43.

Duncan, J. J., N. F. Gordon, et al. (1991). "Women walking for health and fitness. How much is enough?" Jama **266**(23): 3295-9.

Ernst, E. (1991). "Peripheral vascular disease. Benefits of exercise." Sports Med **12**(3): 149-51.

Filipovsky, J., J. Simon, et al. (1991). "Changes of blood pressure and lipid pattern during a physical training course in hypertensive subjects." Cardiology **78**(1): 31-8.

Franklin, B. A. (1991). "Introduction: physiologic adaptations to exercise training in cardiac patients: contemporary issues and concerns." Med Sci Sports Exerc **23**(6): 645-7.

Franklin, B. A., S. Gordon, et al. (1991). "Exercise prescription for hypertensive patients." Ann Med **23**(3): 279-87.

Franz, I. W. (1991). "Blood pressure response to exercise in normotensives and hypertensives." Can J Sport Sci **16**(4): 296-301.

Gordon, N. F. and J. J. Duncan (1991). "Effect of beta-blockers on exercise physiology: implications for exercise training." Med Sci Sports Exerc **23**(6): 668-76.

Gordon, N. F. and C. B. Scott (1991). "The role of exercise in the primary and secondary prevention of coronary artery disease." Clin Sports Med **10**(1): 87-103.

Harris, T. B., D. M. Makuc, et al. (1991). "Is the serum cholesterol-coronary heart disease relationship modified by activity level in older persons?" J Am Geriatr Soc **39**(8): 747-54.

Helmrich, S. P., D. R. Ragland, et al. (1991). "Physical activity and reduced occurrence of non-insulin-dependent diabetes mellitus [see comments]." N Engl J Med **325**(3): 147-52.

Hill, D. W. and S. D. Butler (1991). "Haemodynamic responses to weightlifting exercise." Sports Med **12**(1): 1-7.

Horton, E. S. (1991). "Exercise and decreased risk of NIDDM [editorial] [published erratum appears in N Engl J Med 1991 Oct 17; 325(16):1188] [comment]." N Engl J Med **325**(3): 196-8.

Jennings, G., A. Dart, et al. (1991). "Effects of exercise and other nonpharmacological measures on blood pressure and cardiac hypertrophy." J Cardiovasc Pharmacol **17**(1): S70-4.

Kokkinos, P. F., B. F. Hurley, et al. (1991). "Strength training does not improve lipoprotein-lipid profiles in men at risk for CHD [see comments]." Med Sci Sports Exerc **23**(10): 1134-9.

Manson, J. E., E. B. Rimm, et al. (1991). "Physical activity and incidence of non-insulin-dependent diabetes mellitus in women." Lancet **338**(8770): 774-8.

Marti, B. (1991). "Health effects of recreational running in women. Some epidemiological and preventive aspects." Sports Med **11**(1): 20-51.

Numminen, H., M. Hillbom, et al. (1991). "Effects of exercise and ethanol ingestion on platelet thromboxane release in healthy men." Metabolism **40**(7): 695-701.

O'Connor, D. T. (1991). "The wise for cure on exercise depend [editorial; comment]." Circulation **83**(5): 1822-3.

Pescatello, L. S., A. E. Fargo, et al. (1991). "Short-term effect of dynamic exercise on arterial blood pressure [see comments]." Circulation **83**(5): 1557-61.

Pickering, T. G., P. L. Schnall, et al. (1991). "Can behavioural factors produce a sustained elevation of blood pressure? Some observations and a hypothesis." J Hypertens Suppl **9**(8): S66-8.

Riddoch, C., J. M. Savage, et al. (1991). "Long term health implications of fitness and physical activity patterns." Arch Dis Child **66**(12): 1426-33.

Samitz, G. and N. Bachl (1991). "Physical training programs and their effects on aerobic capacity and coronary risk profile in sedentary individuals. Design of a long-term exercise training program." J Sports Med Phys Fitness **31**(2): 283-93.

Schieken, R. M. (1991). "Effect of exercise on lipids." Ann N Y Acad Sci **623**(1): 269-74.

Segal, K. R., A. Edano, et al. (1991). "Effect of exercise training on insulin sensitivity and glucose metabolism in lean, obese, and diabetic men." J Appl Physiol **71**(6): 2402-11.

Shaper, A. G., G. Wannamethee, et al. (1991). "Physical activity and ischaemic heart disease in middle-aged British men [published erratum appears in Br Heart J 1992 Feb; 67(2):209]." Br Heart J **66**(5): 384-94.

Somers, V. K., J. Conway, et al. (1991). "Effects of endurance training on baroreflex sensitivity and blood pressure in borderline hypertension." Lancet **337**(8754): 1363-8.

Stratton, J. R., W. L. Chandler, et al. (1991). "Effects of physical conditioning on fibrinolytic variables and fibrinogen in young and old healthy adults." Circulation **83**(5): 1692-7.

Stray-Gundersen, J., M. A. Denke, et al. (1991). "Influence of lifetime cross-country skiing on plasma lipids and lipoproteins." Med Sci Sports Exerc **23**(6): 695-702.

Sumimoto, T., M. Hamada, et al. (1991). "Influence of age and severity of hypertension on blood pressure response to isometric handgrip exercise." J Hum Hypertens **5**(5): 399-403.

Summerson, J. H., J. C. Konen, et al. (1991). "Association between exercise and other preventive health behaviors among diabetics." Public Health Rep **106**(5): 543-7.

Superko, H. R. (1991). "Exercise training, serum lipids, and lipoprotein particles: is there a change threshold?" Med Sci Sports Exerc **23**(6): 677-85.

Thompson, P. D., E. M. Cullinane, et al. (1991). "High density lipoprotein metabolism in endurance athletes and sedentary men." Circulation **84**(1): 140-52.

Todd, I. C., M. S. Bradnam, et al. (1991). "Effects of daily high-intensity exercise on myocardial perfusion in angina pectoris." Am J Cardiol **68**(17): 1593-9.

Tremblay, A., J. P. Despres, et al. (1991). "Normalization of the metabolic profile in obese women by exercise and a low fat diet." Med Sci Sports Exerc **23**(12): 1326-31.

Watts, E. J. (1991). "Haemostatic changes in long-distance runners and their relevance to the prevention of ischaemic heart disease." Blood Coagul Fibrinolysis **2**(2): 221-5.

Wood, P. D., M. L. Stefanick, et al. (1991). "The effects on plasma lipoproteins of a prudent weight-reducing diet, with or without exercise, in overweight men and women." N Engl J Med **325**(7): 461-6.

Ades, P. A. and M. H. Grunvald (1990). "Cardiopulmonary exercise testing before and after conditioning in older coronary patients." Am Heart J **120**(3): 585-9.

Blumenthal, J. A., M. Fredrikson, et al. (1990). "Aerobic exercise reduces levels of cardiovascular and sympathoadrenal responses to mental stress in subjects without prior evidence of myocardial ischemia." Am J Cardiol **65**(1): 93-8.

Emery, C. F. and J. A. Blumenthal (1990). "Perceived change among participants in an exercise program for older adults." Gerontologist **30**(4): 516-21.

Johnson, C. and P. Greenland (1990). "Effects of exercise, dietary cholesterol, and dietary fat on blood lipids." Arch Intern Med **150**(1): 137-41.

Kelemen, M. H., M. B. Effron, et al. (1990). "Exercise training combined with antihypertensive drug therapy. Effects on lipids, blood pressure, and left ventricular mass [see comments]." Jama **263**(20): 2766-71.

Kitajima, K., J. Sasaki, et al. (1990). "Prognostic significance of daily physical activity after first acute myocardial infarction." Am Heart J **119**(5): 1193-4.

Reaven, P. D., J. B. McPhillips, et al. (1990). "Leisure time exercise and lipid and lipoprotein levels in an older population." J Am Geriatr Soc **38**(8): 847-54.

Stein, R. A., D. W. Michielli, et al. (1990). "Effects of different exercise training intensities on lipoprotein cholesterol fractions in healthy middle-aged men." Am Heart J **119**(2 Pt 1): 277-83.

Fiber

Levi, F., S. Franceschi, et al. (1993). "Dietary factors and the risk of endometrial cancer." Cancer **71**(11): 3575-81.

Rohan, T. E., G. R. Howe, et al. (1993). "Dietary fiber, vitamins A, C, and E, and risk of breast cancer: a cohort study." Cancer Causes Control **4**(1): 29-37.

(1992). "Dietary fibre: importance of function as well as amount [editorial]." Lancet **340**(8828): 1133-4.

Anderson, J. W. (1992). "Dietary fiber and diabetes: what else do we need to know? [editorial]." Diabetes Res Clin Pract **17**(2): 71-3.

Anderson, J. W., T. F. Garrity, et al. (1992). "Prospective, randomized, controlled comparison of the effects of low-fat and low-fat plus high-fiber diets on serum lipid concentrations." Am J Clin Nutr **56**(5): 887-94.

Anderson, J. W., S. Riddell-Mason, et al. (1992). "Cholesterol-lowering effects of psyllium-enriched cereal as an adjunct to a prudent diet in the treatment of mild to moderate hypercholesterolemia." Am J Clin Nutr **56**(1): 93-8.

Arbman, G., O. Axelson, et al. (1992). "Cereal fiber, calcium, and colorectal cancer." Cancer **69**(8): 2042-8.

Bolton-Smith, C., M. Woodward, et al. (1992). "The Scottish Heart Health Study. Dietary intake by food frequency questionnaire and odds ratios for coronary heart disease risk. II. The antioxidant vitamins and fibre." Eur J Clin Nutr **46**(2): 85-93.

Cara, L., C. Dubois, et al. (1992). "Effects of oat bran, rice bran, wheat fiber, and wheat germ on postprandial lipemia in healthy adults." Am J Clin Nutr **55**(1): 81-8.

Clevidence, B. A., J. T. Judd, et al. (1992). "Plasma lipid and lipoprotein concentrations of men consuming a low-fat, high-fiber diet." Am J Clin Nutr **55**(3): 689-94.

Evans, A. J., R. L. Hood, et al. (1992). "Relationship between structure and function of dietary fibre: a comparative study of the effects of three galactomannans on cholesterol metabolism in the rat." Br J Nutr **68**(1): 217-29.

Fernandez, M. L., E. C. Lin, et al. (1992). "Prickly pear (Opuntia sp.) pectin reverses low density lipoprotein receptor suppression induced by a hypercholesterolemic diet in guinea pigs." J Nutr **122**(12): 2330-40.

Haskell, W. L., G. A. Spiller, et al. (1992). "Role of water-soluble dietary fiber in the management of elevated plasma cholesterol in healthy subjects." Am J Cardiol **69**(5): 433-9.

Heitman, D. W., W. E. Hardman, et al. (1992). "Dietary supplementation with pectin and guar gum on 1,2-dimethylhydrazine-induced colon carcinogenesis in rats." Carcinogenesis **13**(5): 815-8.

Howe, G. R., E. Benito, et al. (1992). "Dietary intake of fiber and decreased risk of cancers of the colon and rectum: evidence from the combined analysis of 13 case-control studies [see comments]." J Natl Cancer Inst **84**(24): 1887-96.

Kashtan, H., H. S. Stern, et al. (1992). "Wheat-bran and oat-bran supplements' effects on blood lipids and lipoproteins." Am J Clin Nutr **55**(5): 976-80.

Keenan, J. M., J. B. Wenz, et al. (1992). "A clinical trial of oat bran and niacin in the treatment of hyperlipidemia." J Fam Pract **34**(3): 313-9.

Krebs-Smith, S. M., F. J. Cronin, et al. (1992). "Food sources of energy, macronutrients, cholesterol, and fiber in diets of women." J Am Diet Assoc **92**(2): 168-74.

Landin, K., G. Holm, et al. (1992). "Guar gum improves insulin sensitivity, blood lipids, blood pressure, and fibrinolysis in healthy men." Am J Clin Nutr **56**(6): 1061-5.

Lepre, F. and S. Crane (1992). "Effect of oatbran on mild hyperlipidaemia." Med J Aust **157**(5): 305-8.

Mackay, S. and M. J. Ball (1992). "Do beans and oat bran add to the effectiveness of a low-fat diet?" Eur J Clin Nutr **46**(9): 641-8.

Martinez, V. M., R. K. Newman, et al. (1992). "Barley diets with different fat sources have hypocholesterolemic effects in chicks." J Nutr **122**(5): 1070-6.

McCall, M. R., T. Mehta, et al. (1992). "Psyllium husk. I: Effect on plasma lipoproteins, cholesterol metabolism, and atherosclerosis in African green monkeys." Am J Clin Nutr **56**(2): 376-84.

McCall, M. R., T. Mehta, et al. (1992). "Psyllium husk. II: Effect on the metabolism of apolipoprotein B in African green monkeys." Am J Clin Nutr **56**(2): 385-93.

Pirich, C., P. Schmid, et al. (1992). "[Lowering cholesterol with Anticholest—a high fiber guar-apple pectin drink]." Wien Klin Wochenschr **104**(11): 314-6.

Reddy, B. S., A. Engle, et al. (1992). "Effect of dietary fiber on colonic bacterial enzymes and bile acids in relation to colon cancer." Gastroenterology **102**(5): 1475-82.

Ripsin, C. M., J. M. Keenan, et al. (1992). "Oat products and lipid lowering. A meta-analysis." Jama **267**(24): 3317-25.

Rock, C. L. and M. E. Swendseid (1992). "Plasma beta-carotene response in humans after meals supplemented with dietary pectin." Am J Clin Nutr **55**(1): 96-9.

Rose, D. P. (1992). "Dietary fiber, phytoestrogens, and breast cancer." Nutrition **8**(1): 47-51.

Sanders, T. A. and S. Reddy (1992). "The influence of rice bran on plasma lipids and lipoproteins in human volunteers." Eur J Clin Nutr **46**(3): 167-72.

Vuorinen-Markkola, H., M. Sinisalo, et al. (1992). "Guar gum in insulin-dependent diabetes: effects on glycemic control and serum lipoproteins." Am J Clin Nutr **56**(6): 1056-60.

Whyte, J. L., R. McArthur, et al. (1992). "Oat bran lowers plasma cholesterol levels in mildly hypercholesterolemic men." J Am Diet Assoc **92**(4): 446-9.

Willett, W. C., D. J. Hunter, et al. (1992). "Dietary fat and fiber in relation to risk of breast cancer. An 8-year follow-up [see comments]." Jama **268**(15): 2037-44.

Anderson, J. W. and A. O. Akanji (1991). "Dietary fiber—an overview." Diabetes Care **14**(12): 1126-31.

Anderson, J. W., T. L. Floore, et al. (1991). "Hypocholesterolemic effects of different bulk-forming hydrophilic fibers as adjuncts to dietary therapy in mild to moderate hypercholesterolemia." Arch Intern Med **151**(8): 1597-602.

Anderson, J. W., N. H. Gilinsky, et al. (1991). "Lipid responses of hypercholesterolemic men to oat-bran and wheat-bran intake." Am J Clin Nutr **54**(4): 678-83.

Anderson, J. W., S. Riddell-Lawrence, et al. (1991). "Bakery products lower serum cholesterol concentrations in hypercholesterolemic men." Am J Clin Nutr **54**(5): 836-40.

Anderson, J. W., N. J. Gustafson, et al. (1990). "Serum lipid response of hypercholesterolemic men to single and divided doses of canned beans." Am J Clin Nutr **51**(6): 1013-9.

Anderson, J. W., B. M. Smith, et al. (1990). "High-fiber diet for diabetes. Safe and effective treatment." Postgrad Med **88**(2): 157-61.

Anderson, J. W., D. B. Spencer, et al. (1990). "Oat-bran cereal lowers serum total and LDL cholesterol in hypercholesterolemic men." Am J Clin Nutr **52**(3): 495-9.

Bell, L. P., K. J. Hectorn, et al. (1990). "Cholesterol-lowering effects of soluble-fiber cereals as part of a prudent diet for patients with mild to moderate hypercholesterolemia." Am J Clin Nutr **52**(6): 1020-6.

Fibrinogen

Elwood, P. C., J. W. Yarnell, et al. (1993). "Exercise, fibrinogen, and other risk factors for ischaemic heart disease. Caerphilly Prospective Heart Disease Study." Br Heart J **69**(2): 183-7.

Wilson, T. W., G. A. Kaplan, et al. (1993). "Association between plasma fibrinogen concentration and five socioeconomic indices in the Kuopio Ischemic Heart Disease Risk Factor Study." Am J Epidemiol **137**(3): 292-300.

Banerjee, A. K., J. Pearson, et al. (1992). "A six year prospective study of fibrinogen and other risk factors associated with mortality in stable claudicants." Thromb Haemost **68**(3): 261-3.

Burr, M. L., R. M. Holliday, et al. (1992). "Haematological prognostic indices after myocardial infarction: evidence from the diet and reinfarction trial (DART)." Eur Heart J **13**(2): 166-70.

Connelly, J. B., J. A. Cooper, et al. (1992). "Strenuous exercise, plasma fibrinogen, and factor VII activity." Br Heart J **67**(5): 351-4.

Ernst, E. (1992). "Fibrinogen: the plot thickens." J Clin Epidemiol **45**(5): 561-2.

Fowkes, F. G., J. M. Connor, et al. (1992). "Fibrinogen genotype and risk of peripheral atherosclerosis." Lancet **339**(8795): 693-6.

Kannel, W. B., et al (1992). "Update on fibrinogen as a cardiovascular risk factor." Ann Epidem **2**: 457-466.

Kelleher, C. C. (1992). "Plasma fibrinogen and factor VII as risk factors for cardiovascular disease." Eur J Epidemiol **8**(1): 79-82.

Kovacs, I. B., C. P. Ratnatunga, et al. (1992). "Significance of plasma fibrinogen in coronary arterial disease: marker or causative risk factor for arterial thrombosis?" Int J Cardiol **35**(1): 57-64.

Krobot, K., H. W. Hense, et al. (1992). "Determinants of plasma fibrinogen: relation to body weight, waist-to-hip ratio, smoking, alcohol, age, and sex. Results from the second MONICA Augsburg survey 1989-1990." Arterioscler Thromb **12**(7): 780-8.

Lee, A. J., G. D. Lowe, et al. (1992). "Plasma fibrinogen: its relationship with oral contraception, the menopause, and hormone replacement therapy." Clin Biochem **25**(5): 403-5.

Matsunaga, A., K. Handa, et al. (1992). "Effects of niceritrol on levels of serum lipids, lipoprotein(a), and fibrinogen in patients with primary hypercholesterolemia." Atherosclerosis **94**(2-3): 241-8.

Resch, K. L., E. Ernst, et al. (1992). "Fibrinogen and viscosity as risk factors for subsequent cardiovascular events in stroke survivors." Ann Intern Med **117**(5): 371-5.

Saynor, R. and T. Gillott (1992). "Changes in blood lipids and fibrinogen with a note on safety in a long term study on the effects of n-3 fatty acids in subjects receiving fish oil supplements and followed for seven years." Lipids **27**(7): 533-8.

Smith, E. B., W. D. Thompson, et al. (1992). "Fibrinogen/fibrin in atherogenesis." Eur J Epidemiol **8**(1): 83-7.

Wosornu, D., W. Allardyce, et al. (1992). "Influence of power and aerobic exercise training on haemostatic factors after coronary artery surgery." Br Heart J **68**(2): 181-6.

Athukorala, T. M. and L. P. Ranjini (1991). "Lipid patterns and fibrinogen levels of smokers and non-smokers." Ceylon Med J **36**(3): 98-101.

Fibrinolysis

Legnani, C., M. Frascaro, et al. (1993). "Effects of a dried garlic preparation on fibrinolysis and platelet aggregation in healthy subjects." Arzneimittelforschung **43**(2): 119-22.

Schneider, D. J., T. K. Nordt, et al. (1993). "Attenuated fibrinolysis and accelerated atherogenesis in type II diabetic patients." Diabetes **42**(1): 1-7.

Andersen, P. (1992). "Hypercoagulability and reduced fibrinolysis in hyperlipidemia: relationship to the metabolic cardiovascular syndrome." J Cardiovasc Pharmacol **20**(1): S29-31.

Fujii, S. and B. E. Sobel (1992). "Direct effects of gemfibrozil on the fibrinolytic system. Diminution of synthesis of plasminogen activator inhibitor type 1." Circulation **85**(5): 1888-93.

Halvorsen, S., O. H. Skjonsberg, et al. (1992). "Does Lp(a) lipoprotein inhibit the fibrinolytic system? (no)." Thromb Res **68**(3): 223-32.

Hegele, R. A. (1992). "Lipoprotein(a) and fibrinolysis." Can J Cardiol **8**(10): 1021-2.

Iacoviello, L., C. Amore, et al. (1992). "Modulation of fibrinolytic response to venous occlusion in humans by a combination of low-dose aspirin and n-3 polyunsaturated fatty acids." Arterioscler Thromb **12**(10): 1191-7.

Landin, K., G. Holm, et al. (1992). "Guar gum improves insulin sensitivity, blood lipids, blood pressure, and fibrinolysis in healthy men." Am J Clin Nutr **56**(6): 1061-5.

Winther, K., W. Hillegass, et al. (1992). "Effects on platelet aggregation and fibrinolytic activity during upright posture and exercise in healthy men." Am J Cardiol **70**(11): 1051-5.

Gadkari, J. V. and V. D. Joshi (1991). "Effect of ingestion of raw garlic on serum cholesterol level, clotting time and fibrinolytic activity in normal subjects." J Postgrad Med **37**(3): 128-31.

Heinrich, J., M. Sandkamp, et al. (1991). "Relationship of lipoprotein(a) to variables of coagulation and fibrinolysis in a healthy population." Clin Chem **37**(11): 1950-4.

Lowe, G. D., D. A. Wood, et al. (1991). "Relationships of plasma viscosity, coagulation and fibrinolysis to coronary risk factors and angina." Thromb Haemost **65**(4): 339-43.

Stratton, J. R., W. L. Chandler, et al. (1991). "Effects of physical conditioning on fibrinolytic variables and fibrinogen in young and old healthy adults." Circulation **83**(5): 1692-7.

Watts, E. J. (1991). "Haemostatic changes in long-distance runners and their relevance to the prevention of ischaemic heart disease." Blood Coagul Fibrinolysis **2**(2): 221-5.

Zalewski, A., Y. Shi, et al. (1991). "Evidence for reduced fibrinolytic activity in unstable angina at rest. Clinical, biochemical, and angiographic correlates." Circulation **83**(5): 1685-91.

Fish/Fish Oil

Chin, J. P., A. P. Gust, et al. (1993). "Marine oils dose-dependently inhibit vasoconstriction of forearm resistance vessels in humans." Hypertension **21**(1): 22-8.

Harker, L. A., A. B. Kelly, et al. (1993). "Interruption of vascular thrombus formation and vascular lesion formation by dietary n-3 fatty acids in fish oil in nonhuman primates." Circulation **87**(3): 1017-29.

Lofgren, R. P., T. J. Wilt, et al. (1993). "The effect of fish oil supplements on blood pressure." Am J Public Health **83**(2): 267-9.

Morris, M. C., J. O. Taylor, et al. (1993). "The effect of fish oil on blood pressure in mild hypertensive subjects: a randomized crossover trial." Am J Clin Nutr **57**(1): 59-64.

Ross, E. (1993). "The role of marine fish oils in the treatment of ulcerative colitis." Nutr Rev **51**(2): 47-9.

Svensson, B. G., B. Akesson, et al. (1993). "Fatty acid composition of serum phosphatidylcholine in healthy subjects consuming varying amounts of fish." Eur J Clin Nutr **47**(2): 132-40.

Wolmarans, P., D. Labadarios, et al. (1993). "The influence of consuming fatty fish instead of red meat on plasma levels of vitamins A, C and E." Eur J Clin Nutr **47**(2): 97-103.

Aslan, A. and G. Triadafilopoulos (1992). "Fish oil fatty acid supplementation in active ulcerative colitis: a double-blind, placebo-controlled, crossover study." Am J Gastroenterol **87**(4): 432-7.

Bairati, I., L. Roy, et al. (1992). "Double-blind, randomized, controlled trial of fish oil supplements in prevention of recurrence of stenosis after coronary angioplasty." Circulation **85**(3): 950-6.

Bairati, I., L. Roy, et al. (1992). "Effects of a fish oil supplement on blood pressure and serum lipids in patients treated for coronary artery disease." Can J Cardiol **8**(1): 41-6.

Bonaa, K. H., K. S. Bjerve, et al. (1992). "Docosahexaenoic and eicosapentaenoic acids in plasma phospholipids are divergently associated with high density lipoprotein in humans." Arterioscler Thromb **12**(6): 675-81.

Bonaa, K. H., K. S. Bjerve, et al. (1992). "Habitual fish consumption, plasma phospholipid fatty acids, and serum lipids: the Tromso study." Am J Clin Nutr **55**(6): 1126-34.

Burr, M. L. (1992). "Fish food, fish oil and cardiovascular disease." Clin Exp Hypertens [a] **14**(1-2): 181-92.

Cobiac, L., P. J. Nestel, et al. (1992). "A low-sodium diet supplemented with fish oil lowers blood pressure in the elderly." J Hypertens **10**(1): 87-92.

Coniglio, J. G. (1992). "How does fish oil lower plasma triglycerides?" Nutr Rev **50**(7): 195-7.

Dallongeville, J., E. Selinger, et al. (1992). "Fish-oil supplementation reduces Ip(a) concentrations in type III dysbetalipoproteinemia [letter]." Clin Chem **38**(8 Pt 1): 1510-1.

Gonzalez, M. J., J. I. Gray, et al. (1992). "Lipid peroxidation products are elevated in fish oil diets even in the presence of added antioxidants." J Nutr **122**(11): 2190-5.

Goodnight, S. H., J. A. Cairns, et al. (1992). "Assessment of the therapeutic use of n-3 fatty acids in vascular disease and thrombosis." Chest **102**(4 Suppl): 374S-384S.

Harker, L. A. (1992). "What are the effects of dietary n-3 fatty acids on vascular thrombus and lesion formation in nonhuman primates?" Am J Clin Nutr **56**(4 Suppl): 817S-818S.

Hawthorne, A. B., T. K. Daneshmend, et al. (1992). "Treatment of ulcerative colitis with fish oil supplementation: a prospective 12 month randomised controlled trial." Gut **33**(7): 922-8.

Iacoviello, L., C. Amore, et al. (1992). "Modulation of fibrinolytic response to venous occlusion in humans by a combination of low-dose aspirin and n-3 polyunsaturated fatty acids." Arterioscler Thromb **12**(10): 1191-7.

Israel, D. H. and R. Gorlin (1992). "Fish oils in the prevention of atherosclerosis." J Am Coll Cardiol **19**(1): 174-85.

Kaul, U., S. Sanghvi, et al. (1992). "Fish oil supplements for prevention of restenosis after coronary angioplasty." Int J Cardiol **35**(1): 87-93.

Kelley, D. S., G. J. Nelson, et al. (1992). "Salmon diet and human immune status." Eur J Clin Nutr **46**(6): 397-404.

Lam, J. Y., J. J. Badimon, et al. (1992). "Cod liver oil alters platelet-arterial wall response to injury in pigs." Circ Res **71**(4): 769-75.

Leaf, A. (1992). "Health claims: omega-3 fatty acids and cardiovascular disease." Nutr Rev **50**(5): 150-4.

Lindsey, S., A. Pronczuk, et al. (1992). "Low density lipoprotein from humans supplemented with n-3 fatty acids depresses both LDL receptor activity and LDLr mRNA abundance in HepG2 cells." J Lipid Res **33**(5): 647-58.

McLennan, P. L., T. M. Bridle, et al. (1992). "Dietary lipid modulation of ventricular fibrillation threshold in the marmoset monkey." Am Heart J **123**(6): 1555-61.

Meydani, M. (1992). "Vitamin E requirement in relation to dietary fish oil and oxidative stress in elderly." Exs **62**(1): 411-8.

Mori, T. A., R. Vandongen, et al. (1992). "Plasma lipid levels and platelet and neutrophil function in patients with vascular disease following fish oil and olive oil supplementation." Metabolism **41**(10): 1059-67.

Morris, M. C., J. E. Mason, et al. (1992). "A prospective study of fish consumption on cardiovascular disease (abstract)." Supplement to Circulation **abstract#1846**(Abstracts from the 65th scientific sessions of the American Heart Association): I-463.

Nenseter, M. S., A. C. Rustan, et al. (1992). "Effect of dietary supplementation with n-3 polyunsaturated fatty acids on physical properties and metabolism of low density lipoprotein in humans." Arterioscler Thromb **12**(3): 369-79.

Notarbartolo, A., I. Catalano, et al. (1992). "Platelets, eicosanoids and aging." Aging **4**(1): 13-20.

O'Connor, G. T., D. J. Malenka, et al. (1992). "A meta-analysis of randomized trials of fish oil in prevention of restenosis following coronary angioplasty." Am J Prev Med **8**(3): 186-92.

Raper, N. R., F. J. Cronin, et al. (1992). "Omega-3 fatty acid content of the US food supply." J Am Coll Nutr **11**(3): 304-8.

Sanders, T. A. and A. Hinds (1992). "The influence of a fish oil high in docosahexaenoic acid on plasma lipoprotein and vitamin E concentrations and haemostatic function in healthy male volunteers." Br J Nutr **68**(1): 163-73.

Saynor, R. and T. Gillott (1992). "Changes in blood lipids and fibrinogen with a note on safety in a long term study on the effects of n-3 fatty acids in subjects receiving fish oil supplements and followed for seven years." Lipids **27**(7): 533-8.

Schmidt, E. B., H. H. Lervang, et al. (1992). "Long-term supplementation with n-3 fatty acids, I: Effect on blood lipids, haemostasis and blood pressure." Scand J Clin Lab Invest **52**(3): 221-8.

Schmidt, E. B., K. Varming, et al. (1992). "Long-term supplementation with n-3 fatty acids, II: Effect on neutrophil and monocyte chemotaxis." Scand J Clin Lab Invest **52**(3): 229-36.

Schmidt, E. B., K. Varming, et al. (1992). "n-3 polyunsaturated fatty acid supplementation (Pikasol) in men with moderate and severe hypertriglyceridaemia: a dose-response study." Ann Nutr Metab **36**(5-6): 283-7.

Seidelin, K. N., B. Myrup, et al. (1992). "n-3 fatty acids in adipose tissue and coronary artery disease are inversely related." Am J Clin Nutr **55**(6): 1117-9.

Stenson, W. F., D. Cort, et al. (1992). "Dietary supplementation with fish oil in ulcerative colitis." Ann Intern Med **116**(8): 609-14.

Fish—Pollution

(1992). Is our fish fit to eat? Consumer reports. 103-120.

Gellert, G. A., J. Ralls, et al. (1992). "Scombroid fish poisoning. Underreporting and prevention among noncommercial recreational fishers." West J Med **157**(6): 645-7.

Gollop, J. H. and E. W. Pon (1992). "Ciguatera: a review [see comments]." Hawaii Med J **51**(4): 91-9.

Jaroff, L. (1992). Is your fish really foul? Time. 70-71.

Lange, W. R., F. R. Snyder, et al. (1992). "Travel and ciguatera fish poisoning." Arch Intern Med **152**(10): 2049-53.

Muller, G. J., J. H. Lamprecht, et al. (1992). "Scombroid poisoning. Case series of 10 incidents involving 22 patients." S Afr Med J **81**(8): 427-30.

(1991). "Seafood safety. Highlights of the Executive Summary of the 1991 report by the Committee on Evaluation of the Safety of Fishery Products of the Food and Nutrition Board, Institute of Medicine, National Academy of Sciences." Nutr Rev **49**(12): 357-63.

Fasano, A., Y. Hokama, et al. (1991). "Diarrhea in ciguatera fish poisoning: preliminary evaluation of pathophysiological mechanisms." Gastroenterology **100**(2): 471-6.

Geller, R. J., K. R. Olson, et al. (1991). "Ciguatera fish poisoning in San Francisco, California, caused by imported barracuda." West J Med **155**(6): 639-42.

Hughes, J. M. and M. E. Potter (1991). "Scombroid-fish poisoning. From pathogenesis to prevention [editorial; comment] [see comments]." N Engl J Med **324**(11): 766-8.

Shukla, V. K. and E. G. Perkins (1991). "The presence of oxidative polymeric materials in encapsulated fish oils." Lipids **26**(1): 23-6.

Svensson, B. G., A. Nilsson, et al. (1991). "Exposure to dioxins and dibenzofurans through the consumption of fish." N Engl J Med **324**(1): 8-12.

Schantz, P. M. (1989). "The dangers of eating raw fish [editorial]." N Engl J Med **320**(17): 1143-5.

Folic Acid

Giovannucci, E., M. J. Stampfer, et al. (1993). "Folate, methionine, and alcohol intake and risk of colorectal adenoma [see comments]." J Natl Cancer Inst **85**(11): 875-84.

Ubbink, J. B., W. J. Vermaak, et al. (1993). "Vitamin B-12, vitamin B-6, and folate nutritional status in men with hyperhomocysteinemia." Am J Clin Nutr **57**(1): 47-53.

Freudenheim, J. L., S. Graham, et al. (1991). "Folate intake and carcinogenesis of the colon and rectum." Int J Epidemiol **20**(2): 368-74.

Kang, S. S., P. W. Wong, et al. (1987). "Homocysteinemia due to folate deficiency." Metabolism **36**(5): 458-62.

Free Radicals

Buettner, G. R. (1993). "The pecking order of free radicals and antioxidants: lipid peroxidation, alpha-tocopherol, and ascorbate." Arch Biochem Biophys **300**(2): 535-43.

Bulkley, G. B. (1993). "Free radicals and other reactive oxygen metabolites: clinical relevance and the therapeutic efficacy of antioxidant therapy." Surgery **113**(5): 479-83.

Davies, S. W., J. P. Duffy, et al. (1993). "Time-course of free radical activity during coronary artery operations with cardiopulmonary bypass." J Thorac Cardiovasc Surg **105**(6): 979-87.

Davies, S. W., K. Ranjadayalan, et al. (1993). "Free radical activity and left ventricular function after thrombolysis for acute infarction." Br Heart J **69**(2): 114-20.

Halliwell, B. (1993). "The role of oxygen radicals in human disease, with particular reference to the vascular system." Haemostasis **23**(1): 118-26.

Kahler, W., B. Kuklinski, et al. (1993). "[Diabetes mellitus—a free radical-associated disease. Results of adjuvant antioxidant supplementation]." Z Gesamte Inn Med **48**(5): 223-32.

Kubow, S. (1993). "Lipid oxidation products in food and atherogenesis." Nutr Rev **51**(2): 33-40.

Niki, E., S. Minamisawa, et al. (1993). "Membrane damage from lipid oxidation induced by free radicals and cigarette smoke." Ann N Y Acad Sci **686**(1): 29-37.

Prasad, K. and J. Kalra (1993). "Oxygen free radicals and hypercholesterolemic atherosclerosis: effect of vitamin E." Am Heart J **125**(4): 958-73.

Sohal, R. S. (1993). "The free radical hypothesis of aging: an appraisal of the current status [see comments]." Aging **5**(1): 3-17.

Taylor, A., P. F. Jacques, et al. (1993). "Oxidation and aging: impact on vision." Toxicol Ind Health **9**(1-2): 349-71.

Barsacchi, R., G. Pelosi, et al. (1992). "Myocardial vitamin E is consumed during cardiopulmonary bypass: indirect evidence of free radical generation in human ischemic heart." Int J Cardiol **37**(3): 339-43.

Bradamante, S., L. Barenghi, et al. (1992). "Free radicals promote modifications in plasma high-density lipoprotein: nuclear magnetic resonance analysis." Free Radic Biol Med **12**(3): 193-203.

Bunker, V. (1992). "Free radicals, antioxidants, and ageing." Med Lab Sci **49**: 299-312.

Csillag, C. and P. Aldhous (1992). "Smoking and health. Signs of damage by radicals [news]." Science **258**(5090): 1875-6.

Dargel, R. (1992). "Lipid peroxidation—a common pathogenetic mechanism?" Exp Toxicol Pathol **44**(4): 169-81.

Halliwell, B., J. M. Gutteridge, et al. (1992). "Free radicals, antioxidants, and human disease: where are we now?" J Lab Clin Med **119**(6): 598-620.

Jayakumari, N., V. Ambikakumari, et al. (1992). "Antioxidant status in relation to free radical production during stable and unstable anginal syndromes." Atherosclerosis **94**(2-3): 183-90.

Kubow, S. (1992). "Routes of formation and toxic consequences of lipid oxidation products in foods." Free Radic Biol Med **12**(1): 63-81.

McMurray, J., M. Chopra, et al. (1992). "Evidence for oxidative stress in unstable angina." Br Heart J **68**(5): 454-7.

Meydani, M. (1992). "Vitamin E requirement in relation to dietary fish oil and oxidative stress in elderly." Exs **62**(1): 411-8.

Meydani, M., W. Evans, et al. (1992). "Antioxidant response to exercise-induced oxidative stress and protection by vitamin E." Ann N Y Acad Sci **669**(1): 363-4.

Mozsik, G., M. Fiegler, et al. (1992). "Oxygen free radicals, lipid metabolism, and whole blood and plasma viscosity in the prevention and treatment of human cardiovascular diseases." Bibl Nutr Dieta **49**: 111-24.

Murphy, M. E., R. Kolvenbach, et al. (1992). "Antioxidant depletion in aortic crossclamping ischemia: increase of the plasma alpha-tocopheryl quinone/alpha-tocopherol ratio." Free Radic Biol Med **13**(2): 95-100.

Murthy, V. K., J. C. Shipp, et al. (1992). "Delayed onset and decreased incidence of diabetes in BB rats fed free radical scavengers." Diabetes Res Clin Pract **18**(1): 11-6.

Niki, E. (1992). "Free radical pathology and antioxidants: overview." J Nutr Sci Vitaminol **1**(40): 538-40.

Prasad, K., J. Kalra, et al. (1992). "Increased oxygen free radical activity in patients on cardiopulmonary bypass undergoing aortocoronary bypass surgery." Am Heart J **123**(1): 37-45.

Sharma, R. C., D. W. Crawford, et al. (1992). "Immunolocalization of native antioxidant scavenger enzymes in early hypertensive and atherosclerotic arteries. Role of oxygen free radicals." Arterioscler Thromb **12**(4): 403-15.

Witt, E. H., A. Z. Reznick, et al. (1992). "Exercise, oxidative damage and effects of antioxidant manipulation." J Nutr **122**(3 Suppl): 766-73.

Belch, J. J., A. B. Bridges, et al. (1991). "Oxygen free radicals and congestive heart failure." Br Heart J **65**(5): 245-8.

Bertelli, A., A. Conte, et al. (1991). "Protective effect of propionyl carnitine against peroxidative damage to arterial endothelium membranes." Int J Tissue React **13**(1): 41-3.

Bridges, A. B., N. A. Scott, et al. (1991). "Probucol, a superoxide free radical scavenger in vitro." Atherosclerosis **89**(2-3): 263-5.

Carpenter, K. L., C. E. Brabbs, et al. (1991). "Oxygen radicals and atherosclerosis." Klin Wochenschr **69**(21-23): 1039-45.

Clemens, M. R. (1991). "Free radicals in chemical carcinogenesis." Klin Wochenschr **69**(21-23): 1123-34.

Crawford, D. W. and D. H. Blankenhorn (1991). "Arterial wall oxygenation, oxyradicals, and atherosclerosis." Atherosclerosis **89**(2-3): 97-108.

Cutler, R. G. (1991). "Antioxidants and aging." Am J Clin Nutr **53**(1 Suppl): 373S-379S.

Duthie, G. G., J. R. Arthur, et al. (1991). "Effects of smoking and vitamin E on blood antioxidant status." Am J Clin Nutr **53**(4 Suppl): 1061S-1063S.

Ferrari, R. (1991). "The role of free radicals in the ischemic myocardium." Bratisl Lek Listy **92**(2): 108-12.

Ferrari, R., C. Ceconi, et al. (1991). "Oxygen free radicals and myocardial damage: protective role of thiol-containing agents." Am J Med **91**(3C):

Flaherty, J. T. (1991). "Myocardial injury mediated by oxygen free radicals." Am J Med **91**(3C): 79S-85S.

Halliwell, B. (1991). "Drug antioxidant effects. A basis for drug selection?" Drugs **42**(4): 569-605.

Halliwell, B. (1991). "Reactive oxygen species in living systems: source, biochemistry, and role in human disease." Am J Med **91**(3C): 14S-22S.

Halliwell, B. and C. E. Cross (1991). "Reactive oxygen species, antioxidants, and acquired immunodeficiency syndrome. Sense or speculation?" Arch Intern Med **151**(1): 29-31.

Hodis, H. N., D. W. Crawford, et al. (1991). "Cholesterol feeding increases plasma and aortic tissue cholesterol oxide levels in parallel: further evidence for the role of cholesterol oxidation in atherosclerosis." Atherosclerosis **89**(2-3): 117-26.

Kourounakis, P. N. and E. A. Rekka (1991). "Effect on active oxygen species of alliin and Allium sativum (garlic) powder." Res Commun Chem Pathol Pharmacol **74**(2): 249-52.

Menger, M. D., H. A. Lehr, et al. (1991). "Role of oxygen radicals in the microcirculatory manifestations of postischemic injury [published erratum appears in Klin Wochenschr 1990 Dec 30; 69(24):1185]." Klin Wochenschr **69**(21-23): 1050-5.

Mulholland, C. W. and J. J. Strain (1991). "Serum total free radical trapping ability in acute myocardial infarction." Clin Biochem **24**(5): 437-41.

Niki, E., Y. Yamamoto, et al. (1991). "Membrane damage due to lipid oxidation." Am J Clin Nutr **53**(1 Suppl): 201S-205S.

Packer, L., M. Valenza, et al. (1991). "Free radical scavenging is involved in the protective effect of L-propionyl-carnitine against ischemia-reperfusion injury of the heart." Arch Biochem Biophys **288**(2): 533-7.

Panasenko, O. M., T. V. Vol'nova, et al. (1991). "Free-radical generation by monocytes and neutrophils: a possible cause of plasma lipoprotein modification." Biomed Sci **2**(6): 581-9.

Pryor, W. A. and S. S. Godber (1991). "Noninvasive measures of oxidative stress status in humans." Free Radic Biol Med **10**(3-4): 177-84.

Pryor, W. A. and S. S. Godber (1991). "Oxidative stress status: an introduction." Free Radic Biol Med **10**(3-4): 173.

Reizenstein, P. (1991). "Iron, free radicals and cancer." Med Oncol Tumor Pharmacother **8**(4): 229-33.

Ruuge, E. K., A. N. Ledenev, et al. (1991). "Free radical metabolites in myocardium during ischemia and reperfusion." Am J Physiol **261**(4 Suppl): 81-6.

Santamaria, L. and A. Bianchi-Santamaria (1991). "Free radicals as carcinogens and their quenchers as anticarcinogens." Med Oncol Tumor Pharmacother **8**(3): 121-40.

Sies, H. (1991). "Oxidative stress: from basic research to clinical application." Am J Med **91**(3C): 31S-38S.

Taylor, C. G. and T. M. Bray (1991). "Effect of hyperoxia on oxygen free radical defense enzymes in the lung of zinc-deficient rats." J Nutr **121**(4): 460-6.

Troll, W. (1991). "Prevention of cancer by agents that suppress oxygen radical formation." Free Radic Res Commun **13**(1): 751-7.

Weitz, Z. W., A. J. Birnbaum, et al. (1991). "High breath pentane concentrations during acute myocardial infarction [see comments]." Lancet **337**(8747): 933-5.

Babiy, A. V., J. M. Gebicki, et al. (1990). "Vitamin E content and low density lipoprotein oxidizability induced by free radicals." Atherosclerosis **81**(3): 175-82.

Fruits and Vegetables

Chug-Ahuja, J. K., J. M. Holden, et al. (1993). "The development and application of a carotenoid database for fruits, vegetables, and selected multicomponent foods." J Am Diet Assoc **93**(3): 318-23.

Chung, F. L., M. A. Morse, et al. (1993). "Inhibition of tobacco-specific nitrosamine-induced lung tumorigenesis by compounds derived from cruciferous vegetables and green tea." Ann N Y Acad Sci **686**(1): 186-201.

Levi, F., S. Franceschi, et al. (1993). "Dietary factors and the risk of endometrial cancer." Cancer **71**(11): 3575-81.

Mangels, A. R., J. M. Holden, et al. (1993). "Carotenoid content of fruits and vegetables: an evaluation of analytic data." J Am Diet Assoc **93**(3): 284-96.

Singh, R. B., S. S. Rastogi, et al. (1993). "Can guava fruit intake decrease blood pressure and blood lipids?" J Hum Hypertens **7**(1): 33-8.

Block, G., B. Patterson, et al. (1992). "Fruit, vegetables, and cancer prevention: a review of the epidemiological evidence." Nutr Cancer **18**(1): 1-29.

Chow, W. H., L. M. Schuman, et al. (1992). "A cohort study of tobacco use, diet, occupation, and lung cancer mortality." Cancer Causes Control **3**(3): 247-54.

Correa, P. (1992). "Diet modification and gastric cancer prevention." Monogr Natl Cancer Inst **12**: 75-8.

Shibata, A., A. Paganini-Hill, et al. (1992). "Intake of vegetables, fruits, beta-carotene, vitamin C and vitamin supplements and cancer incidence among the elderly: a prospective study." Br J Cancer **66**(4): 673-9.

Singh, R. B., S. Ghosh, et al. (1992). "Effects on serum lipids of adding fruits and vegetables to prudent diet in the Indian Experiment of Infarct Survival (IEIS)." Cardiology **80**(3-4): 283-93.

Singh, R. B., S. S. Rastogi, et al. (1992). "Effect of fat-modified and fruit- and vegetable-enriched diets on blood lipids in the Indian Diet Heart Study." Am J Cardiol **70**(9): 869-74.

Singh, R. B., S. S. Rastogi, et al. (1992). "Effects of guava intake on serum total and high-density lipoprotein cholesterol levels and on systemic blood pressure." Am J Cardiol **70**(15): 1287-91.

Thun, M. J., E. E. Calle, et al. (1992). "Risk factors for fatal colon cancer in a large prospective study." J Natl Cancer Inst **84**(19): 1491-500.

Negri, E., C. La Vecchia, et al. (1991). "Vegetable and fruit consumption and cancer risk." Int J Cancer **48**(3): 350-4.

Steinmetz, K. A. and J. D. Potter (1991). "Vegetables, fruit, and cancer. I. Epidemiology." Cancer Causes Control **2**(5): 325-57.

Ziegler, R. G. (1991). "Vegetables, fruits, and carotenoids and the risk of cancer." Am J Clin Nutr **53**(1 Suppl): 251S-259S.

Garlic

Dorant, E., P. A. van den Brandt, et al. (1993). "Garlic and its significance for the prevention of cancer in humans: a critical view." Br J Cancer **67**(3): 424-9.

Guo, N. L., D. P. Lu, et al. (1993). "Demonstration of the anti-viral activity of garlic extract against human cytomegalovirus in vitro." Chin Med J **106**(2): 93-6.

Isensee, H., B. Rietz, et al. (1993). "Cardioprotective actions of garlic (Allium sativum)." Arzneimittelforschung **43**(2): 94-8.

Jain, A. K., R. Vargas, et al. (1993). "Can garlic reduce levels of serum lipids? A controlled clinical study." Am J Med **94**(6): 632-5.

Kiesewetter, H., F. Jung, et al. (1993). "Effects of garlic coated tablets in peripheral arterial occlusive disease." Clin Investig **71**(5): 383-6.

Legnani, C., M. Frascaro, et al. (1993). "Effects of a dried garlic preparation on fibrinolysis and platelet aggregation in healthy subjects." Arzneimittelforschung **43**(2): 119-22.

Phelps, S. and W. S. Harris (1993). "Garlic supplementation and lipoprotein oxidation susceptibility." Lipids **28**(5): 475-7.

Randerson, K. (1993). "Cardiology update. Garlic and the healthy heart." Nurs Stand **7**(30): 51.

Rietz, B., H. Isensee, et al. (1993). "Cardioprotective actions of wild garlic (allium ursinum) in ischemia and reperfusion." Mol Cell Biochem **119**(1-2): 143-50.

Apitz-Castro, R., J. J. Badimon, et al. (1992). "Effect of ajoene, the major antiplatelet compound from garlic, on platelet thrombus formation." Thromb Res **68**(2): 145-55.

Chen, J. (1992). "The antimutagenic and anticarcinogenic effects of tea, garlic and other natural foods in China: a review." Biomed Environ Sci **5**(1): 1-17.

Holzgartner, H., U. Schmidt, et al. (1992). "Comparison of the efficacy and tolerance of a garlic preparation vs. bezafibrate." Arzneimittelforschung **42**(12): 1473-7.

Ip, C., D. J. Lisk, et al. (1992). "Mammary cancer prevention by regular garlic and selenium-enriched garlic." Nutr Cancer **17**(3): 279-86.

Lawson, L. D., D. K. Ransom, et al. (1992). "Inhibition of whole blood platelet-aggregation by compounds in garlic clove extracts and commercial garlic products." Thromb Res **65**(2): 141-56.

Rotzsch, W., V. Richter, et al. (1992). "[Postprandial lipemia under treatment with Allium sativum. Controlled double-blind study of subjects with reduced HDL2-cholesterol]." Arzneimittelforschung **42**(10): 1223-7.

Sendl, A., G. Elbl, et al. (1992). "Comparative pharmacological investigations of Allium ursinum and Allium sativum." Planta Med **58**(1): 1-7.

Sendl, A., M. Schliack, et al. (1992). "Inhibition of cholesterol synthesis in vitro by extracts and isolated compounds prepared from garlic and wild garlic." Atherosclerosis **94**(1): 79-85.

Sheela, C. G. and K. T. Augusti (1992). "Antidiabetic effects of S-allyl cysteine sulphoxide isolated from garlic Allium sativum Linn." Indian J Exp Biol **30**(6): 523-6.

Weber, N. D., D. O. Andersen, et al. (1992). "In vitro virucidal effects of Allium sativum (garlic) extract and compounds." Planta Med **58**(5): 417-23.

Gadkari, J. V. and V. D. Joshi (1991). "Effect of ingestion of raw garlic on serum cholesterol level, clotting time and fibrinolytic activity in normal subjects." J Postgrad Med **37**(3): 128-31.

Gebhardt, R. (1991). "Inhibition of cholesterol biosynthesis by a water-soluble garlic extract in primary cultures of rat hepatocytes." Arzneimittelforschung **41**(8): 800-4.

Kiesewetter, H., F. Jung, et al. (1991). "Effect of garlic on thrombocyte aggregation, microcirculation, and other risk factors." Int J Clin Pharmacol Ther Toxicol **29**(4): 151-5.

Kourounakis, P. N. and E. A. Rekka (1991). "Effect on active oxygen species of alliin and Allium sativum (garlic) powder." Res Commun Chem Pathol Pharmacol **74**(2): 249-52.

Lata, S., K. K. Saxena, et al. (1991). "Beneficial effects of Allium sativum, Allium cepa and Commiphora mukul on experimental hyperlipidemia and atherosclerosis—a comparative evaluation." J Postgrad Med **37**(3): 132-5.

Lau, B. H., T. Yamasaki, et al. (1991). "Garlic compounds modulate macrophage and T-lymphocyte functions." Mol Biother **3**(2): 103-7.

Mansell, P. and J. P. Reckless (1991). "Garlic [editorial] [see comments]." Bmj **303**(6799): 379-80.

Mirhadi, S. A., S. Singh, et al. (1991). "Effect of garlic supplementation to cholesterol-rich diet on development of atherosclerosis in rabbits." Indian J Exp Biol **29**(2): 162-8.

Pantoja, C. V., L. C. Chiang, et al. (1991). "Diuretic, natriuretic and hypotensive effects produced by Allium sativum (garlic) in anaesthetized dogs." J Ethnopharmacol **31**(3): 325-31.

HDL

(1993). "NIH Consensus conference. Triglyceride, high-density lipoprotein, and coronary heart disease. NIH Consensus Development Panel on Triglyceride, High-Density Lipoprotein, and Coronary Heart Disease." Jama **269**(4): 505-10.

Eden, S., O. Wiklund, et al. (1993). "Growth hormone treatment of growth hormone-deficient adults results in a marked increase in Lp(a) and HDL cholesterol concentrations." Arterioscler Thromb **13**(2): 296-301.

French, J. K., J. M. Elliott, et al. (1993). "Association of angiographically detected coronary artery disease with low levels of high-density lipoprotein cholesterol and systemic hypertension." Am J Cardiol **71**(7): 505-10.

Klimov, A. N., V. S. Gurevich, et al. (1993). "Antioxidative activity of high density lipoproteins in vivo." Atherosclerosis **100**(1): 13-8.

Kreisberg, R. A. (1993). "Low high-density lipoprotein cholesterol: what does it mean, what can we do about it, and what should we do about it? [editorial; comment]." Am J Med **94**(1): 1-6.

Maislos, M., N. Khamaysi, et al. (1993). "Marked increase in plasma high-density-lipoprotein cholesterol after prolonged fasting during Ramadan." Am J Clin Nutr **57**(5): 640-2.

Rubins, H. B., S. J. Robins, et al. (1993). "Rationale and design of the Department of Veterans Affairs High-Density Lipoprotein Cholesterol Intervention Trial (HIT) for secondary prevention of coronary artery disease in men with low high-density lipoprotein cholesterol and desirable low-density lipoprotein cholesterol." Am J Cardiol **71**(1): 45-52.

Taylor, P. A. and A. Ward (1993). "Women, high-density lipoprotein cholesterol, and exercise." Arch Intern Med **153**(10): 1178-84.

Taylor, P. A. and A. Ward (1993). "Women, High-density lipoprotein cholesterol, and exercise." Arch Intern Med **153**: 1178-1184.

(1992). "Triglyceride, high density lipoprotein, and coronary heart disease." Consens Statement **10**(2): 1-28.

Assmann, G. and H. Schulte (1992). "Relation of high-density lipoprotein cholesterol and triglycerides to incidence of atherosclerotic coronary artery disease (the PROCAM experience). Prospective Cardiovascular Munster study." Am J Cardiol **70**(7): 733-7.

Badimon, J. J., V. Fuster, et al. (1992). "Role of high density lipoproteins in the regression of atherosclerosis." Circulation **86**(6 Suppl): III86-94.

Bainton, D., N. E. Miller, et al. (1992). "Plasma triglyceride and high density lipoprotein cholesterol as predictors of ischaemic heart disease in British men. The Caerphilly and Speedwell Collaborative Heart Disease Studies." Br Heart J **68**(1): 60-6.

Bowry, V. W., K. K. Stanley, et al. (1992). "High density lipoprotein is the major carrier of lipid hydroperoxides in human blood plasma from fasting donors." Proc Natl Acad Sci U S A **89**(21): 10316-20.

Bradamante, S., L. Barenghi, et al. (1992). "Free radicals promote modifications in plasma high-density lipoprotein: nuclear magnetic resonance analysis." Free Radic Biol Med **12**(3): 193-203.

Buring, J. E., G. T. O'Connor, et al. (1992). "Decreased HDL2 and HDL3 cholesterol, Apo A-I and Apo A-II, and increased risk of myocardial infarction." Circulation **85**(1): 22-9.

Cohen, J. C. and S. M. Grundy (1992). "Normal postprandial lipemia in men with low plasma HDL concentrations." Arterioscler Thromb **12**(8): 972-5.

Drexel, H., F. W. Amann, et al. (1992). "Relation of the level of high-density lipoprotein subfractions to the presence and extent of coronary artery disease." Am J Cardiol **70**(4): 436-40.

Genest, J., Jr., S. S. Martin-Munley, et al. (1992). "Familial lipoprotein disorders in patients with premature coronary artery disease." Circulation **85**(6): 2025-33.

Hargreaves, A. D., R. L. Logan, et al. (1992). "Glucose tolerance, plasma insulin, HDL cholesterol and obesity: 12-year follow-up and development of coronary heart disease in Edinburgh men." Atherosclerosis **94**(1): 61-9.

Jacques, P. F. (1992). "Effects of vitamin C on high-density lipoprotein cholesterol and blood pressure." J Am Coll Nutr **11**(2): 139-44.

Johansson, J., G. Walldius, et al. (1992). "Close correlation between high-density lipoprotein and triglycerides in normotriglyceridaemia." J Intern Med **232**(1): 43-51.

Kannel, W. B. (1992). "Low high-density lipoprotein cholesterol and what to do about it [editorial]." Am J Cardiol **70**(7): 810-4.

Kannel, W. B. and P. W. Wilson (1992). "Efficacy of lipid profiles in prediction of coronary disease." Am Heart J **124**(3): 768-74.

Kokkinos, P., J. Holland, et al. (1992). "Exercise threshold for favorable HDL changes in middle-aged men. (abstract)." J Am Coll Cardiol **19**(3): 346A #825-6.

Laws, A. and G. M. Reaven (1992). "Evidence for an independent relationship between insulin resistance and fasting plasma HDL-cholesterol, triglyceride and insulin concentrations." J Intern Med **231**(1): 25-30.

Miller, M., A. Seidler, et al. (1992). "Long-term predictors of subsequent cardiovascular events with coronary artery disease and 'desirable' levels of plasma total cholesterol [see comments]." Circulation **86**(4): 1165-70.

Miyazaki, A., A. T. Rahim, et al. (1992). "High density lipoprotein mediates selective reduction in cholesteryl esters from macrophage foam cells." Biochim Biophys Acta **1126**(1): 73-80.

Rotzsch, W., V. Richter, et al. (1992). "[Postprandial lipemia under treatment with Allium sativum. Controlled double-blind study of subjects with reduced HDL2-cholesterol]." Arzneimittelforschung **42**(10): 1223-7.

Rubins, H. B., G. Schectman, et al. (1992). "Distribution of lipid phenotypes in community-living men with coronary heart disease. High prevalence of isolated low levels of high-density lipoprotein cholesterol." Arch Intern Med **152**(12): 2412-6.

Sacks, F. M. (1992). "Desirable serum total cholesterol with low HDL cholesterol levels. An undesirable situation in coronary heart disease [editorial; comment]." Circulation **86**(4): 1341-4.

Schmidt, K., P. Klatt, et al. (1992). "High-density lipoprotein antagonizes the inhibitory effects of oxidized low-density lipoprotein and lysolecithin on soluble guanylyl cyclase." Biochem Biophys Res Commun **182**(1): 302-8.

Shah, P. K. and J. Amin (1992). "Low high density lipoprotein level is associated with increased restenosis rate after coronary angioplasty [see comments]." Circulation **85**(4): 1279-85.

Simons, L. A., J. Simons, et al. (1992). "Dubbo Study of the elderly: hypertension and lipid levels." Atherosclerosis **92**(1): 59-65.

Squires, R. W., T. G. Allison, et al. (1992). "Low-dose, time-release nicotinic acid: effects in selected patients with low concentrations of high-density lipoprotein cholesterol." Mayo Clin Proc **67**(9): 855-60.

Stensvold, I., P. Urdal, et al. (1992). "High-density lipoprotein cholesterol and coronary, cardiovascular and all cause mortality among middle-aged Norwegian men and women." Eur Heart J **13**(9): 1155-63.

Suh, I., B. J. Shaten, et al. (1992). "Alcohol use and mortality from coronary heart disease: the role of high-density lipoprotein cholesterol. The Multiple Risk Factor Intervention Trial Research Group." Ann Intern Med **116**(11): 881-7.

Weitzman, J. B. and A. O. Vladutiu (1992). "Very high values of serum high-density lipoprotein cholesterol." Arch Pathol Lab Med **116**(8): 831-6.

Arntzenius, A. C. (1991). "Regression of atherosclerosis. Benefit can be expected from low LDL-C and high HDL-C levels [editorial]." Acta Cardiol **46**(4): 431-8.

Barth, J. D. and A. C. Arntzenius (1991). "Progression and regression of atherosclerosis, what roles for LDL-cholesterol and HDL-cholesterol: a perspective." Eur Heart J **12**(8): 952-7.

Roeback, J. J., K. M. Hla, et al. (1991). "Effects of chromium supplementation on serum high-density lipoprotein cholesterol levels in men taking beta-blockers. A randomized, controlled trial [see comments]." Ann Intern Med **115**(12): 917-24.

Heart Attack/Myocardial Infarction

Axford-Gately, R. A. and G. J. Wilson (1993). "Myocardial infarct size reduction by single high dose or repeated low dose vitamin E supplementation in rabbits [see comments]." Can J Cardiol **9**(1): 94-8.

Becker, R. C. (1993). "Antiplatelet therapy in coronary heart disease. Emerging strategies for the treatment and prevention of acute myocardial infarction." Arch Pathol Lab Med **117**(1): 89-96.

Davies, S. W., K. Ranjadayalan, et al. (1993). "Free radical activity and left ventricular function after thrombolysis for acute infarction." Br Heart J **69**(2): 114-20.

Yusuf, S., K. Teo, et al. (1993). "Intravenous magnesium in acute myocardial infarction. An effective, safe, simple and inexpensive intervention. (Editorial)." Circulation **87**: 2043-2046.

(1992). "Morning peak in the incidence of myocardial infarction: experience in the ISIS-2 trial. ISIS-2 (Second International Study of Infarct Survival) Collaborative Group." Eur Heart J **13**(5): 594-8.

Ambrose, J. A. (1992). "Plaque disruption and the acute coronary syndromes of unstable angina and myocardial infarction: if the substrate is similar, why is the clinical presentation different? [editorial]." J Am Coll Cardiol **19**(7): 1653-8.

Cohen, M. C. and J. E. Muller (1992). "Onset of acute myocardial infarction—circadian variation and triggers." Cardiovasc Res **26**(9): 831-8.

Juul-Moller, S., N. Edvardsson, et al. (1992). "Double-blind trial of aspirin in primary prevention of myocardial infarction in patients with stable chronic angina pectoris. The Swedish Angina Pectoris Aspirin Trial (SAPAT) Group." Lancet **340**(8833): 1421-5.

Mueller, H. S., L. S. Cohen, et al. (1992). "Predictors of early morbidity and mortality after thrombolytic therapy of acute myocardial infarction. Analyses of patient subgroups in the Thrombolysis in Myocardial Infarction (TIMI) trial, phase II." Circulation **85**(4): 1254-64.

Shechter, M., E. Kaplinsky, et al. (1992). "The rationale of magnesium supplementation in acute myocardial infarction. A review of the literature." Arch Intern Med **152**(11): 2189-96.

Tan, I. K., K. S. Chua, et al. (1992). "Serum magnesium, copper, and zinc concentrations in acute myocardial infarction." J Clin Lab Anal **6**(5): 324-8.

Tofler, G. H., J. E. Muller, et al. (1992). "Modifiers of timing and possible triggers of acute myocardial infarction in the Thrombolysis in Myocardial Infarction Phase II (TIMI II) Study Group." J Am Coll Cardiol **20**(5): 1049-55.

Woods, K. L., S. Fletcher, et al. (1992). "Modification of the circadian rhythm of onset of acute myocardial infarction by long-term antianginal treatment." Br Heart J **68**(5): 458-61.

Woods, K. L., S. Fletcher, et al. (1992). "Intravenous magnesium sulphate in suspected acute myocardial infarction: results of the second Leicester Intravenous Magnesium Intervention Trial (LIMIT-2)." Lancet **339**(8809): 1553-8.

Axford-Gatley, R. A. and G. J. Wilson (1991). "Reduction of experimental myocardial infarct size by oral administration of alpha tocopherol." Cardiovasc Res **25**(2): 89-92.

Horowitz, J. D. (1991). "Thiol-containing agents in the management of unstable angina pectoris and acute myocardial infarction." Am J Med **91**(3C): 113S-117S.

Nattel, S., N. Turmel, et al. (1991). "Actions of intravenous magnesium on ventricular arrhythmias caused by acute myocardial infarction." J Pharmacol Exp Ther **259**(2): 939-46.

Ridker, P. M. and C. H. Hennekens (1991). "Hemostatic risk factors for coronary heart disease [editorial; comment]." Circulation **83**(3): 1098-100.

Ridker, P. M., J. E. Manson, et al. (1991). "Clinical characteristics of nonfatal myocardial infarction among individuals on prophylactic low-dose aspirin therapy." Circulation **84**(2): 708-11.

Ridker, P. M., J. E. Manson, et al. (1991). "The effect of chronic platelet inhibition with low-dose aspirin on atherosclerotic progression and acute thrombosis: clinical evidence from the Physicians' Health Study." Am Heart J **122**(6): 1588-92.

Ridker, P. M., J. E. Manson, et al. (1991). "Low-dose aspirin therapy for chronic stable angina. A randomized, placebo-controlled clinical trial." Ann Intern Med **114**(10): 835-9.

Ridker, P. M., S. N. Willich, et al. (1991). "Aspirin, platelet aggregation, and the circadian variation of acute thrombotic events." Chronobiol Int **8**(5): 327-35.

Weitz, Z. W., A. J. Birnbaum, et al. (1991). "High breath pentane concentrations during acute myocardial infarction [see comments]." Lancet **337**(8747): 933-5.

Woods, K. L. (1991). "Possible pharmacological actions of magnesium in acute myocardial infarction." Br J Clin Pharmacol **32**(1): 3-10.

Ridker, P. M., J. E. Manson, et al. (1990). "Circadian variation of acute myocardial infarction and the effect of low-dose aspirin in a randomized trial of physicians." Circulation **82**(3): 897-902.

Davies, M. J. and A. C. Thomas (1985). "Plaque fissuring—the cause of acute myocardial infarction, sudden ischaemic death, and crescendo angina." Br Heart J **53**(4): 363-73.

Herbs

Dragsted, L. O., M. Strube, et al. (1993). "Cancer-protective factors in fruits and vegetables: biochemical and biological background." Pharmacol Toxicol **72**(1): 116-35.

Reddy, A. C. and B. R. Lokesh (1992). "Studies on spice principles as antioxidants in the inhibition of lipid peroxidation of rat liver microsomes." Mol Cell Biochem **111**(1-2): 117-24.

Sharma, H. M., A. N. Hanna, et al. (1992). "Inhibition of human low-density lipoprotein oxidation in vitro by Maharishi Ayur-Veda herbal mixtures." Pharmacol Biochem Behav **43**(4): 1175-82.

Lata, S., K. K. Saxena, et al. (1991). "Beneficial effects of Allium sativum, Allium cepa and Commiphora mukul on experimental hyperlipidemia and atherosclerosis—a comparative evaluation." J Postgrad Med **37**(3): 132-5.

Sambaiah, K. and K. Srinivasan (1991). "Effect of cumin, cinnamon, ginger, mustard and tamarind in induced hypercholesterolemic rats (no effect)." Nahrung **35**(1): 47-51.

Sauvaire, Y., G. Ribes, et al. (1991). "Implication of steroid saponins and sapogenins in the hypocholesterolemic effect of fenugreek." Lipids **26**(3): 191-7.

Heredity/Genetic/Familial

Grech, E. D., D. R. Ramsdale, et al. (1992). "Family history as an independent risk factor of coronary artery disease." Eur Heart J **13**(10): 1311-5.

Roncaglioni, M. C., L. Santoro, et al. (1992). "Role of family history in patients with myocardial infarction. An Italian case-control study. GISSI-EFRIM Investigators." Circulation **85**(6): 2065-72.

Colditz, G. A., E. B. Rimm, et al. (1991). "A prospective study of parental history of myocardial infarction and coronary artery disease in men [see comments]." Am J Cardiol **67**(11): 933-8.

High Blood Pressure

(1993). "The fifth report of the Joint National Committee on Detection, Evaluation, and Treatment of High Blood Pressure (JNC V) [see comments]." Arch Intern Med **153**(2): 154-83.

(1993). "National High Blood Pressure Education Program Working Group report on primary prevention of hypertension [see comments]." Arch Intern Med **153**(2): 186-208.

Chin, J. P., A. P. Gust, et al. (1993). "Marine oils dose-dependently inhibit vasoconstriction of forearm resistance vessels in humans." Hypertension **21**(1): 22-8.

Fetkovska, N., Z. Jakubovska, et al. (1993). "Treatment of hypertension with calcium antagonists and aspirin. Effects on 24-h platelet activity." Am J Hypertens **6**(3 Pt 2): 98S-101S.

French, J. K., J. M. Elliott, et al. (1993). "Association of angiographically detected coronary artery disease with low levels of high-density lipoprotein cholesterol and systemic hypertension." Am J Cardiol **71**(7): 505-10.

Galloe, A. M., N. Graudal, et al. (1993). "Effect of oral calcium supplementation on blood pressure in patients with previously untreated hypertension: a randomised, double-blind, placebo-controlled, crossover study." J Hum Hypertens **7**(1): 43-5.

Gillman, M. W. and R. C. Ellison (1993). "Childhood prevention of essential hypertension." Pediatr Clin North Am **40**(1): 179-94.

Hatton, D. C., K. E. Scrogin, et al. (1993). "Dietary calcium modulates blood pressure through alpha 1-adrenergic receptors." Am J Physiol **264**(2 Pt 2): F234-8.

Hebert, P. R., M. Moser, et al. (1993). "Recent evidence on drug therapy of mild to moderate hypertension and decreased risk of coronary heart disease." Arch Intern Med **153**(5): 578-81.

Jiang, X., S. R. Srinivasan, et al. (1993). "Association of fasting insulin with blood pressure in young individuals. The Bogalusa Heart Study [see comments]." Arch Intern Med **153**(3): 323-8.

Kaplan, N. M. (1993). "The promises and perils of treating the elderly hypertensive." Am J Med Sci **305**(3): 183-97.

Kochar, M. S. (1993). "Hypertension in obese patients." Postgrad Med **93**(4): 193-5.

Lind, L., H. Lithell, et al. (1993). "Calcium metabolism and sodium sensitivity in hypertensive subjects." J Hum Hypertens **7**(1): 53-7.

Lofgren, R. P., T. J. Wilt, et al. (1993). "The effect of fish oil supplements on blood pressure." Am J Public Health **83**(2): 267-9.

Moran, J. P., L. Cohen, et al. (1993). "Plasma ascorbic acid concentrations relate inversely to blood pressure in human subjects." Am J Clin Nutr **57**(2): 213-7.

Morris, M. C., J. O. Taylor, et al. (1993). "The effect of fish oil on blood pressure in mild hypertensive subjects: a randomized crossover trial." Am J Clin Nutr **57**(1): 59-64.

Sabate, J., G. E. Fraser, et al. (1993). "Effects of walnuts on serum lipid levels and blood pressure in normal men." N Engl J Med **328**(9): 603-7.

Singh, R. B., S. S. Rastogi, et al. (1993). "Can guava fruit intake decrease blood pressure and blood lipids?" J Hum Hypertens **7**(1): 33-8.

Stamler, J., R. Stamler, et al. (1993). "Blood pressure, systolic and diastolic, and cardiovascular risks. US population data." Arch Intern Med **153**(5): 598-615.

Sutton-Tyrrell, K., H. G. Alcorn, et al. (1993). "Predictors of carotid stenosis in older adults with and without isolated systolic hypertension." Stroke **24**(3): 355-61.

Ueshima, H., K. Mikawa, et al. (1993). "Effect of reduced alcohol consumption on blood pressure in untreated hypertensive men." Hypertension **21**(2): 248-52.

Widman, L., P. O. Wester, et al. (1993). "The dose-dependent reduction in blood pressure through administration of magnesium. A double blind placebo controlled cross-over study." Am J Hypertens **6**(1): 41-5.

Wylie-Rosett, J., S. Wassertheil-Smoller, et al. (1993). "Trial of antihypertensive intervention and management: greater efficacy with weight reduction than with a sodium-potassium intervention." J Am Diet Assoc **93**(4): 408-15.

(1992). "Calcium supplementation prevents hypertensive disorders of pregnancy." Nutr Rev **50**(8): 233-6.

(1992). "The effects of nonpharmacologic interventions on blood pressure of persons with high normal levels. Results of the Trials of Hypertension Prevention, Phase I [published erratum appears in JAMA 1992 May 6; 267(17):2330] [see comments]." Jama **267**(9): 1213-20.

Applegate, W. B., S. T. Miller, et al. (1992). "Nonpharmacologic intervention to reduce blood pressure in older patients with mild hypertension." Arch Intern Med **152**(6): 1162-6.

Applegate, W. B. and G. H. Rutan (1992). "Advances in management of hypertension in older persons." J Am Geriatr Soc **40**(11): 1164-74.

Arauz-Pacheco, C. and P. Raskin (1992). "Management of hypertension in diabetes." Endocrinol Metab Clin North Am **21**(2): 371-94.

Arroll, B. and R. Beaglehole (1992). "Does physical activity lower blood pressure: a critical review of the clinical trials." J Clin Epidemiol **45**(5): 439-47.

Ascherio, A., E. B. Rimm, et al. (1992). "A prospective study of nutritional factors and hypertension among US men [see comments]." Circulation **86**(5): 1475-84.

Bairati, I., L. Roy, et al. (1992). "Effects of a fish oil supplement on blood pressure and serum lipids in patients treated for coronary artery disease." Can J Cardiol **8**(1): 41-6.

Beilin, L. J. and I. B. Puddey (1992). "Alcohol and hypertension." Clin Exp Hypertens [a] **14**(1-2): 119-38.

Benotti, P. N., B. Bistrain, et al. (1992). "Heart disease and hypertension in severe obesity: the benefits of weight reduction." Am J Clin Nutr **55**(2 Suppl): 586S-590S.

Blaufox, M. D., H. B. Lee, et al. (1992). "Renin predicts diastolic blood pressure response to nonpharmacologic and pharmacologic therapy." Jama **267**(9): 1221-5.

Cappuccio, F. P. (1992). "The epidemiology of diet and blood pressure [editorial; comment]." Circulation **86**(5): 1651-3.

Cobiac, L., P. J. Nestel, et al. (1992). "A low-sodium diet supplemented with fish oil lowers blood pressure in the elderly." J Hypertens **10**(1): 87-92.

Davis, B. R., A. Oberman, et al. (1992). "Effect of antihypertensive therapy on weight loss. The Trial of Antihypertensive Interventions and Management Research Group." Hypertension **19**(4): 393-9.

Digiesi, V., F. Cantini, et al. (1992). "Mechanisum of action of coenzyme Q10 in essential hypertension." Curr Ther Res **51**(5): 668-672.

Durlach, J., V. Durlach, et al. (1992). "Magnesium and blood pressure. II. Clinical studies." Magnes Res **5**(2): 147-53.

Feldman, E. B., S. Gold, et al. (1992). "Ascorbic acid supplements and blood pressure. A four-week pilot study." Ann N Y Acad Sci **669**(1): 342-4.

Ferrara, L. A., R. Iannuzzi, et al. (1992). "Long-term magnesium supplementation in essential hypertension." Cardiology **81**(1): 25-33.

Frohlich, E. D., C. Apstein, et al. (1992). "The heart in hypertension." N Engl J Med **327**(14): 998-1008.

Gillman, M. W., S. A. Oliveria, et al. (1992). "Inverse association of dietary calcium with systolic blood pressure in young children." Jama **267**(17): 2340-3.

Grassi, G., G. Seravalle, et al. (1992). "Physical exercise in essential hypertension." Chest **101**(5 Suppl): 312S-314S.

Gupta, R., K. D. Gupta, et al. (1992). "Influence of mild to moderate treated hypertension on 9-11 year mortality in patients with pre-existing coronary heart disease." J Hum Hypertens **6**(4): 313-6.

Haennel, R. G., G. D. Snydmiller, et al. (1992). "Changes in blood pressure and cardiac output during maximal isokinetic exercise." Arch Phys Med Rehabil **73**(2): 150-5.

Hamet, P., M. Daignault-Gelinas, et al. (1992). "Epidemiological evidence of an interaction between calcium and sodium intake impacting on blood pressure. A Montreal study." Am J Hypertens **5**(6 Pt 1): 378-85.

Hebert, P. R., J. E. Manson, et al. (1992). "Pharmacologic therapy of mild to moderate hypertension: possible generalizability to diabetics." J Am Soc Nephrol **3**(4 Suppl): S135-9.

Hishikawa, K., T. Nakaki, et al. (1992). "L-arginine as an antihypertensive agent." J Cardiovasc Pharmacol **20**(1): S196-7.

Jacques, P. F. (1992). "A cross-sectional study of vitamin C intake and blood pressure in the elderly." Int J Vitam Nutr Res **62**(3): 252-5.

Jacques, P. F. (1992). "Effects of vitamin C on high-density lipoprotein cholesterol and blood pressure." J Am Coll Nutr **11**(2): 139-44.

Jacques, P. F. (1992). "Relationship of vitamin C status to cholesterol and blood pressure." Ann N Y Acad Sci **669**(1): 205-13.

Kaplan, N. M. (1992). "The appropriate goals of antihypertensive therapy: neither too much nor too little." Ann Intern Med **116**(8): 686-90.

Kaplan, N. M. (1992). "Effects of antihypertensive therapy on insulin resistance." Hypertension **19**(1 Suppl): I116-8.

Kaplan, N. M. (1992). "Management of hypertension." Dis Mon **38**(11): 769-838.

Kaplan, N. M. (1992). "A new era in hypertension therapy. Protecting patients from premature cardiovascular disease." Postgrad Med **91**(8): 225-6.

Keli, S., B. Bloemberg, et al. (1992). "Predictive value of repeated systolic blood pressure measurements for stroke risk. The Zutphen Study." Stroke **23**(3): 347-51.

Knight, K. B. and R. E. Keith (1992). "Calcium supplementation on normotensive and hypertensive pregnant women." Am J Clin Nutr **55**(4): 891-5.

Kochar, M. S. (1992). "Hypertension in elderly patients. The special concerns in this growing population." Postgrad Med **91**(4): 393-400.

Krakoff, L. R. (1992). "What is the best therapy? [editorial]." Am J Hypertens **5**(9): 670.

Landin, K., G. Holm, et al. (1992). "Guar gum improves insulin sensitivity, blood lipids, blood pressure, and fibrinolysis in healthy men." Am J Clin Nutr **56**(6): 1061-5.

Laragh, J. H. (1992). "Lewis K. Dahl Memorial Lecture. The renin system and four lines fo hypertension research. Nephron heterogeneity, the calcium connection, the prorenin vasodilator limb, and plasma renin and heart attack." Hypertension **20**(3): 267-79.

Lee, L. and R. C. Webb (1992). "Endothelium-dependent relaxation and L-arginine metabolism in genetic hypertension." Hypertension **19**(5): 435-41.

Levenson, J., M. Del Pino, et al. (1992). "Hypercholesterolaemia alters arterial and blood factors related to atherosclerosis in hypertension." Atherosclerosis **95**(2-3): 171-9.

Lind, L., H. Lithell, et al. (1992). "Metabolic cardiovascular risk factors and sodium sensitivity in hypertensive subjects." Am J Hypertens **5**(8): 502-5.

Lund-Johansen, P. (1992). "Treatment of hypertension in the elderly—what have we learned from the recent trials?" Cardiovasc Drugs Ther **6**(6): 571-3.

Maheswaran, R., M. Beevers, et al. (1992). "Effectiveness of advice to reduce alcohol consumption in hypertensive patients." Hypertension **19**(1): 79-84.

McCloskey, L. W., B. M. Psaty, et al. (1992). "Level of blood pressure and risk of myocardial infarction among treated hypertensive patients [see comments]." Arch Intern Med **152**(3): 513-20.

Menard, J., M. Day, et al. (1992). "Some lessons from systolic hypertension in the elderly program (SHEP)." Am J Hypertens **5**(5 Pt 1): 325-30.

Mervaala, E. M., J. J. Himberg, et al. (1992). "Beneficial effects of a potassium- and magnesium-enriched salt alternative." Hypertension **19**(6 Pt 1): 535-40.

Morgenstern, N. and R. L. Byyny (1992). "Epidemiology of hypertension in the elderly." Drugs Aging **2**(3): 222-42.

Morris, C. D. and D. A. McCarron (1992). "Effect of calcium supplementation in an older population with mildly increased blood pressure." Am J Hypertens **5**(4 Pt 1): 230-7.

Mutanen, M., P. Kleemola, et al. (1992). "Lack of effect on blood pressure by polyunsaturated and monounsaturated fat diets." Eur J Clin Nutr **46**(1): 1-6.

Petrovitch, H., T. M. Vogt, et al. (1992). "Isolated systolic hypertension: lowering the risk of stroke in older patients. SHEP Cooperative Research Group." Geriatrics **47**(3): 30-2.

Pickering, T. G. (1992). "Predicting the response to nonpharmacologic treatment in mild hypertension [editorial; comment]." Jama **267**(9): 1256-7.

Preuss, H. G., J. J. Knapka, et al. (1992). "High sucrose diets increase blood pressure of both salt-sensitive and salt-resistant rats." Am J Hypertens **5**(9): 585-91.

Psaty, B. M., C. D. Furberg, et al. (1992). "Isolated systolic hypertension and subclinical cardiovascular disease in the elderly. Initial findings from the Cardiovascular Health Study." Jama **268**(10): 1287-91.

Puddey, I. B., M. Parker, et al. (1992). "Effects of alcohol and caloric restrictions on blood pressure and serum lipids in overweight men." Hypertension **20**(4): 533-41.

Resnick, L. M. (1992). "Cellular calcium and magnesium metabolism in the pathophysiology and treatment of hypertension and related metabolic disorders." Am J Med **93**(2A): 11S-20S.

Resnick, L. M. (1992). "Cellular ions in hypertension, insulin resistance, obesity, and diabetes: a unifying theme." J Am Soc Nephrol **3**(4 Suppl): S78-85.

Robertson, J. I. (1992). "The case for antihypertensive drug treatment in subjects over the age of 60." Cardiovasc Drugs Ther **6**(6): 579-83.

Schnall, P. L., J. E. Schwartz, et al. (1992). "Relation between job strain, alcohol, and ambulatory blood pressure." Hypertension **19**(5): 488-94.

Schoenberger, J. A. (1992). "Effects of antihypertensive agents on coronary artery disease risk factors." Am J Cardiol **69**(10): 33C-39C.

Siegel, D., D. M. Black, et al. (1992). "Circadian variation in ventricular arrhythmias in hypertensive men." Am J Cardiol **69**(4): 344-7.

Siegel, D., S. B. Hulley, et al. (1992). "Diuretics, serum and intracellular electrolyte levels, and ventricular arrhythmias in hypertensive men." Jama **267**(8): 1083-9.

Simons, L. A., J. Simons, et al. (1992). "Dubbo Study of the elderly: hypertension and lipid levels." Atherosclerosis **92**(1): 59-65.

Simopoulos, A. P. (1992). "Dietary risk factors for hypertension." Compr Ther **18**(10): 26-30.

Stern, M. P. (1992). "'Syndrome X': is it a significant cause of hypertension? Affirmative [see comments]." Hosp Pract **27**(1): 37-40.

Tanji, J. L. (1992). "Exercise and the hypertensive athlete." Clin Sports Med **11**(2): 291-302.

Vanhoutte, P. M. (1992). "Role of calcium and endothelium in hypertension, cardiovascular disease, and subsequent vascular events." J Cardiovasc Pharmacol **19**(1): S6-10.

Wassertheil-Smoller, S., M. D. Blaufox, et al. (1992). "The Trial of Antihypertensive Interventions and Management (TAIM) study. Adequate weight loss, alone and combined with drug therapy in the treatment of mild hypertension." Arch Intern Med **152**(1): 131-6.

Winterfeld, H. J., H. Siewert, et al. (1992). "[Potential use of the sauna in the long-term treatment of hypertensive cardiovascular circulation disorders—a comparison with kinesiotherapy]." Schweiz Rundsch Med Prax **81**(35): 1016-20.

Yeater, R. A. and I. H. Ullrich (1992). "Hypertension and exercise. Where do we stand?" Postgrad Med **91**(5): 429-36.

Yue, T. L., P. J. McKenna, et al. (1992). "Carvedilol, a new antihypertensive, prevents oxidation of human low density lipoprotein by macrophages and copper." Atherosclerosis **97**(2-3): 209-16.

(1991). "National Education Programs Working Group report on the management of patients with hypertension and high blood cholesterol." Ann Intern Med **114**(3): 224-37.

(1991). "Prevention of stroke by antihypertensive drug treatment in older persons with isolated systolic hypertension. Final results of the Systolic Hypertension in the Elderly Program (SHEP). SHEP Cooperative Research Group [see comments]." Jama **265**(24): 3255-64.

(1991). "The treatment of mild hypertension study. A randomized, placebo-controlled trial of a nutritional-hygienic regimen along with various drug monotherapies. The Treatment of Mild Hypertension Research Group." Arch Intern Med **151**(7): 1413-23.

Altura, B. M. and B. T. Altura (1991). "Cardiovascular risk factors and magnesium: relationships to atherosclerosis, ischemic heart disease and hypertension." Magnes Trace Elem **10**(2-4): 182-92.

Ascherio, A., M. J. Stampfer, et al. (1991). "Nutrient intakes and blood pressure in normotensive males." Int J Epidemiol **20**(4): 886-91.

Chen, P. Y. and P. W. Sanders (1991). "L-arginine abrogates salt-sensitive hypertension in Dahl/Rapp rats." J Clin Invest **88**(5): 1559-67.

Drueke, T. B. and M. Muntzel (1991). "Heterogeneity of blood pressure responses to salt restriction and salt appetite in rats." Klin Wochenschr **69**(1): 73-8.

Dustan, H. P. (1991). "Hypertension and obesity." Prim Care **18**(3): 495-507.

Dustan, H. P. (1991). "A perspective on the salt-blood pressure relation." Hypertension **17**(1 Suppl): I166-9.

Elmer, P. J., R. Grimm Jr., et al. (1991). "Dietary sodium reduction for hypertension prevention and treatment." Hypertension **17**(1 Suppl): I182-9.

Kaplan, N. M. (1991). "Hypertension and hyperinsulinemia." Prim Care **18**(3): 483-94.

Kaplan, N. M. (1991). "Long-term effectiveness of nonpharmacological treatment of hypertension." Hypertension **18**(3 Suppl): I153-60.

Kaplan, N. M. (1991). "New approaches to the treatment of hypertension." Cardiovasc Drugs Ther **5**(6): 973-8.

Kaplan, N. M. (1991). "Treating hypertension to prevent coronary disease [see comments]." Cleve Clin J Med **58**(5): 432-43.

Krakoff, L. R. (1991). "Is reduction of dietary salt a treatment for hypertension? [editorial] [published erratum appears in Am J Hypertens 1991 Jul; 4(7 Pt 1):644] [comment]." Am J Hypertens **4**(5 Pt 1): 481-2.

Krishna, G. G. and S. C. Kapoor (1991). "Potassium depletion exacerbates essential hypertension." Ann Intern Med **115**(2): 77-83.

Kuller, L. H. (1991). "Research and policy directions. Salt and blood pressure." Hypertension **17**(1 Suppl): I211-5.

Langford, H. G. (1991). "Sodium-potassium interaction in hypertension and hypertensive cardiovascular disease." Hypertension **17**(1 Suppl): I155-7.

Langford, H. G., B. R. Davis, et al. (1991). "Effect of drug and diet treatment of mild hypertension on diastolic blood pressure. The TAIM Research Group." Hypertension **17**(2): 210-7.

Lind, L., H. Lithell, et al. (1991). "Blood pressure response during long-term treatment with magnesium is dependent on magnesium status. A double-blind, placebo-controlled study in essential hypertension and in subjects with high-normal blood pressure." Am J Hypertens **4**(8): 674-9.

McCarron, D. A. (1991). "A consensus approach to electrolytes and blood pressure. Could we all be right?" Hypertension **17**(1 Suppl): I170-2.

McCarron, D. A. (1991). "Epidemiological evidence and clinical trials of dietary calcium's effect on blood pressure." Contrib Nephrol **90**(1): 2-10.

McCarron, D. A., C. D. Morris, et al. (1991). "Dietary calcium and blood pressure: modifying factors in specific populations." Am J Clin Nutr **54**(1 Suppl): 215S-219S.

Xu, C. P., S. Glagov, et al. (1991). "Hypertension sustains plaque progression despite reduction of hypercholesterolemia." Hypertension **18**(2): 123-9.

Kaplan, N. M. (1990). "The potential benefits of nonpharmacological therapy." Am J Hypertens **3**(5 Pt 1): 425-7.

Wing, L. M., P. J. Nestel, et al. (1990). "Lack of effect of fish oil supplementation on blood pressure in treated hypertensives." J Hypertens **8**(4): 339-43.

Knapp, H. R. and G. A. Fitz Gerald (1989). "The antihypertensive effects of fish oil. A controlled study of polyunsaturated fatty acid supplements in essential hypertension [see comments]." N Engl J Med **320**(16): 1037-43.

Homocysteine

Hajjar, K. A. (1993). "Homocysteine-induced modulation of tissue plasminogen activator binding to its endothelial cell membrane receptor." J Clin Invest **91**(6): 2873-9.

Malinow, M. R., F. J. Nieto, et al. (1993). "Carotid artery intimal-medial wall thickening and plasma homocyst(e)ine in asymptomatic adults. The atherosclerosis risk in communities study." Circulation **87**: 1107-1113.

Stamler, J. S., J. A. Osborne, et al. (1993). "Adverse vascular effects of homocysteine are modulated by endothelium-derived relaxing factor and related oxides of nitrogen." J Clin Invest **91**(1): 308-18.

Ubbink, J. B., W. J. Vermaak, et al. (1993). "Vitamin B-12, vitamin B-6, and folate nutritional status in men with hyperhomocysteinemia." Am J Clin Nutr **57**(1): 47-53.

Beaumont, V., M. R. Malinow, et al. (1992). "Hyperhomocyst(e)inemia, anti-estrogen antibodies and other risk factors for thrombosis in women on oral contraceptives." Atherosclerosis **94**(2-3): 147-52.

Brattstrom, L., A. Lindgren, et al. (1992). "Hyperhomocysteinaemia in stroke: prevalence, cause, and relationships to type of stroke and stroke risk factors." Eur J Clin Invest **22**(3): 214-21.

Harpel, P. C., V. T. Chang, et al. (1992). "Homocysteine and other sulfhydryl compounds enhance the binding of lipoprotein(a) to fibrin: a potential biochemical link between thrombosis, atherogenesis, and sulfhydryl compound metabolism." Proc Natl Acad Sci U S A **89**(21): 10193-7.

Kang, S. S., P. W. Wong, et al. (1992). "Hyperhomocyst(e)inemia as a risk factor for occlusive vascular disease." Annu Rev Nutr **12**(1): 279-98.

Klevay, L. M. (1992). "The homocysteine theory of arteriosclerosis [letter]." Nutr Rev **50**(5): 155.

Mason, J. B. and J. W. Miller (1992). "The effects of vitamins B12, B6, and folate on blood homocysteine levels." Ann N Y Acad Sci **669**(1): 197-203.

McCully, K. S. (1992). "Homocystinuria, arteriosclerosis, methylmalonic aciduria, and methyltransferase deficiency: a key case revisited." Nutr Rev **50**(1): 7-12.

Miller, J. W., M. J. Ribaya, et al. (1992). "Effect of vitamin B-6 deficiency on fasting plasma homocysteine concentrations." Am J Clin Nutr **55**(6): 1154-60.

Molgaard, J., M. R. Malinow, et al. (1992). "Hyperhomocyst(e)inaemia: an independent risk factor for intermittent claudication." J Intern Med **231**(3): 273-9.

Stamler, J. S. and J. Loscalzo (1992). "Endothelium-derived relaxing factor modulates the atherothrombogenic effects of homocysteine." J Cardiovasc Pharmacol **20**(1): S202-4.

Stampfer, M. J., M. R. Malinow, et al. (1992). "A prospective study of plasma homocyst(e)ine and risk of myocardial infarction in US physicians." Jama **268**(7): 877-81.

Clarke, R., L. Daly, et al. (1991). "Hyperhomocysteinemia: an independent risk factor for vascular disease [see comments]." N Engl J Med **324**(17): 1149-55.

Genest, J., Jr., J. R. McNamara, et al. (1991). "Prevalence of familial hyperhomocyst(e)inemia in men with premature coronary artery disease." Arterioscler Thromb **11**(5): 1129-36.

Olszewski, A. J. (1991). "Homocysteine content of plasma in ischemic heart disease, the reducing effect of pyridoxine, folate, cobalamin, choline, riboflavin and troxerutin. Correction of a calculation error [letter]." Atherosclerosis **88**(1): 97-8.

Olszewski, A. J. and K. S. McCully (1991). "Homocysteine content of lipoproteins in hypercholesterolemia." Atherosclerosis **88**(1): 61-8.

Taylor, L. J., F. R. De, et al. (1991). "The association of elevated plasma homocyst(e)ine with progression of symptomatic peripheral arterial disease." J Vasc Surg **13**(1): 128-36.

Ubbink, J. B., W. J. Vermaak, et al. (1991). "The prevalence of homocysteinemia and hypercholesterolemia in angiographically defined coronary heart disease." Klin Wochenschr **69**(12): 527-34.

Genest, J. J., J. R. McNamara, et al. (1990). "Plasma homocyst(e)ine levels in men with premature coronary artery disease." J Am Coll Cardiol **16**(5): 1114-9.

McCully, K. S. (1990). "Atherosclerosis, serum cholesterol and the homocysteine theory: a study of 194 consecutive autopsies." Am J Med Sci **299**(4): 217-21.

Malinow, M. R., S. S. Kang, et al. (1989). "Prevalence of hyperhomocyst(e)inemia in patients with peripheral arterial occlusive disease." Circulation **79**(6): 1180-8.

Olszewski, A. J., W. B. Szostak, et al. (1989). "Reduction of plasma lipid and homocysteine levels by pyridoxine, folate, cobalamin, choline, riboflavin, and troxerutin in atherosclerosis [published erratum appears in Atherosclerosis 1991 May; 88(1):978]." Atherosclerosis **75**(1): 1-6.

Ueland, P. M. and H. Refsum (1989). "Plasma homocysteine, a risk factor for vascular disease: plasma levels in health, disease, and drug therapy." J Lab Clin Med **114**(5): 473-501.

Israelsson, B., L. E. Brattstrom, et al. (1988). "Homocysteine and myocardial infarction." Atherosclerosis **71**(2-3): 227-33.

Kang, S. S., P. W. Wong, et al. (1987). "Homocysteinemia due to folate deficiency." Metabolism **36**(5): 458-62.

Kang, S. S., P. W. Wong, et al. (1986). "Protein-bound homocyst(e)ine. A possible risk factor for coronary artery disease." J Clin Invest **77**(5): 1482-6.

Hypercholesterolemia

Denke, M. A., T. S. Christopher, et al. (1993). "Excess body weight: An unrecognized contributor to high blood cholesterol levels in white american men." Arch Intern Med **153**: 1093-1103.

Giles, W. H., R. F. Anda, et al. (1993). "Recent trends in the identification and treatment of high blood cholesterol by physicians. Progress and missed opportunities." Jama **269**(9): 1133-8.

Godin, D. V. and D. M. Dahlman (1993). "Effects of hypercholesterolemia on tissue antioxidant status in two species differing in susceptibility to atherosclerosis." Res Commun Chem Pathol Pharmacol **79**(2): 151-66.

Klag, M. J., D. E. Ford, et al. (1993). "Serum cholesterol in young men and subsequent cardiovascular disease." N Engl J Med **328**(5): 313-8.

Barr, S. L., R. Ramakrishnan, et al. (1992). "Reducing total dietary fat without reducing saturated fatty acids does not significantly lower total plasma cholesterol concentrations in normal males." Am J Clin Nutr **55**(3): 675-81.

Barrett-Connor, E. (1992). "Lower endogenous androgen levels and dyslipidemia in men with non-insulin-dependent diabetes mellitus [see comments]." Ann Intern Med **117**(10): 807-11.

Colyvas, N., J. H. Rapp, et al. (1992). "Relation of plasma lipid and apoprotein levels to progressive intimal hyperplasia after arterial endarterectomy [see comments]." Circulation **85**(4): 1286-92.

Genest, J., Jr., J. R. McNamara, et al. (1992). "Lipoprotein cholesterol, apolipoprotein A-I and B and lipoprotein (a) abnormalities in men with premature coronary artery disease." J Am Coll Cardiol **19**(4): 792-802.

Hemila, H. (1992). "Vitamin C and plasma cholesterol." Crit Rev Food Sci Nutr **32**(1): 33-57.

Henkin, Y., J. A. Como, et al. (1992). "Secondary dyslipidemia. Inadvertent effects of drugs in clinical practice." Jama **267**(7): 961-8.

Kannel, W. B. and P. W. Wilson (1992). "Efficacy of lipid profiles in prediction of coronary disease." Am Heart J **124**(3): 768-74.

Levenson, J., M. Del Pino, et al. (1992). "Hypercholesterolaemia alters arterial and blood factors related to atherosclerosis in hypertension." Atherosclerosis **95**(2-3): 171-9.

Miller, M., A. Seidler, et al. (1992). "Long-term predictors of subsequent cardiovascular events with coronary artery disease and 'desirable' levels of plasma total cholesterol [see comments]." Circulation **86**(4): 1165-70.

(1991). "National Education Programs Working Group report on the management of patients with hypertension and high blood cholesterol." Ann Intern Med **114**(3): 224-37.

Bak, A. A. and D. E. Grobbee (1991). "Caffeine, blood pressure, and serum lipids." Am J Clin Nutr **53**(4): 971-5.

Bolton-Smith, C., M. Woodward, et al. (1991). "Dietary and non-dietary predictors of serum total and HDL-cholesterol in men and women: results from the Scottish Heart Health Study." Int J Epidemiol **20**(1): 95-104.

Burke, G. L., J. M. Sprafka, et al. (1991). "Trends in serum cholesterol levels from 1980 to 1987. The Minnesota Heart Survey." N Engl J Med **324**(14): 941-6.

Criqui, M. H. (1991). "Cholesterol, primary and secondary prevention, and all-cause mortality." Ann Intern Med **115**(12): 973-6.

Dalen, J. E. (1991). "Detection and treatment of elevated blood cholesterol. What have we learned? [comment]." Arch Intern Med **151**(1): 25-8.

Gadkari, J. V. and V. D. Joshi (1991). "Effect of ingestion of raw garlic on serum cholesterol level, clotting time and fibrinolytic activity in normal subjects." J Postgrad Med **37**(3): 128-31.

Gotto, A., Jr. (1991). "Hypercholesterolemia: new findings and clinical applications. Introduction." Am J Med **91**(1B): 1S-2S.

Grundy, S. M. (1991). "George Lyman Duff Memorial Lecture. Multifactorial etiology of hypercholesterolemia. Implications for prevention of coronary heart disease." Arterioscler Thromb **11**(6): 1619-35.

Gwynne, J. T. (1991). "Measuring and knowing. The trouble with cholesterol and decision making [editorial; comment]." Jama **266**(12): 1696-8.

Harris, T. B., D. M. Makuc, et al. (1991). "Is the serum cholesterol-coronary heart disease relationship modified by activity level in older persons?" J Am Geriatr Soc **39**(8): 747-54.

Phinney, S. D., A. B. Tang, et al. (1991). "The transient hypercholesterolemia of major weight loss." Am J Clin Nutr **53**(6): 1404-10.

Ubbink, J. B., W. J. Vermaak, et al. (1991). "The prevalence of homocysteinemia and hypercholesterolemia in angiographically defined coronary heart disease." Klin Wochenschr **69**(12): 527-34.

Vasilieva, E. J., A. V. Shpector, et al. (1991). "Platelet function and plasma lipid levels in patients with stable and unstable angina pectoris." Am J Cardiol **68**(9): 959-61.

Vega, G. L., M. A. Denke, et al. (1991). "Metabolic basis of primary hypercholesterolemia." Circulation **84**(1): 118-28.

Vega, G. L. and S. M. Grundy (1991). "Influence of lovastatin therapy on metabolism of low density lipoproteins in mixed hyperlipidaemia." J Intern Med **230**(4): 341-50.

Wong, N. D., P. W. Wilson, et al. (1991). "Serum cholesterol as a prognostic factor after myocardial infarction: the Framingham Study [see comments]." Ann Intern Med **115**(9): 687-93.

(1990). "Relationship of atherosclerosis in young men to serum lipoprotein cholesterol concentrations and smoking. A preliminary report from the Pathobiological Determinants of Atherosclerosis in Youth (PDAY) Research Group [see comments]." Jama **264**(23): 3018-24.

Press, R. I., J. Geller, et al. (1990). "The effect of chromium picolinate on serum cholesterol and apolipoprotein fractions in human subjects [see comments]." West J Med **152**(1): 41-5.

Olson, R. E. (1989). "A critique of the report of the National Institutes of Health Expert Panel on detection, evaluation, and treatment of high blood cholesterol [comment]." Arch Intern Med **149**(7): 1501-3.

Connor, S. L., J. R. Gustafson, et al. (1986). "The cholesterol/saturated-fat index: an indication of the hypercholesterolaemic and atherogenic potential of food." Lancet **1**(8492): 1229-32.

Immune System

De Simone, C., S. Tzantzoglou, et al. (1993). "High dose L-carnitine improves immunologic and metabolic parameters in AIDS patients." Immunopharmacol Immunotoxicol **15**(1): 1-12.

Folkers, K., M. Morita, et al. (1993). "The activities of coenzyme Q10 and vitamin B6 for immune responses." Biochem Biophys Res Commun **193**(1): 88-92.

van Poppel, G., S. Spanhaak, et al. (1993). "Effect of beta-carotene on immunological indexes in healthy male smokers." Am J Clin Nutr **57**(3): 402-7.

Chandra, R. K. (1992). "Effect of vitamin and trace-element supplementation on immune responses and infection in elderly subjects." Lancet **340**(8828): 1124-7.

Chandra, R. K. (1992). "Nutrition and immunity in the elderly." Nutr Rev **50**(12): 367-71.

Chandra, R. K. (1992). "Nutrition and immunoregulation. Significance for host resistance to tumors and infectious diseases in humans and rodents." J Nutr **122**(3 Suppl): 754-7.

Kelley, D. S., G. J. Nelson, et al. (1992). "Salmon diet and human immune status." Eur J Clin Nutr **46**(6): 397-404.

Khoo, J. C., E. Miller, et al. (1992). "Monoclonal antibodies against LDL further enhance macrophage uptake of LDL aggregates." Arterioscler Thromb **12**(11): 1258-66.

Kowdley, K. V., J. B. Mason, et al. (1992). "Vitamin E deficiency and impaired cellular immunity related to intestinal fat malabsorption." Gastroenterology **102**(6): 2139-42.

Libby, P. (1992). "Do vascular wall cytokines promote atherogenesis?" Hosp Pract **27**(10): 51-8.

Meydani, S. N., M. Hayek, et al. (1992). "Influence of vitamins E and B6 on immune response." Ann N Y Acad Sci **669**(1): 125-39.

Middleton, E., Jr. and C. Kandaswami (1992). "Effects of flavonoids on immune and inflammatory cell functions." Biochem Pharmacol **43**(6): 1167-79.

Jacob, R. A., D. S. Kelley, et al. (1991). "Immunocompetence and oxidant defense during ascorbate depletion of healthy men." Am J Clin Nutr **54**(6 Suppl): 1302S-1309S.

Kramer, T. R., N. Schoene, et al. (1991). "Increased vitamin E intake restores fish-oil-induced suppressed blastogenesis of mitogen-stimulated T lymphocytes." Am J Clin Nutr **54**(5): 896-902.

Lau, B. H., T. Yamasaki, et al. (1991). "Garlic compounds modulate macrophage and T-lymphocyte functions." Mol Biother **3**(2): 103-7.

Meydani, S. N., S. Endres, et al. (1991). "Effect of oral n-3 fatty acid supplementation on the immune response of young and older women." Adv Prostaglandin Thromboxane Leukot Res **1**: 245-8.

Meydani, S. N., J. D. Ribaya-Mercado, et al. (1991). "Vitamin B-6 deficiency impairs interleukin 2 production and lymphocyte proliferation in elderly adults." Am J Clin Nutr **53**(5): 1275-80.

Schmidt, K. (1991). "Antioxidant vitamins and beta-carotene: effects on immunocompetence." Am J Clin Nutr **53**(1 Suppl): 383S-385S.

Meydani, S. N., M. P. Barklund, et al. (1990). "Vitamin E supplementation enhances cell-mediated immunity in healthy elderly subjects [see comments]." Am J Clin Nutr **52**(3): 557-63.

Iron/Ferritin

Chevion, M., Y. Jiang, et al. (1993). "Copper and iron are mobilized following myocardial ischemia: possible predictive criteria for tissue injury." Proc Natl Acad Sci U S A **90**(3): 1102-6.

Cooper, R. S. and Y. Liao (1993). "Iron stores and coronary heart disease: Negative findings in the NHANES I epidemiologic follow-up study. (abstract)." Circulation **87**(2): 686.

Morel, I., G. Lescoat, et al. (1993). "Antioxidant and iron-chelating activities of the flavonoids catechin, quercetin and diosmetin on iron-loaded rat hepatocyte cultures." Biochem Pharmacol **45**(1): 13-9.

Rimm, E. B., A. Ascherio, et al. (1993). "Dietary iron intake and risk of coronary disease among men. (abstract)." Circulation **87**(2): 692.

Shivaswamy, V., C. K. Kurup, et al. (1993). "Ferrous-iron induces lipid peroxidation with little damage to energy transduction in mitochondria." Mol Cell Biochem **120**(2): 141-9.

Stampfer, M. J., F. Grodstein, et al. (1993). "A prospective study of plasma ferritin and risk of myocardial infarction in US physicians. (abstract)." Circulation **87**(2): 688.

Abdalla, D. S., A. Campa, et al. (1992). "Low density lipoprotein oxidation by stimulated neutrophils and ferritin." Atherosclerosis **97**(2-3): 149-59.

Ani, M. and A. A. Moshtaghie (1992). "The effect of chromium on parameters related to iron metabolism." Biol Trace Elem Res **32**(1): 57-64.

Dasgupta, A., T. Zdunek, et al. (1992). "Differential effects of transition metal ions on in vitro lipid peroxidation of human serum and protein precipitated from serum." Clin Physiol Biochem **9**(1): 7-10.

Moreno, J. J., M. Foroozesh, et al. (1992). "Release of iron from ferritin by aqueous extracts of cigarette smoke." Chem Res Toxicol **5**(1): 116-23.Reznick, A. Z., V. E. Kagan, et al. (1992). "Antiradical effects in L-propionyl carnitine protection of the heart against ischemia-reperfusion injury: the possible role of iron chelation." Arch Biochem Biophys **296**(2): 394-401.

Ryan, T. P. and S. D. Aust (1992). "The role of iron in oxygen-mediated toxicities." Crit Rev Toxicol **22**(2): 119-41.

Salonen, J. T., K. Nyyssonen, et al. (1992). "High stored iron levels are associated with excess risk of myocardial infarction in eastern Finnish men [see comments]." Circulation **86**(3): 803-11.

Sullivan, J. L. (1992). "Ferritin cannot release iron in vivo if there is no ferritin present [letter]." Free Radic Biol Med **13**(6): 703-4.

Sullivan, J. L. (1992). "Stored iron and ischemic heart disease. Empirical support for a new paradigm [editorial; comment]." Circulation **86**(3): 1036-7.

Hann, H. W., M. W. Stahlhut, et al. (1991). "Iron enhances tumor growth. Observation on spontaneous mammary tumors in mice." Cancer **68**(11): 2407-10.

Kuzuya, M., K. Yamada, et al. (1991). "Oxidation of low-density lipoprotein by copper and iron in phosphate buffer." Biochim Biophys Acta **1084**(2): 198-201.

Lauffer, R. B. (1991). "Iron stores and the international variation in mortality from coronary artery disease." Med Hypotheses **35**(2): 96-102.

McCord, J. M. (1991). "Is iron sufficiency a risk factor in ischemic heart disease? [editorial; comment]." Circulation **83**(3): 1112-4.

Reizenstein, P. (1991). "Iron, free radicals and cancer." Med Oncol Tumor Pharmacother **8**(4): 229-33.

Sakurai, T., S. Kimura, et al. (1991). "Oxidative modification of glycated low density lipoprotein in the presence of iron." Biochem Biophys Res Commun **177**(1): 433-9.

Sullivan, J. L. (1991). "Blood donation may be good for the donor. Iron, heart disease, and donor recruitment." Vox Sang **61**(3): 161-4.

L-arginine

Luscher, T. F. and W. E. Haefeli (1993). "L-arginine in the clinical arena: tool or ready. (Editorial)." Circulation **87**(5): 1746-1748.

McNamara, D. B., B. Bedi, et al. (1993). "L-arginine inhibits balloon catheter-induced intimal hyperplasia." Biochem Biophys Res Commun **193**(1): 291-6.

Mittal, C. K. (1993). "Nitric oxide synthase: involvement of oxygen radicals in conversion of L-arginine to nitric oxide." Biochem Biophys Res Commun **193**(1): 126-32.

Cooke, J. P., A. H. Singer, et al. (1992). "Antiatherogenic effects of L-arginine in the hypercholesterolemic rabbit." J Clin Invest **90**(3): 1168-72.

Creager, M. A., S. J. Gallagher, et al. (1992). "L-arginine improves endothelium-dependent vasodilation in hypercholesterolemic humans." J Clin Invest **90**(4): 1248-53.

Dubois-Rande, J. L., R. Zelinsky, et al. (1992). "Effects of infusion of L-arginine into the left anterior descending coronary artery on acetylcholine-induced vasoconstriction of human atheromatous coronary arteries." Am J Cardiol **70**(15): 1269-75.

Hishikawa, K., T. Nakaki, et al. (1992). "L-arginine as an antihypertensive agent." J Cardiovasc Pharmacol **20**(1): S196-7.

Kuo, L., M. J. Davis, et al. (1992). "Pathophysiological consequences of atherosclerosis extend into the coronary microcirculation. Restoration of endothelium-dependent responses by L-arginine." Circ Res **70**(3): 465-76.

Lee, L. and R. C. Webb (1992). "Endothelium-dependent relaxation and L-arginine metabolism in genetic hypertension." Hypertension **19**(5): 435-41.

Matheis, G., M. P. Sherman, et al. (1992). "Role of L-arginine-nitric oxide pathway in myocardial reoxygenation injury." Am J Physiol **262**(2 Pt 2): H616-20.

Park, K. G., S. D. Heys, et al. (1992). "Stimulation of human breast cancers by dietary L-arginine." Clin Sci **82**(4): 413-7.

Weyrich, A. S., X. L. Ma, et al. (1992). "The role of L-arginine in ameliorating reperfusion injury after myocardial ischemia in the cat." Circulation **86**(1): 279-88.

Chen, P. Y. and P. W. Sanders (1991). "L-arginine abrogates salt-sensitive hypertension in Dahl/Rapp rats." J Clin Invest **88**(5): 1559-67.

Drexler, H., A. M. Zeiher, et al. (1991). "Correction of endothelial dysfunction in coronary microcirculation of hypercholesterolaemic patients by L-arginine." Lancet **338**(8782-8783): 1546-50.

Park, K. G., P. D. Hayes, et al. (1991). "Stimulation of lymphocyte natural cytotoxicity by L-arginine." Lancet **337**(8742): 645-6.

Rubanyi, G. M. (1991). "Reversal of hypercholesterolemia-induced endothelial dysfunction by L-arginine [editorial; comment]." Circulation **83**(3): 1118-20.

L-carnitine

Broderick, T. L., H. A. Quinney, et al. (1993). "Beneficial effect of carnitine on mechanical recovery of rat hearts reperfused after a transient period of global ischemia is accompanied by a stimulation of glucose oxidation." Circulation **87**(3): 972-81.

De Simone, C., S. Tzantzoglou, et al. (1993). "High dose L-carnitine improves immunologic and metabolic parameters in AIDS patients." Immunopharmacol Immunotoxicol **15**(1): 1-12.

Micheletti, R., E. D. Di Paola, et al. (1993). "Propionyl-L-carnitine limits chronic ventricular dilation after myocardial infarction in rats." Am J Physiol **264**(4 Pt 2): H1111-7.

Palazzuoli, V., S. Mondillo, et al. (1993). "[The evaluation of the antiarrhythmic activity of L-carnitine and propafenone in ischemic cardiopathy]." Clin Ter **142**(2): 155-9.

Saltin, B. and P. O. Astrand (1993). "Free fatty acids and exercise." Am J Clin Nutr **57**(5 Suppl): 757S-758S.

Arduini, A. (1992). "Carnitine and its acyl esters as secondary antioxidants? [letter]." Am Heart J **123**(6): 1726-7.

Bartels, G. L., W. J. Remme, et al. (1992). "Acute improvement of cardiac function with intravenous L-propionylcarnitine in humans." J Cardiovasc Pharmacol **20**(1): 157-64.

Brevetti, G., S. Perna, et al. (1992). "Superiority of L-propionylcarnitine vs L-carnitine in improving walking capacity in patients with peripheral vascular disease: an acute, intravenous, double-blind, cross-over study." Eur Heart J **13**(2): 251-5.

Corbucci, G. G., A. Menichetti, et al. (1992). "Metabolic aspects of acute tissue hypoxia during extracorporeal circulation and their modification induced by L-carnitine treatment." Int J Clin Pharmacol Res **12**(3): 149-57.

Coto, V., L. D'Alessandro, et al. (1992). "Evaluation of the therapeutic efficacy and tolerability of levocarnitine propionyl in the treatment of chronic obstructive arteriopathies of the lower extremities: a multicentre controlled study vs. placebo." Drugs Exp Clin Res **18**(1): 29-36.

Davini, P., A. Bigalli, et al. (1992). "Controlled study on L-carnitine therapeutic efficacy in post-infarction." Drugs Exp Clin Res **18**(8): 355-65.

Fernandez, C. and C. Proto (1992). "[L-carnitine in the treatment of chronic myocardial ischemia. An analysis of 3 multicenter studies and a bibliographic review]." Clin Ter **140**(4): 353-77.

Greco, A. V., G. Mingrone, et al. (1992). "Effect of propionyl-L-carnitine in the treatment of diabetic angiopathy: controlled double blind trial versus placebo." Drugs Exp Clin Res **18**(2): 69-80.

Guarnieri, G., M. Fonda, et al. (1992). "Effects of L-carnitine supplementation in the dialysate on serum lipoprotein composition of hemodialysis patients." Contrib Nephrol **98**(1): 36-43.

Kobayashi, A., Y. Masumura, et al. (1992). "L-carnitine treatment for congestive heart failure—experimental and clinical study." Jpn Circ J **56**(1): 86-94.

Lagioia, R., D. Scrutinio, et al. (1992). "Propionyl-L-carnitine: a new compound in the metabolic approach to the treatment of effort angina." Int J Cardiol **34**(2): 167-72.

Li, B., M. L. Lloyd, et al. (1992). "The effect of enteral carnitine administration in humans." Am J Clin Nutr **55**(4): 838-45.

Pasini, E., A. Cargnoni, et al. (1992). "Effect of prolonged treatment with propionyl-L-carnitine on erucic acid-induced myocardial dysfunction in rats." Mol Cell Biochem **112**(2): 117-23.

Pasini, E., L. Comini, et al. (1992). "Effect of propionyl-L-carnitine on experimental induced cardiomyopathy in rats." Am J Cardiovasc Pathol **4**(3): 216-22.

Pasini, E., L. Comini, et al. (1992). "Effect of propionyl-L-carnitine on experimental induced cardiomyopathy in rats." Am J Cardiovasc Pathol **4**(3): 216-22.

Paulson, D. J., A. L. Shug, et al. (1992). "Protection of the ischemic diabetic heart by L-propionylcarnitine therapy." Mol Cell Biochem **116**(1-2): 131-7.

Pucciarelli, G., M. Mastursi, et al. (1992). "[The clinical and hemodynamic effects of propionyl-L-carnitine in the treatment of congestive heart failure]." Clin Ter **141**(11): 379-84.

Rebouche, C. J. (1992). "Carnitine function and requirements during the life cycle." Faseb J **6**(15): 3379-86.

Reznick, A. Z., V. E. Kagan, et al. (1992). "Antiradical effects in L-propionyl carnitine protection of the heart against ischemia-reperfusion injury: the possible role of iron chelation." Arch Biochem Biophys **296**(2): 394-401.

Savica, V., G. Bellinghieri, et al. (1992). "[The hypotriglyceridemic action of the combination of L-carnitine + simvastatin vs. L-carnitine and vs. simvastatin]." Clin Ter **140**(1 Pt 2): 17-22.

Tonda, M. E. and L. L. Hart (1992). "N,N dimethylglycine and L-carnitine as performance enhancers in athletes." Ann Pharmacother **26**(7-8): 935-7.

van Es, A., F. C. Henny, et al. (1992). "Amelioration of cardiac function by L-carnitine administration in patients on haemodialysis." Contrib Nephrol **98**(1): 28-35.

(1991). "A role for carnitine in medium-chain fatty acid metabolism?" Nutr Rev **49**(8): 243-5.

Bertelli, A., A. Conte, et al. (1991). "Protective effect of propionyl carnitine against peroxidative damage to arterial endothelium membranes." Int J Tissue React **13**(1): 41-3.

Bolukoglu, H., A. M. Eggleston, et al. (1991). "Effects of propionyl-L-carnitine in chronically hypoperfused ("hibernating") myocardium." Cardioscience **2**(4): 245-55.

Brevetti, G., C. Angelini, et al. (1991). "Muscle carnitine deficiency in patients with severe peripheral vascular disease." Circulation **84**(4): 1490-5.

Cacciatore, L., R. Cerio, et al. (1991). "The therapeutic effect of L-carnitine in patients with exercise-induced stable angina: a controlled study." Drugs Exp Clin Res **17**(4): 225-35.

Chiddo, A., A. Gaglione, et al. (1991). "Hemodynamic study of intravenous propionyl-L-carnitine in patients with ischemic heart disease and normal left ventricular function." Cardiovasc Drugs Ther **5**(1): 107-11.

Corbucci, G. G. and B. Lettieri (1991). "Cardiogenic shock and L-carnitine: clinical data and therapeutic perspectives." Int J Clin Pharmacol Res **11**(6): 283-93.

Di Biase, M., M. Tritto, et al. (1991). "Electrophysiologic evaluation of intravenous L-propionyl-carnitine in man." Int J Cardiol **30**(3): 329-33.

Ferrari, R., C. Ceconi, et al. (1991). "The effect of propionyl-L-carnitine on the ischemic and reperfused intact myocardium and on their derived mitochondria." Cardiovasc Drugs Ther **5**(1): 57-65.

Fritz, I. B., K. Wong, et al. (1991). "Clustering of erythrocytes by fibrinogen is inhibited by carnitine: evidence that sulfhydryl groups on red blood cell membranes are involved in carnitine actions." J Cell Physiol **149**(2): 269-76.

Fujiwara, M., T. Nakano, et al. (1991). "[Effect of L-carnitine in patients with ischemic heart disease]." J Cardiol **21**(2): 493-504.

Hulsmann, W. C. (1991). "Biochemical profile of propionyl-L-carnitine." Cardiovasc Drugs Ther **5**(1): 7-9.

Keene, B. W. (1991). "L-carnitine supplementation in the therapy of canine dilated cardiomyopathy." Vet Clin North Am Small Anim Pract **21**(5): 1005-9.

Leasure, J. E. and K. Kordenat (1991). "Effect of propionyl-L-carnitine on experimental myocardial infarction in dogs." Cardiovasc Drugs Ther **5**(1): 85-95.

Leipala, J. A., R. Bhatnagar, et al. (1991). "Protection of the reperfused heart by L-propionyl-carnitine." J Appl Physiol **71**(4): 1518-22.

Packer, L., M. Valenza, et al. (1991). "Free radical scavenging is involved in the protective effect of L-propionyl-carnitine against ischemia-reperfusion injury of the heart." Arch Biochem Biophys **288**(2): 533-7.

Pepine, C. J. (1991). "The therapeutic potential of carnitine in cardiovascular disorders." Clin Ther **13**(1): 2-21.

Pregant, P., G. Schernthaner, et al. (1991). "[Decreased plasma carnitine in Type I diabetes mellitus]." Klin Wochenschr **69**(12): 511-6.

Rebouche, C. J. (1991). "Ascorbic acid and carnitine biosynthesis." Am J Clin Nutr **54**(6 Suppl): 1147S-1152S.

Rebouche, C. J. (1991). "Quantitative estimation of absorption and degradation of a carnitine supplement by human adults." Metabolism **40**(12): 1305-10.

Rossle, C., Y. A. Carpentier, et al. (1991). "[Parenterally administered medium-chain triglyceride-induced changes in carnitine metabolism]." Infusionstherapie **18**(4): 167-71.

Shug, A., D. Paulson, et al. (1991). "Protective effects of propionyl-L-carnitine during ischemia and reperfusion." Cardiovasc Drugs Ther **5**(1): 77-83.

Siliprandi, N., F. Di Lisa, et al. (1991). "Propionyl-L-carnitine: biochemical significance and possible role in cardiac metabolism." Cardiovasc Drugs Ther **5**(1): 11-5.

Demeyere, R., P. Lormans, et al. (1990). "Cardioprotective effects of carnitine in extensive aortocoronary bypass grafting: a double-blind, randomized, placebo-controlled clinical trial." Anesth Analg **71**(5): 520-8.

Regitz, V., A. L. Shug, et al. (1990). "Defective myocardial carnitine metabolism in congestive heart failure secondary to dilated cardiomyopathy and to coronary, hypertensive and valvular heart diseases." Am J Cardiol **65**(11): 755-60.

Demeyere, R., P. Lormans, et al. (1989). "Cardioprotective effects of carnitine in extensive aorto-coronary bypass grafting." J Cardiothorac Anesth **3**(5 Suppl 1):

Siliprandi, N., L. F. Di, et al. (1984). "Biochemical derangements in ischemic myocardium: the role of carnitine." G Ital Cardiol **14**(10): 804-8.

LDL

Boyden, T. W., R. W. Pamenter, et al. (1993). "Resistance exercise training is associated with decreases in serum low-density lipoprotein cholesterol levels in premenopausal women." Arch Intern Med **153**(1): 97-100.

Campos, H., J. Genest Jr., et al. (1992). "Low density lipoprotein particle size and coronary artery disease." Arterioscler Thromb **12**(2): 187-95.

Kannel, W. B. and P. W. Wilson (1992). "Efficacy of lipid profiles in prediction of coronary disease." Am Heart J **124**(3): 768-74.

Arntzenius, A. C. (1991). "Regression of atherosclerosis. Benefit can be expected from low LDL-C and high HDL-C levels [editorial]." Acta Cardiol **46**(4): 431-8.

Barth, J. D. and A. C. Arntzenius (1991). "Progression and regression of atherosclerosis, what roles for LDL-cholesterol and HDL-cholesterol: a perspective." Eur Heart J **12**(8): 952-7.

Brown, S. A., J. Morrisett, et al. (1991). "Influence of short term dietary cholesterol and fat on human plasma Lp[a] and LDL levels." J Lipid Res **32**(8): 1281-9.

Dieber-Rotheneder, M., H. Puhl, et al. (1991). "Effect of oral supplementation with D-alpha-tocopherol on the vitamin E content of human low density lipoproteins and resistance to oxidation." J Lipid Res **32**(8): 1325-32.

Mensink, R. P. and M. B. Katan (1990). "Effect of dietary trans fatty acids on high-density and low-density lipoprotein cholesterol levels in healthy subjects [see comments]." N Engl J Med **323**(7): 439-45.

Wilson, P. W. (1990). "High-density lipoprotein, low-density lipoprotein and coronary artery disease." Am J Cardiol **66**(6): 7A-10A.

LDL Apheresis

Lane, D. M., W. J. McConathy, et al. (1993). "Weekly treatment of diet/drug-resistant hypercholesterolemia with the heparin-induced extracorporeal low-density lipoprotein precipitation (HELP) system by selective plasma low-density lipoprotein removal." Am J Cardiol **71**(10): 816-22.

Mimura, Y., M. Kuriyama, et al. (1993). "Treatment of cerebrotendinous xanthomatosis with low-density lipoprotein (LDL)-apheresis." J Neurol Sci **114**(2): 227-30.

Suzuki, H., E. Mutoh, et al. (1993). "[Arteriosclerosis obliterans that was improved by LDL apheresis]." Hokkaido Igaku Zasshi **68**(1): 126-31.

Gordon, B. R., S. F. Kelsey, et al. (1992). "Treatment of refractory familial hypercholesterolemia by low-density lipoprotein apheresis using an automated dextran sulfate cellulose adsorption system. The Liposorber Study Group." Am J Cardiol **70**(11): 1010-6.

Lasuncion, M. A., J. L. Teruel, et al. (1992). "[Serum lipoprotein (a) levels during treatment with LDL apheresis for homozygous familial hypercholesterolemia]." Med Clin **99**(14): 541-4.

Maher, V. M., Y. Kitano, et al. (1992). "Effective reduction of plasma LDL levels by LDL apheresis in familial defective apolipoprotein B-100." Atherosclerosis **95**(2-3): 231-4.

Nomura, S., R. Kouzuma, et al. (1992). "[A case of heterozygous familial hypercholesterolemia showing the regression of coronary atherosclerosis by LDL-apheresis]." Kokyu To Junkan **40**(3): 299-302.

Tatami, R., N. Inoue, et al. (1992). "Regression of coronary atherosclerosis by combined LDL-apheresis and lipid-lowering drug therapy in patients with familial hypercholesterolemia: a multicenter study. The LARS Investigators." Atherosclerosis **95**(1): 1-13.

Uauy, R., R. J. Zwiener, et al. (1992). "Treatment of children with homozygous familial hypercholesterolemia: safety and efficacy of low-density lipoprotein apheresis." J Pediatr **120**(6): 892-8.

Wenke, K., J. Thiery, et al. (1992). "Treatment of hypercholesterolemia and prevention of coronary artery disease after heart transplantation by combination of low-dose simvastatin and HELP-LDL-apheresis." Transplant Proc **24**(6): 2674-6.

LDL/HDL-Cholesterol Ratio

Gohlke, H. (1992). "[Effect of the LDL/HDL-cholesterol quotient on progression and regression of arteriosclerotic lesions. An analysis of controlled angiographic intervention studies]." Wien Klin Wochenschr **104**(11): 309-13.

Hong, M. K., P. A. Romm, et al. (1991). "Usefulness of the total cholesterol to high-density lipoprotein cholesterol ratio in predicting angiographic coronary artery disease in women." Am J Cardiol **68**(17): 1646-50.

Luria, M. H., J. Erel, et al. (1991). "Cardiovascular risk factor clustering and ratio of total cholesterol to high-density lipoprotein cholesterol in angiographically documented coronary artery disease." Am J Cardiol **67**(1): 31-6.

Lecithin

Knuiman, J. T., A. C. Beynen, et al. (1989). "Lecithin intake and serum cholesterol." Am J Clin Nutr **49**(2): 266-8.

Longevity/Aging/Mortality

Cullen, K. J., M. W. Knuiman, et al. (1993). "Alcohol and mortality in Busselton, Western Australia." Am J Epidemiol **137**(2): 242-8.

Gunby, P. (1993). "Two new reports help put nation's No. 1 killer disease challenges into perspective for 1993 [news]." Jama **269**(4): 449-50.

Paffenbarger, R., Jr., R. T. Hyde, et al. (1993). "The association of changes in physical-activity level and other lifestyle characteristics with mortality among men [see comments]." N Engl J Med **328**(8): 538-45.

Sandvik, L., J. Erikssen, et al. (1993). "Physical fitness as a predictor of mortality among healthy, middle-aged Norwegian men [see comments]." N Engl J Med **328**(8): 533-7.

Sohal, R. S. (1993). "The free radical hypothesis of aging: an appraisal of the current status [see comments]." Aging **5**(1): 3-17.

Stamler, J., O. Vaccaro, et al. (1993). "Diabetes, other risk factors, and 12-yr cardiovascular mortality for men screened in the Multiple Risk Factor Intervention Trial." Diabetes Care **16**(2): 434-44.

Bunker, V. (1992). "Free radicals, antioxidants, and ageing." Med Lab Sci **49**: 299-312.

Criqui, M. H., R. D. Langer, et al. (1992). "Mortality over a period of 10 years in patients with peripheral arterial disease." N Engl J Med **326**(6): 381-6.

de Labry, L. O., R. J. Glynn, et al. (1992). "Alcohol consumption and mortality in an American male population: recovering the U-shaped curve—findings from the normative Aging Study." J Stud Alcohol **53**(1): 25-32.

Deucher, G. P. (1992). "Antioxidant therapy in the aging process." Exs **62**(1): 428-37.

Enstrom, J. E., L. E. Kanim, et al. (1992). "Vitamin C intake and mortality among a sample of the United States population [see comments]." Epidemiology **3**(3): 194-202.

Evans, W. J. (1992). "Exercise, nutrition and aging." J Nutr **122**(3 Suppl): 796-801.

Grover, S. A., M. Abrahamowicz, et al. (1992). "The benefits of treating hyperlipidemia to prevent coronary heart disease. Estimating changes in life expectancy and morbidity." Jama **267**(6): 816-22.

Gunby, P. (1992). "Cardiovascular diseases remain nation's leading cause of death [news]." Jama **267**(3): 335-6.

Gupta, R., K. D. Gupta, et al. (1992). "Influence of mild to moderate treated hypertension on 9-11 year mortality in patients with pre-existing coronary heart disease." J Hum Hypertens **6**(4): 313-6.

Harris, T., J. J. Feldman, et al. (1992). "The low cholesterol-mortality association in a national cohort." J Clin Epidemiol **45**(6): 595-601.

Lee, I. M. and R. Paffenbarger Jr. (1992). "Change in body weight and longevity." Jama **268**(15): 2045-9.

Lindberg, G., L. Rastam, et al. (1992). "Low serum cholesterol concentration and short term mortality from injuries in men and women." Bmj **305**(6848): 277-9.

Mueller, H. S., L. S. Cohen, et al. (1992). "Predictors of early morbidity and mortality after thrombolytic therapy of acute myocardial infarction. Analyses of patient subgroups in the Thrombolysis in Myocardial Infarction (TIMI) trial, phase II." Circulation **85**(4): 1254-64.

Neaton, J. D., H. Blackburn, et al. (1992). "Serum cholesterol level and mortality findings for men screened in the Multiple Risk Factor Intervention Trial. Multiple Risk Factor Intervention Trial Research Group." Arch Intern Med **152**(7): 1490-500.

Nerbrand, C., K. Svardsudd, et al. (1992). "Cardiovascular mortality and morbidity in seven counties in Sweden in relation to water hardness and geological settings. The project: myocardial infarction in mid-Sweden." Eur Heart J **13**(6): 721-7.

Notarbartolo, A., I. Catalano, et al. (1992). "Platelets, eicosanoids and aging." Aging **4**(1): 13-20.

Oliver, M. F. (1992). "Cholesterol and coronary disease—outstanding questions." Cardiovasc Drugs Ther **6**(2): 131-6.

Owens, J. F., K. A. Matthews, et al. (1992). "Can physical activity mitigate the effects of aging in middle-aged women?" Circulation **85**(4): 1265-70.

Pekkanen, J., A. Nissinen, et al. (1992). "Short- and long-term association of serum cholesterol with mortality. The 25-year follow-up of the Finnish cohorts of the seven countries study." Am J Epidemiol **135**(11): 1251-8.

Ravnskov, U. (1992). "Cholesterol lowering trials in coronary heart disease: frequency of citation and outcome." Bmj **305**(6844): 15-9.

Scherr, P. A., A. Z. La Croix, et al. (1992). "Light to moderate alcohol consumption and mortality in the elderly." J Am Geriatr Soc **40**(7): 651-7.

Simonoff, M., C. Sergeant, et al. (1992). "Antioxidant status (selenium, vitamins A and E) and aging." Exs **62**(1): 368-97.

Skelton, N. K. and W. 3. Skelton (1992). "Medical implications of obesity. Losing pounds, gaining years." Postgrad Med **92**(1): 151-6.

Stengard, J. H., J. Tuomilehto, et al. (1992). "Diabetes mellitus, impaired glucose tolerance and mortality among elderly men: the Finnish cohorts of the Seven Countries Study." Diabetologia **35**(8): 760-5.

Suh, I., B. J. Shaten, et al. (1992). "Alcohol use and mortality from coronary heart disease: the role of high-density lipoprotein cholesterol. The Multiple Risk Factor Intervention Trial Research Group." Ann Intern Med **116**(11): 881-7.

Berg, K. and O. C. Ro (1991). "Lp(a) lipoprotein level and longevity." Ann Genet **34**(3-4): 264-9.

Criqui, M. H. (1991). "Cholesterol, primary and secondary prevention, and all-cause mortality." Ann Intern Med **115**(12): 973-6.

Cutler, R. G. (1991). "Antioxidants and aging." Am J Clin Nutr **53**(1 Suppl): 373S-379S.

Menotti, A., A. Keys, et al. (1991). "Blood pressure changes as predictors of future mortality in the seven countries study." J Hum Hypertens **5**(3): 137-44.

Menotti, A., A. Keys, et al. (1991). "All cause mortality and its determinants in middle aged men in Finland, The Netherlands, and Italy in a 25 year follow up." J Epidemiol Community Health **45**(2): 125-30.

Oliver, M. F. (1991). "Might treatment of hypercholesterolaemia increase non-cardiac mortality? [see comments]." Lancet **337**(8756): 1529-31.

Shaten, B. J., L. H. Kuller, et al. (1991). "Association between baseline risk factors, cigarette smoking, and CHD mortality after 10.5 years. MRFIT Research Group." Prev Med **20**(5): 655-9.

Stemmermann, G. N., P. H. Chyou, et al. (1991). "Serum cholesterol and mortality among Japanese-American men. The Honolulu (Hawaii) Heart Program." Arch Intern Med **151**(5): 969-72.

Strandberg, T. E., V. V. Salomaa, et al. (1991). "Long-term mortality after 5-year multifactorial primary prevention of cardiovascular diseases in middle-aged men [see comments]." Jama **266**(9): 1225-9.

Thaulow, E., J. Erikssen, et al. (1991). "Blood platelet count and function are related to total and cardiovascular death in apparently healthy men [see comments]." Circulation **84**(2): 613-7.

Tsevat, J., M. C. Weinstein, et al. (1991). "Expected gains in life expectancy from various coronary heart disease risk factor modifications [published erratum appears in Circulation 1991 Dec; 84(6):2610] [see comments]." Circulation **83**(4): 1194-201.

Warram, J. H., L. M. Laffel, et al. (1991). "Excess mortality associated with diuretic therapy in diabetes mellitus [see comments]." Arch Intern Med **151**(7): 1350-6.

Wolf, P. H., J. H. Madans, et al. (1991). "Reduction of cardiovascular disease-related mortality among postmenopausal women who use hormones: evidence from a national cohort." Am J Obstet Gynecol **164**(2): 489-94.

Wong, N. D., P. W. Wilson, et al. (1991). "Serum cholesterol as a prognostic factor after myocardial infarction: the Framingham Study [see comments]." Ann Intern Med **115**(9): 687-93.

Pekkanen, J., S. Linn, et al. (1990). "Ten-year mortality from cardiovascular disease in relation to cholesterol level among men with and without preexisting cardiovascular disease [see comments]." N Engl J Med **322**(24): 1700-7.

Lowfat Diet

Anderson, J. W., T. F. Garrity, et al. (1992). "Prospective, randomized, controlled comparison of the effects of low-fat and low-fat plus high-fiber diets on serum lipid concentrations." Am J Clin Nutr **56**(5): 887-94.

Clevidence, B. A., J. T. Judd, et al. (1992). "Plasma lipid and lipoprotein concentrations of men consuming a low-fat, high-fiber diet." Am J Clin Nutr **55**(3): 689-94.

Clifton, P. M., M. B. Wight, et al. (1992). "Is fat restriction needed with HMGCoA reductase inhibitor treatment?" Atherosclerosis **93**(1-2): 59-70.

Cobb, M. M., H. Teitlebaum, et al. (1992). "Influence of dietary fat, apolipoprotein E phenotype, and sex on plasma lipoprotein levels." Circulation **86**(3): 849-57.

Garg, A. and S. M. Grundy (1992). "High-carbohydrate, low-fat diet? Negative [comment]." Hosp Pract (Off Ed) **27**(1): 11-4.

Schuler, G., R. Hambrecht, et al. (1992). "Myocardial perfusion and regression of coronary artery disease in patients on a regimen of intensive physical exercise and low fat diet." J Am Coll Cardiol **19**(1): 34-42.

Schuler, G., R. Hambrecht, et al. (1992). "Regular physical exercise and low-fat diet. Effects on progression of coronary artery disease." Circulation **86**(1): 1-11.

Seim, H. C. and K. B. Holtmeier (1992). "Effects of a six-week, low-fat diet on serum cholesterol, body weight, and body measurements." Fam Pract Res J **12**(4): 411-9.

Bonanome, A., A. Visona, et al. (1991). "Carbohydrate and lipid metabolism in patients with non-insulin-dependent diabetes mellitus: effects of a low-fat, high-carbohydrate diet vs a diet high in monounsaturated fatty acids." Am J Clin Nutr **54**(3): 586-90.

Browner, W. S., J. Westenhouse, et al. (1991). "What if Americans ate less fat? A quantitative estimate of the effect on mortality [see comments]." Jama **265**(24): 3285-91.

Cobb, M. M., H. S. Teitelbaum, et al. (1991). "Lovastatin efficacy in reducing low-density lipoprotein cholesterol levels on high- vs low-fat diets." Jama **265**(8): 997-1001.

Kendall, A., D. A. Levitsky, et al. (1991). "Weight loss on a low-fat diet: consequence of the imprecision of the control of food intake in humans." Am J Clin Nutr **53**(5): 1124-9.

Ruoff, G. E. (1991). "Reducing fat intake with fat substitutes." Am Fam Physician **43**(4): 1235-42.

Sheppard, L., A. R. Kristal, et al. (1991). "Weight loss in women participating in a randomized trial of low-fat diets." Am J Clin Nutr **54**(5): 821-8.

Singh, R. B., R. Verma, et al. (1991). "The effect of diet and aspirin on patient outcome after myocardial infarction." Nutrition **7**(2): 125-9.

Stacpoole, P. W., K. von Bergmann, et al. (1991). "Nutritional regulation of cholesterol synthesis and apolipoprotein B kinetics: studies in patients with familial hypercholesterolemia and normal subjects treated with a high carbohydrate, low fat diet." J Lipid Res **32**(11): 1837-48.

Stacpoole, P. W., K. von Bergmann, et al. (1991). "Nutritional regulation of cholesterol synthesis and apolipoprotein B kinetics: studies in patients with familial hypercholesterolemia and normal subjects treated with a high carbohydrate, low fat diet." J Lipid Res **32**(11): 1837-48.

Tremblay, A., J. P. Despres, et al. (1991). "Normalization of the metabolic profile in obese women by exercise and a low fat diet." Med Sci Sports Exerc **23**(12): 1326-31.

Ullmann, D., W. E. Connor, et al. (1991). "Will a high-carbohydrate, low-fat diet lower plasma lipids and lipoproteins without producing hypertriglyceridemia?" Arterioscler Thromb **11**(4): 1059-67.

Blankenhorn, D. H., R. L. Johnson, et al. (1990). "The influence of diet on the appearance of new lesions in human coronary arteries [see comments]." Jama **263**(12): 1646-52.

Edington, J., M. Geekie, et al. (1987). "Effect of dietary cholesterol on plasma cholesterol concentration in subjects following reduced fat, high fibre diet." Br Med J **294**(6568): 333-6.

Lp(a)

Di Lorenzo, M., P. Salvini, et al. (1993). "Acute reduction of lipoprotein(a) by tissue-type plasminogen activator [letter]." Circulation **87**(3): 1052-3.

Eden, S., O. Wiklund, et al. (1993). "Growth hormone treatment of growth hormone-deficient adults results in a marked increase in Lp(a) and HDL cholesterol concentrations." Arterioscler Thromb **13**(2): 296-301.

Jenner, J. L., J. M. Ordovas, et al. (1993). "Effects of age, sex, and menopausal status on plasma lipoprotein(a) levels. The Framingham offspring study." Circulation **87**: 1135-1141.

Tennant, M. and J. K. McGeachie (1993). "Lipoprotein(a) and its role in occlusive vascular disease." Ann R Coll Surg Engl **75**(1): 3-7.

Averna, M. R., C. M. Barbagallo, et al. (1992). "Lp(a) levels in patients undergoing aorto-coronary bypass surgery." Eur Heart J **13**(10): 1405-9.

Bihari-Varga, M., G. Kostner, et al. (1992). "Lp(a) and the risk of coronary heart disease." Eur J Epidemiol **8**(1): 33-5.

Cambillau, M., A. Simon, et al. (1992). "Serum Lp(a) as a discriminant marker of early atherosclerotic plaque at three extracoronary sites in hypercholesterolemic men. The PCVMETRA Group." Arterioscler Thromb **12**(11): 1346-52.

Cressman, M. D., R. J. Heyka, et al. (1992). "Lipoprotein(a) is an independent risk factor for cardiovascular disease in hemodialysis patients." Circulation **86**(2): 475-82.

Crook, D., M. Sidhu, et al. (1992). "Lipoprotein Lp(a) levels are reduced by danazol, an anabolic steroid." Atherosclerosis **92**(1): 41-7.

Dallongeville, J., E. Selinger, et al. (1992). "Fish-oil supplementation reduces Ip(a) concentrations in type III dysbetalipoproteinemia [letter]." Clin Chem **38**(8 Pt 1): 1510-1.

Edelberg, J. and S. V. Pizzo (1992). "Why is lipoprotein(a) relevant to thrombosis?" Am J Clin Nutr **56**(4 Suppl):

Fulcher, G. (1992). "Lipoprotein(a): a new independent risk factor for atherosclerosis [editorial; comment]." Aust N Z J Med **22**(4): 326-8.

Genest, J., Jr., S. S. Martin-Munley, et al. (1992). "Familial lipoprotein disorders in patients with premature coronary artery disease." Circulation **85**(6): 2025-33.

Genest, J., Jr., J. R. McNamara, et al. (1992). "Lipoprotein cholesterol, apolipoprotein A-I and B and lipoprotein (a) abnormalities in men with premature coronary artery disease." J Am Coll Cardiol **19**(4): 792-802.

Haberland, M. E., G. M. Fless, et al. (1992). "Malondialdehyde modification of lipoprotein(a) produces avid uptake by human monocyte-macrophages." J Biol Chem **267**(6): 4143-51.

Haffner, S. M., S. E. Moss, et al. (1992). "Lack of association between lipoprotein (a) concentrations and coronary heart disease mortality in diabetes: the Wisconsin Epidemiologic Study of Diabetic Retinopathy." Metabolism **41**(2): 194-7.

Haffner, S. M., K. R. Tuttle, et al. (1992). "Lack of change of lipoprotein (a) concentration with improved glycemic control in subjects with type II diabetes." Metabolism **41**(2): 116-20.

Halvorsen, S., O. H. Skjonsberg, et al. (1992). "Does Lp(a) lipoprotein inhibit the fibrinolytic system? (no)." Thromb Res **68**(3): 223-32.

Harpel, P. C., V. T. Chang, et al. (1992). "Homocysteine and other sulfhydryl compounds enhance the binding of lipoprotein(a) to fibrin: a potential biochemical link between thrombosis, atherogenesis, and sulfhydryl compound metabolism." Proc Natl Acad Sci U S A **89**(21): 10193-7.

Hearn, J. A., B. C. Donohue, et al. (1992). "Usefulness of serum lipoprotein (a) as a predictor of restenosis after percutaneous transluminal coronary angioplasty." Am J Cardiol **69**(8): 736-9.

Hegele, R. A. (1992). "Lipoprotein(a) and fibrinolysis." Can J Cardiol **8**(10): 1021-2.

Hiraga, T., K. Harada, et al. (1992). "Reduction of serum lipoprotein(a) using estrogen in a man with familial hypercholesterolemia [letter]." Jama **267**(17): 2328.

Klausen, I. C., L. U. Gerdes, et al. (1992). "Differences in apolipoprotein (a) polymorphism in west Greenland Eskimos and Caucasian Danes." Hum Genet **89**(4): 384-8.

Kraft, H. G., C. Sandholzer, et al. (1992). "Apolipoprotein (a) alleles determine lipoprotein (a) particle density and concentration in plasma." Arterioscler Thromb **12**(3): 302-6.

Lasuncion, M. A., J. L. Teruel, et al. (1992). "[Serum lipoprotein (a) levels during treatment with LDL apheresis for homozygous familial hypercholesterolemia]." Med Clin **99**(14): 541-4.

Lawn, R. M. (1992). "Lipoprotein(a) in heart disease." Sci Am **266**(6): 54-60.

Lepre, F., B. Campbell, et al. (1992). "Low-dose sustained release nicotinic acid (Tri-B3) and lipoprotein (a) [letter]." Am J Cardiol **70**(1): 133.

Leren, T. P., I. Hjermann, et al. (1992). "Long-term effect of lovastatin alone and in combination with cholestyramine on lipoprotein (a) level in familial hypercholesterolemic subjects." Clin Investig **70**(8): 711-8.

Lobo, R. A., M. Notelovitz, et al. (1992). "Lp(a) lipoprotein: relationship to cardiovascular disease risk factors, exercise, and estrogen." Am J Obstet Gynecol **166**(4): 1182-8.

Matsunaga, A., K. Handa, et al. (1992). "Effects of niceritrol on levels of serum lipids, lipoprotein(a), and fibrinogen in patients with primary hypercholesterolemia." Atherosclerosis **94**(2-3): 241-8.

Mensink, R. P., P. L. Zock, et al. (1992). "Effect of dietary cis and trans fatty acids on serum lipoprotein[a] levels in humans." J Lipid Res **33**(10): 1493-501.

Naruszewicz, M., E. Selinger, et al. (1992). "Oxidative modification of lipoprotein(a) and the effect of beta-carotene." Metabolism **41**(11): 1215-24.

Naruszewicz, M., E. Selinger, et al. (1992). "Probucol protects lipoprotein (a) against oxidative modification." Metabolism **41**(11): 1225-8.

Nestel, P., M. Noakes, et al. (1992). "Plasma lipoprotein lipid and Lp[a] changes with substitution of elaidic acid for oleic acid in the diet." J Lipid Res **33**(7): 1029-36.

Rader, D. J. and H. Brewer Jr. (1992). "Lipoprotein(a). Clinical approach to a unique atherogenic lipoprotein [clinical conference] [published erratum appears in JAMA 1992 Apr 8; 267(14):1922]." Jama **267**(8): 1109-12.

Ramirez, L. C., C. Arauz-Pacheco, et al. (1992). "Lipoprotein (a) levels in diabetes mellitus: relationship to metabolic control." Ann Intern Med **117**(1): 42-7.

Sandholzer, C., E. Boerwinkle, et al. (1992). "Apolipoprotein(a) phenotypes, Lp(a) concentration and plasma lipid levels in relation to coronary heart disease in a Chinese population: evidence for the role of the apo(a) gene in coronary heart disease." J Clin Invest **89**(3): 1040-6.

Sandholzer, C., N. Saha, et al. (1992). "Apo(a) isoforms predict risk for coronary heart disease. A study in six populations." Arterioscler Thromb **12**(10): 1214-26.

Scanu, A. M. (1992). "Genetic basis and pathophysiological implications of high plasma Lp(a) levels." J Intern Med **231**(6): 679-83.

Scanu, A. M. (1992). "Lipoprotein(a). A genetic risk factor for premature coronary heart disease." Jama **267**(24): 3326-9.

Scanu, A. M. (1992). "Lipoprotein(a): its inheritance and molecular basis of its atherothrombotic role." Mol Cell Biochem **113**(2): 127-31.

Scanu, A. M. (1992). "Lp(a): a link between thrombosis and atherosclerosis." Eur J Epidemiol **8**(1): 76-8.

Scanu, A. M., D. Pfaffinger, et al. (1992). "Attenuation of immunologic reactivity of lipoprotein(a) by thiols and cysteine-containing compounds. Structural implications." Arterioscler Thromb **12**(4): 424-9.

Magnesium

Hwang, D. L., C. F. Yen, et al. (1993). "Insulin increases intracellular magnesium transport in human platelets." J Clin Endocrinol Metab **76**(3): 549-53.

Matz, R. (1993). "Magnesium: deficiencies and therapeutic uses." Hosp Pract **28**(4A): 79-82.

Nadler, J. L., T. Buchanan, et al. (1993). "Magnesium deficiency produces insulin resistance and increased thromboxane synthesis." Hypertension **21**: 1024-1029.

Rayssiguier, Y., E. Gueux, et al. (1993). "Dietary magnesium affects susceptibility of lipoproteins and tissues to peroxidation in rats." J Am Coll Nutrt **12**(2): 133-137.

Widman, L., P. O. Wester, et al. (1993). "The dose-dependent reduction in blood pressure through administration of magnesium. A double blind placebo controlled cross-over study." Am J Hypertens **6**(1): 41-5.

Yusuf, S., K. Teo, et al. (1993). "Intravenous magnesium in acute myocardial infarction. An effective, safe, simple, and inexpensive intervention [editorial]." Circulation **87**(6): 2043-6.

(1992). "Magnesium supplementation in the treatment of diabetes. American Diabetes Association." Diabetes Care **15**(8): 1065-7.

Brilla, L. R. and T. F. Haley (1992). "Effect of magnesium supplementation on strength training in humans." J Am Coll Nutr **11**(3): 326-9.

Durlach, J. (1992). "Commentary on recent clinical advances: almonds, monounsaturated fats, magnesium and hypolipidaemic diets." Magnes Res **5**(4): 315.

Durlach, J., V. Durlach, et al. (1992). "Magnesium and blood pressure. II. Clinical studies." Magnes Res **5**(2): 147-53.

Eisenberg, M. J. (1992). "Magnesium deficiency and sudden death [editorial]." Am Heart J **124**(2): 544-9.

England, M. R., G. Gordon, et al. (1992). "Magnesium administration and dysrhythmias after cardiac surgery. A placebo-controlled, double-blind, randomized trial." Jama **268**(17): 2395-402.

Ferrara, L. A., R. Iannuzzi, et al. (1992). "Long-term magnesium supplementation in essential hypertension." Cardiology **81**(1): 25-33.

Garland, H. O. (1992). "New experimental data on the relationship between diabetes mellitus and magnesium." Magnes Res **5**(3): 193-202.

Gettes, L. S. (1992). "Electrolyte abnormalities underlying lethal and ventricular arrhythmias." Circulation **85**(1 Suppl): I70-6.

Grafton, G. and M. A. Baxter (1992). "The role of magnesium in diabetes mellitus. A possible mechanism for the development of diabetic complications." J Diabetes Complications **6**(2): 143-9.

Grafton, G., C. M. Bunce, et al. (1992). "Effect of Mg2+ on Na(+)-dependent inositol transport. Role for Mg2+ in etiology of diabetic complications." Diabetes **41**(1): 35-9.

Horner, S. M. (1992). "Efficacy of intravenous magnesium in acute myocardial infarction in reducing arrhythmias and mortality. Meta-analysis of magnesium in acute myocardial infarction." Circulation **86**(3): 774-9.

Hsieh, S. T., H. Sano, et al. (1992). "Magnesium supplementation prevents the development of alcohol-induced hypertension." Hypertension **19**(2): 175-82.

Hwang, D. L., C. F. Yen, et al. (1992). "Effect of extracellular magnesium on platelet activation and intracellular calcium mobilization." Am J Hypertens **5**(10): 700-6.

Mervaala, E. M., J. J. Himberg, et al. (1992). "Beneficial effects of a potassium- and magnesium-enriched salt alternative." Hypertension **19**(6 Pt 1): 535-40.

Millane, T. A. and A. J. Camm (1992). "Magnesium and the myocardium [editorial]." Br Heart J **68**(5): 441-2.

Nadler, J. L., S. Malayan, et al. (1992). "Intracellular free magnesium deficiency plays a key role in increased platelet reactivity in type II diabetes mellitus." Diabetes Care **15**(7): 835-41.

Ott, P. and P. Fenster (1992). "Should magnesium be part of the routine therapy for acute myocardial infarction? [editorial]." Am Heart J **124**(4): 1113-8.

Paolisso, G., G. Di Maro, et al. (1992). "Chronic magnesium administration enhances oxidative glucose metabolism in thiazide treated hypertensive patients." Am J Hypertens **5**(10): 681-6.

Paolisso, G., S. Sgambato, et al. (1992). "Daily magnesium supplements improve glucose handling in elderly subjects." Am J Clin Nutr **55**(6): 1161-7.

Resnick, L. M. (1992). "Cellular calcium and magnesium metabolism in the pathophysiology and treatment of hypertension and related metabolic disorders." Am J Med **93**(2A): 11S-20S.

Resnick, L. M. (1992). "Cellular ions in hypertension, insulin resistance, obesity, and diabetes: a unifying theme." J Am Soc Nephrol **3**(4 Suppl): S78-85.

Rude, R. K. (1992). "Magnesium deficiency and diabetes mellitus. Causes and effects." Postgrad Med **92**(5): 217-9.

Schnack, C., I. Bauer, et al. (1992). "Hypomagnesaemia in type 2 (non-insulin-dependent) diabetes mellitus is not corrected by improvement of long-term metabolic control." Diabetologia **35**(1): 77-9.

Shechter, M., E. Kaplinsky, et al. (1992). "The rationale of magnesium supplementation in acute myocardial infarction. A review of the literature." Arch Intern Med **152**(11): 2189-96.

Stendig-Lindberg, G. (1992). "Sudden death of athletes: is it due to long-term changes in serum magnesium, lipids and blood sugar?" J Basic Clin Physiol Pharmacol **3**(2): 153-64.

Tan, I. K., K. S. Chua, et al. (1992). "Serum magnesium, copper, and zinc concentrations in acute myocardial infarction." J Clin Lab Anal **6**(5): 324-8.

Weglicki, W. B., S. Bloom, et al. (1992). "Antioxidants and the cardiomyopathy of Mg-deficiency." Am J Cardiovasc Pathol **4**(3): 210-5.

Whang, R., D. D. Whang, et al. (1992). "Refractory potassium repletion. A consequence of magnesium deficiency." Arch Intern Med **152**(1): 40-5.

Woods, K. L., S. Fletcher, et al. (1992). "Intravenous magnesium sulphate in suspected acute myocardial infarction: results of the second Leicester Intravenous Magnesium Intervention Trial (LIMIT-2)." Lancet **339**(8809): 1553-8.

Altura, B. M. and B. T. Altura (1991). "Cardiovascular risk factors and magnesium: relationships to atherosclerosis, ischemic heart disease and hypertension." Magnes Trace Elem **10**(2-4): 182-92.

Dzurik, R., K. Stefikova, et al. (1991). "The role of magnesium deficiency in insulin resistance: an in vitro study." J Hypertens Suppl **9**(6): S312-3.

Mediterranean Diet/French Paradox

Frankel, E. N., J. Kanner, et al. (1993). "Inhibition of oxidation of human low-density lipoprotein by phenolic substances in red wine." Lancet **341**(8843): 454-7.

Lindholm, L. H., A. D. Koutis, et al. (1992). "Risk factors for ischaemic heart disease in a Greek population. A cross-sectional study of men and women living in the village of Spili in Crete." Eur Heart J **13**(3): 291-8.

Mariani-Costantini, A. and G. Ligabue (1992). "Did Columbus also open the exploration of the modern diet?" Nutr Rev **50**(11): 313-9.

Renaud, S. and M. de Lorgeril (1992). "Wine, alcohol, platelets, and the French paradox for coronary heart disease." Lancet **339**(8808): 1523-6.

Vialettes, B. (1992). "[Mediterranean nutrition: a model for the world?]." Arch Mal Coeur Vaiss **85**(1): 135-8.

Buzina, R., K. Suboticanec, et al. (1991). "Diet patterns and health problems: diet in southern Europe." Ann Nutr Metab **35**(1): 32-40.

Katsouyanni, K., Y. Skalkidis, et al. (1991). "Diet and peripheral arterial occlusive disease: the role of poly-, mono-, and saturated fatty acids." Am J Epidemiol **133**(1): 24-31.

Masana, L., M. Camprubi, et al. (1991). "The Mediterranean-type diet: is there a need for further modification?" Am J Clin Nutr **53**(4): 886-9.

Minerals

Nerbrand, C., K. Svardsudd, et al. (1992). "Cardiovascular mortality and morbidity in seven counties in Sweden in relation to water hardness and geological settings. The project: myocardial infarction in mid-Sweden." Eur Heart J **13**(6): 721-7.

Neve, J. (1992). "Clinical implications of trace elements in endocrinology." Biol Trace Elem Res **32**(1): 173-85.

Karppanen, H. (1991). "Minerals and blood pressure." Ann Med **23**(3): 299-305.

Luft, F. C. and D. A. McCarron (1991). "Heterogeneity of hypertension: the diverse role of electrolyte intake." Annu Rev Med **42**(1): 347-55.

McCarron, D. A. (1991). "A consensus approach to electrolytes and blood pressure. Could we all be right?" Hypertension **17**(1 Suppl): I170-2.

N-acetyl-cysteine

Boesgaard, S., H. E. Poulsen, et al. (1993). "Acute effects of nitroglycerin depend on both plasma and intracellular sulfhydryl compound levels in vivo. Effect of agents with different sulfhydryl-modulating properties." Circulation **87**(2): 547-53.

Boesgaard, S., J. Aldershvile, et al. (1992). "Preventive administration of intravenous N-acetylcysteine and development of tolerance to isosorbide dinitrate in patients with angina pectoris." Circulation **85**(1): 143-9.

Ghio, S., S. de Servi, et al. (1992). "Different susceptibility to the development of nitroglycerin tolerance in the arterial and venous circulation in humans. Effects of N-acetylcysteine administration." Circulation **86**(3): 798-802.

Kleinveld, H. A., P. N. Demacker, et al. (1992). "Failure of N-acetylcysteine to reduce low-density lipoprotein oxidizability in healthy subjects." Eur J Clin Pharmacol **43**(6): 639-42.

Boesgaard, S., J. Aldershvile, et al. (1991). "Continuous oral N-acetylcysteine treatment and development of nitrate tolerance in patients with stable angina pectoris." J Cardiovasc Pharmacol **17**(6): 889-93.

Boesgaard, S., J. S. Petersen, et al. (1991). "Nitrate tolerance: effect of thiol supplementation during prolonged nitroglycerin infusion in an in vivo rat model." J Pharmacol Exp Ther **258**(3): 851-6.

Cotgreave, I., P. Moldeus, et al. (1991). "The metabolism of N-acetylcysteine by human endothelial cells." Biochem Pharmacol **42**(1): 13-6.

Di Mascio, P., M. E. Murphy, et al. (1991). "Antioxidant defense systems: the role of carotenoids, tocopherols, and thiols." Am J Clin Nutr **53**(1 Suppl): 194S-200S.

Ferrari, R., C. Ceconi, et al. (1991). "Oxygen free radicals and myocardial damage: protective role of thiol-containing agents." Am J Med **91**(3C):

Gavish, D. and J. L. Breslow (1991). "Lipoprotein(a) reduction by N-acetylcysteine [see comments]." Lancet **337**(8735): 203-4.

Horowitz, J. D. (1991). "Thiol-containing agents in the management of unstable angina pectoris and acute myocardial infarction." Am J Med **91**(3C): 113S-117S.

Kroon, A. A., P. N. Demacker, et al. (1991). "N-acetylcysteine and serum concentrations of lipoprotein(a)." J Intern Med **230**(6): 519-26.

Natural Heart Therapies

(1993). "Mighty vitamins. Vitamins emerging as disease fighters, not just supplements. (Cover story)." Medical World News **34**(1): 24-32.

(1992). "The effects of nonpharmacologic interventions on blood pressure of persons with high normal levels. Results of the Trials of Hypertension Prevention, Phase I [published erratum appears in JAMA 1992 May 6; 267(17):2330] [see comments]." Jama **267**(9): 1213-20.

Applegate, W. B., S. T. Miller, et al. (1992). "Nonpharmacologic intervention to reduce blood pressure in older patients with mild hypertension." Arch Intern Med **152**(6): 1162-6.

Ascherio, A., E. B. Rimm, et al. (1992). "A prospective study of nutritional factors and hypertension among US men [see comments]." Circulation **86**(5): 1475-84.

Hishikawa, K., T. Nakaki, et al. (1992). "L-arginine as an antihypertensive agent." J Cardiovasc Pharmacol **20**(1): S196-7.

Winterfeld, H. J., H. Siewert, et al. (1992). "[Potential use of the sauna in the long-term treatment of hypertensive cardiovascular circulation disorders—a comparison with kinesiotherapy]." Schweiz Rundsch Med Prax **81**(35): 1016-20.

(1991). "The treatment of mild hypertension study. A randomized, placebo-controlled trial of a nutritional-hygienic regimen along with various drug monotherapies. The Treatment of Mild Hypertension Research Group." Arch Intern Med **151**(7): 1413-23.

Ascherio, A., M. J. Stampfer, et al. (1991). "Nutrient intakes and blood pressure in normotensive males." Int J Epidemiol **20**(4): 886-91.

Beretz, A. and J. P. Cazenave (1991). "Old and new natural products as the source of modern antithrombotic drugs." Planta Med **57**(7): S68-72.

Blake, G. H. and D. K. Beebe (1991). "Management of hypertension. Useful nonpharmacologic measures." Postgrad Med **90**(1): 151-4.

Cappuccio, F. P. and G. A. Mac Gregor (1991). "Does potassium supplementation lower blood pressure? A meta-analysis of published trials." J Hypertens **9**(5): 465-73.

Elmer, P. J., R. Grimm Jr., et al. (1991). "Dietary sodium reduction for hypertension prevention and treatment." Hypertension **17**(1 Suppl): I182-9.

Kaplan, N. M. (1991). "Long-term effectiveness of nonpharmacological treatment of hypertension." Hypertension **18**(3 Suppl): I153-60.

Kotchen, T. A., J. M. Kotchen, et al. (1991). "Nutrition and hypertension prevention." Hypertension **18**(3 Suppl): I115-20.

Tjoa, H. I. and N. M. Kaplan (1991). "Nonpharmacological treatment of hypertension in diabetes mellitus." Diabetes Care **14**(6): 449-60.

Kaplan, N. M. (1990). "The potential benefits of nonpharmacological therapy." Am J Hypertens **3**(5 Pt 1): 425-7.

NCEP (National Cholesterol Education Program)

Kummerow, F. A. (1993). "Viewpoint on the Report of the National Cholesterol Education Program Expert Panel on Detection, Evaluation and Treatment of High Blood Cholesterol in Adults." J Am Coll Nutr **12**(1): 2-13.

(1992). "Highlights of the report of the expert panel on blood cholesterol levels in children and adolescents. National Cholesterol Education Program Expert Panel on Blood Cholesterol Levels in Children and Adolescents." Am Fam Physician **45**(5): 2127-36.

(1992). "National Cholesterol Education Program (NCEP): highlights of the report of the Expert Panel on Blood Cholesterol Levels in Children and Adolescents [see comments]." Pediatrics **89**(3): 495-501.

Fix, K. N. and A. Oberman (1992). "Barriers to following National Cholesterol Educational Program guidelines. An appraisal of poor physician compliance [editorial; comment]." Arch Intern Med **152**(12): 2385-7.

Headrick, L. A., T. Speroff, et al. (1992). "Efforts to improve compliance with the National Cholesterol Education Program guidelines. Results of a randomized controlled trial [see comments]." Arch Intern Med **152**(12): 2490-6.

Rosenthal, S. L., S. Knauer-Black, et al. (1992). "The National Cholesterol Education Program pediatric guidelines: behavioral considerations." J Dev Behav Pediatr **13**(4): 288-9.

Niacin

Jacobson, E. L. and M. K. Jacobson (1993). "A biomarker for the assessment of niacin nutriture as a potential preventive factor in carcinogenesis." J Intern Med **233**(1): 59-62.

Schmidt, E. B., D. R. Illingworth, et al. (1993). "Hypolipidemic effects of nicotinic acid in patients with familial defective apolipoprotein B-100." Metabolism **42**(2): 137-9.

Dalton, T. A. and R. S. Berry (1992). "Hepatotoxicity associated with sustained-release niacin." Am J Med **93**(1): 102-4.

Dearing, B. D., C. J. Lavie, et al. (1992). "Niacin-induced clotting factor synthesis deficiency with coagulopathy." Arch Intern Med **152**(4): 861-3.

Keenan, J. M., C. Y. Bae, et al. (1992). "Treatment of hypercholesterolemia: comparison of younger versus older patients using wax-matrix sustained-release niacin." J Am Geriatr Soc **40**(1): 12-8.

Keenan, J. M., J. B. Wenz, et al. (1992). "A clinical trial of oat bran and niacin in the treatment of hyperlipidemia." J Fam Pract **34**(3): 313-9.

Lavie, C. J., L. Mailander, et al. (1992). "Marked benefit with sustained-release niacin therapy in patients with "isolated" very low levels of high-density lipoprotein cholesterol and coronary artery disease." Am J Cardiol **69**(12): 1083-5.

Lepre, F., B. Campbell, et al. (1992). "Low-dose sustained release nicotinic acid (Tri-B3) and lipoprotein (a) [letter]." Am J Cardiol **70**(1): 133.

Rader, J. I., R. J. Calvert, et al. (1992). "Hepatic toxicity of unmodified and time-release preparations of niacin." Am J Med **92**(1): 77-81.

Squires, R. W., T. G. Allison, et al. (1992). "Low-dose, time-release nicotinic acid: effects in selected patients with low concentrations of high-density lipoprotein cholesterol." Mayo Clin Proc **67**(9): 855-60.

Stern, R. H., D. Freeman, et al. (1992). "Differences in metabolism of time-release and unmodified nicotinic acid: explanation of the differences in hypolipidemic action?" Metabolism **41**(8): 879-81.

Superko, H. R. and R. M. Krauss (1992). "Differential effects of nicotinic acid in subjects with different LDL subclass patterns." Atherosclerosis **95**(1): 69-76.

Whelan, A. M., S. O. Price, et al. (1992). "The effect of aspirin on niacin-induced cutaneous reactions [see comments]." J Fam Pract **34**(2): 165-8.

Berge, K. G. and P. L. Canner (1991). "Coronary drug project: experience with niacin. Coronary Drug Project Research Group." Eur J Clin Pharmacol **40**(1): S49-51.

Di Palma, J. R. and W. S. Thayer (1991). "Use of niacin as a drug." Annu Rev Nutr **11**(1): 169-87.

Drood, J. M., P. J. Zimetbaum, et al. (1991). "Nicotinic acid for the treatment of hyperlipoproteinemia." J Clin Pharmacol **31**(7): 641-50.

Frost, P. H. (1991). "All niacin is not the same [letter]." Ann Intern Med **114**(12): 1065.

Gorrell, R. L. (1991). "Niacin caution." Postgrad Med **89**(4): 262.

Henkin, Y., A. Oberman, et al. (1991). "Niacin revisited: clinical observations on an important but underutilized drug." Am J Med **91**(3): 239-46.

Keenan, J. M., P. L. Fontaine, et al. (1991). "Niacin revisited. A randomized, controlled trial of wax-matrix sustained-release niacin in hypercholesterolemia." Arch Intern Med **151**(7): 1424-32.

Malloy, M. J., P. H. Frost, et al. (1991). "Niacin—the long and the short of it [editorial; comment] [see comments]." West J Med **155**(4): 424-6.

Palumbo, P. J. (1991). "Rediscovery of crystalline niacin [editorial; comment]." Mayo Clin Proc **66**(1): 112-3.

Pasternak, R. C. and B. S. Kolman (1991). "Unstable myocardial ischemia after the initiation of niacin therapy." Am J Cardiol **67**(9): 904-6.

Stern, R. H., J. D. Spence, et al. (1991). "Tolerance to nicotinic acid flushing." Clin Pharmacol Ther **50**(1): 66-70.

Garg, A. and S. M. Grundy (1990). "Nicotinic acid as therapy for dyslipidemia in non-insulin-dependent diabetes mellitus [see comments]." Jama **264**(6): 723-6.

Henkin, Y., K. C. Johnson, et al. (1990). "Rechallenge with crystalline niacin after drug-induced hepatitis from sustained-release niacin." Jama **264**(2): 241-3.

Alderman, J. D., R. C. Pasternak, et al. (1989). "Effect of a modified, well-tolerated niacin regimen on serum total cholesterol, high density lipoprotein cholesterol and the cholesterol to high density lipoprotein ratio." Am J Cardiol **64**(12): 725-9.

Urberg, M., J. Benyi, et al. (1988). "Hypocholesterolemic effects of nicotinic acid and chromium supplementation." J Fam Pract **27**(6): 603-6.

Canner, P. L., K. G. Berge, et al. (1986). "Fifteen year mortality in Coronary Drug Project patients: long-term benefit with niacin." J Am Coll Cardiol **8**(6): 1245-55.

Gurakar, A., J. M. Hoeg, et al. (1985). "Levels of lipoprotein Lp(a) decline with neomycin and niacin treatment." Atherosclerosis **57**(2-3): 293-301.

Nitroglycerine

Boesgaard, S., H. E. Poulsen, et al. (1993). "Acute effects of nitroglycerin depend on both plasma and intracellular sulfhydryl compound levels in vivo. Effect of agents with different sulfhydryl-modulating properties." Circulation **87**(2): 547-53.

Harrison, D. G. and J. N. Bates (1993). "The Nitrovasodilators. New ideas about old drugs." Circulation **87**: 1461-1467.

Karlberg, K. E., J. Ahlner, et al. (1993). "Effects of nitroglycerin on platelet aggregation beyond the effects of acetylsalicylic acid in healthy subjects." Am J Cardiol **71**(4): 361-4.

(1992). Optimizing antianginal therapy: a consensus conference. Am J Cardiology.

(1992). A symposium: Third North American conference on nitroglycerine therapy. AM J Cardiology.

Boesgaard, S., J. Aldershvile, et al. (1992). "Preventive administration of intravenous N-acetylcysteine and development of tolerance to isosorbide dinitrate in patients with angina pectoris." Circulation **85**(1): 143-9.

Chirkov, Y. Y., J. I. Naujalis, et al. (1992). "Reversal of human platelet aggregation by low concentrations of nitroglycerin in vitro in normal subjects." Am J Cardiol **70**(7): 802-6.

Ghio, S., S. de Servi, et al. (1992). "Different susceptibility to the development of nitroglycerin tolerance in the arterial and venous circulation in humans. Effects of N-acetylcysteine administration." Circulation **86**(3): 798-802.

Horowitz, J. D. (1992). "Role of nitrates in unstable angina pectoris." Am J Cardiol **70**(8): 64B-71B.

Boesgaard, S., J. Aldershvile, et al. (1991). "Continuous oral N-acetylcysteine treatment and development of nitrate tolerance in patients with stable angina pectoris." J Cardiovasc Pharmacol **17**(6): 889-93.

Boesgaard, S., J. S. Petersen, et al. (1991). "Nitrate tolerance: effect of thiol supplementation during prolonged nitroglycerin infusion in an in vivo rat model." J Pharmacol Exp Ther **258**(3): 851-6.

Nuts and Avocados

Sabate, J., G. E. Fraser, et al. (1993). "Effects of walnuts on serum lipid levels and blood pressure in normal men." N Engl J Med **328**(9): 603-7.

Castelli, W. P. (1992). "Concerning the possibility of a nut... [editorial; comment]." Arch Intern Med **152**(7): 1371-2.

Colquhoun, D. M., D. Moores, et al. (1992). "Comparison of the effects on lipoproteins and apolipoproteins of a diet high in monounsaturated fatty acids, enriched with avocado, and a high-carbohydrate diet." Am J Clin Nutr **56**(4): 671-7.

Durlach, J. (1992). "Commentary on recent clinical advances: almonds, monounsaturated fats, magnesium and hypolipidaemic diets." Magnes Res **5**(4): 315.

Fraser, G. E., J. Sabate, et al. (1992). "A possible protective effect of nut consumption on risk of coronary heart disease. The Adventist Health Study [see comments]." Arch Intern Med **152**(7): 1416-24.

Spiller, G. A., D. J. Jenkins, et al. (1992). "Effect of a diet high in monounsaturated fat from almonds on plasma cholesterol and lipoproteins." J Am Coll Nutr **11**(2): 126-30.

Olive Oil/Monounsaturated Fatty Acids (MUFA)

Aviram, M. and K. Eias (1993). "Dietary olive oil reduces low-density lipoprotein uptake by macrophages and decreases the susceptibility of the lipoprotein to undergo lipid peroxidation." Ann Nutr Metab **37**(2): 75-84.

Aviram, M. and E. Kassem (1993). "[Olive oil dietary supplementation decreases susceptibility of LDL to oxidation and its uptake by macrophages]." Harefuah **124**(1): 1-4.

Reaven, P., S. Parthasarathy, et al. (1993). "Effects of oleate-rich and linoleate-rich diets on the susceptibility of low density lipoprotein to oxidative modification in mildly hypercholesterolemic subjects." J Clin Invest **91**(2): 668-76.

Berry, E. M., S. Eisenberg, et al. (1992). "Effects of diets rich in monounsaturated fatty acids on plasma lipoproteins—the Jerusalem Nutrition Study. II. Monounsaturated fatty acids vs carbohydrates." Am J Clin Nutr **56**(2): 394-403.

Bonanome, A., A. Pagnan, et al. (1992). "Effect of dietary monounsaturated and polyunsaturated fatty acids on the susceptibility of plasma low density lipoproteins to oxidative modification." Arterioscler Thromb **12**(4): 529-33.

Bosaeus, I., L. Belfrage, et al. (1992). "Olive oil instead of butter increases net cholesterol excretion from the small bowel." Eur J Clin Nutr **46**(2): 111-5.

Colquhoun, D. M., D. Moores, et al. (1992). "Comparison of the effects on lipoproteins and apolipoproteins of a diet high in monounsaturated fatty acids, enriched with avocado, and a high-carbohydrate diet." Am J Clin Nutr **56**(4): 671-7.

Durlach, J. (1992). "Commentary on recent clinical advances: almonds, monounsaturated fats, magnesium and hypolipidaemic diets." Magnes Res **5**(4): 315.

Foley, M., M. Ball, et al. (1992). "Should mono- or poly-unsaturated fats replace saturated fat in the diet?" Eur J Clin Nutr **46**(6): 429-36.

Gatti, E., D. Noe, et al. (1992). "Differential effect of unsaturated oils and butter on blood glucose and insulin response to carbohydrate in normal volunteers." Eur J Clin Nutr **46**(3): 161-6.

Gustafsson, I. B., B. Vessby, et al. (1992). "Effects of lipid-lowering diets enriched with monounsaturated and polyunsaturated fatty acids on serum lipoprotein composition in patients with hyperlipoproteinaemia." Atherosclerosis **96**(2-3): 109-18.

Khosla, P. and K. C. Hayes (1992). "Comparison between the effects of dietary saturated (16:0), monounsaturated (18:1), and polyunsaturated (18:2) fatty acids on plasma lipoprotein metabolism in cebus and rhesus monkeys fed cholesterol-free diets." Am J Clin Nutr **55**(1): 51-62.

Mata, P., L. A. Alvarez-Sala, et al. (1992). "Effects of long-term monounsaturated- vs polyunsaturated-enriched diets on lipoproteins in healthy men and women." Am J Clin Nutr **55**(4): 846-50.

Mata, P., J. A. Garrido, et al. (1992). "Effect of dietary monounsaturated fatty acids on plasma lipoproteins and apolipoproteins in women." Am J Clin Nutr **56**(1): 77-83.

Mori, T. A., R. Vandongen, et al. (1992). "Plasma lipid levels and platelet and neutrophil function in patients with vascular disease following fish oil and olive oil supplementation." Metabolism **41**(10): 1059-67.

Mutanen, M., P. Kleemola, et al. (1992). "Lack of effect on blood pressure by polyunsaturated and monounsaturated fat diets." Eur J Clin Nutr **46**(1): 1-6.

Pagnan, A. and A. Bonanome (1992). "Position statement: monounsaturated fatty acids in human nutrition." J Am Coll Nutr **11**(1): 79S-81S.

Parillo, M., A. A. Rivellese, et al. (1992). "A high-monounsaturated-fat/low-carbohydrate diet improves peripheral insulin sensitivity in non-insulin-dependent diabetic patients." Metabolism **41**(12): 1373-8.

Scaccini, C., M. Nardini, et al. (1992). "Effect of dietary oils on lipid peroxidation and on antioxidant parameters of rat plasma and lipoprotein fractions." J Lipid Res **33**(5): 627-33.

Spiller, G. A., D. J. Jenkins, et al. (1992). "Effect of a diet high in monounsaturated fat from almonds on plasma cholesterol and lipoproteins." J Am Coll Nutr **11**(2): 126-30.

Valsta, L. M., M. Jauhiainen, et al. (1992). "Effects of a monounsaturated rapeseed oil and a polyunsaturated sunflower oil diet on lipoprotein levels in humans." Arterioscler Thromb **12**(1): 50-7.

Wahrburg, U., H. Martin, et al. (1992). "Comparative effects of a recommended lipid-lowering diet vs a diet rich in monounsaturated fatty acids on serum lipid profiles in healthy young adults." Am J Clin Nutr **56**(4): 678-83.

Berry, E. M., S. Eisenberg, et al. (1991). "Effects of diets rich in monounsaturated fatty acids on plasma lipoproteins—the Jerusalem Nutrition Study: high MUFAs vs high PUFAs." Am J Clin Nutr **53**(4): 899-907.

Bierenbaum, M. L., R. P. Reichstein, et al. (1991). "Effects of canola oil on serum lipids in humans." J Am Coll Nutr **10**(3): 228-33.

Bonanome, A., A. Visona, et al. (1991). "Carbohydrate and lipid metabolism in patients with non-insulin-dependent diabetes mellitus: effects of a low-fat, high-carbohydrate diet vs a diet high in monounsaturated fatty acids." Am J Clin Nutr **54**(3): 586-90.

Katsouyanni, K., Y. Skalkidis, et al. (1991). "Diet and peripheral arterial occlusive disease: the role of poly-, mono-, and saturated fatty acids." Am J Epidemiol **133**(1): 24-31.

McDonald, B. E. (1991). "Monounsaturated fatty acids and heart health." Can Med Assoc J **145**(5): 473.

Mori, T. A., R. Vandongen, et al. (1991). "Comparison of diets supplemented with fish oil or olive oil on plasma lipoproteins in insulin-dependent diabetics." Metabolism **40**(3): 241-6.

Reaven, P., S. Parthasarathy, et al. (1991). "Feasibility of using an oleate-rich diet to reduce the susceptibility of low-density lipoprotein to oxidative modification in humans." Am J Clin Nutr **54**(4): 701-6.

Trevisan, M., V. Krogh, et al. (1990). "Consumption of olive oil, butter, and vegetable oils and coronary heart disease risk factors. The Research Group ATS-RF2 of the Italian National Research Council [published erratum appears in JAMA 1990 Apr;263(13):1768]." Jama **263**(5): 688-92.

Mensink, R. P. and M. B. Katan (1989). "Effect of a diet enriched with monounsaturated or polyunsaturated fatty acids on levels of low-density and high-density lipoprotein cholesterol in healthy women and men [see comments]." N Engl J Med **321**(7): 436-41.

Oxidized LDL

Abbey, M., G. B. Belling, et al. (1993). "Oxidation of low-density lipoproteins: intraindividual variability and the effect of dietary linoleate supplementation." Am J Clin Nutr **57**(3): 391-8.

Aviram, M. (1993). "Modified forms of low density lipoprotein and atherosclerosis." Atherosclerosis **98**(1): 1-9.

Aviram, M. and K. Eias (1993). "Dietary olive oil reduces low-density lipoprotein uptake by macrophages and decreases the susceptibility of the lipoprotein to undergo lipid peroxidation." Ann Nutr Metab **37**(2): 75-84.

Aviram, M. and E. Kassem (1993). "[Olive oil dietary supplementation decreases susceptibility of LDL to oxidation and its uptake by macrophages]." Harefuah **124**(1): 1-4.

Buettner, G. R. (1993). "The pecking order of free radicals and antioxidants: lipid peroxidation, alpha-tocopherol, and ascorbate." Arch Biochem Biophys **300**(2): 535-43.

Chen, Y., M. Zhou, et al. (1993). "Lipoperoxidative damage in experimental rabbits with atherosclerosis." Chin Med J **106**(2): 110-4.

Corboy, J., W. H. Sutherland, et al. (1993). "Fatty acid composition and the oxidation of low-density lipoproteins." Biochem Med Metab Biol **49**(1): 25-35.

Davidson, M. H. (1993). "Antioxidants and lipid metabolism. Implications for the present and direction for the future." Am J Cardiol **71**(6): 32B-36B.

Davies, S. W., J. P. Duffy, et al. (1993). "Time-course of free radical activity during coronary artery operations with cardiopulmonary bypass." J Thorac Cardiovasc Surg **105**(6): 979-87.

Dejager, S., E. Bruckert, et al. (1993). "Dense low density lipoprotein subspecies with diminished oxidative resistance predominate in combined hyperlipidemia." J Lipid Res **34**(2): 295-308.

Duthie, G. G., J. R. Arthur, et al. (1993). "Cigarette smoking, antioxidants, lipid peroxidation, and coronary heart disease." Ann N Y Acad Sci **686**(1): 120-9.

Ferns, G. A., M. Konneh, et al. (1993). "Vitamin E: the evidence for an anti-atherogenic role." Artery **20**(2): 61-94.

Frankel, E. N., J. Kanner, et al. (1993). "Inhibition of oxidation of human low-density lipoprotein by phenolic substances in red wine." Lancet **341**(8843): 454-7.

Giroux, L. M., J. Davignon, et al. (1993). "Simvastatin inhibits the oxidation of low-density lipoproteins by activated human monocyte-derived macrophages." Biochim Biophys Acta **1165**(3): 335-8.

Gottlieb, K., E. J. Zarling, et al. (1993). "Beta-carotene decreases markers of lipid peroxidation in healthy volunteers." Nutr Cancer **19**(2): 207-12.

Halliwell, B. and S. Chirico (1993). "Lipid peroxidation: its mechanism, measurement, and significance." Am J Clin Nutr **57**(5 Suppl): 724S-725S.

Ingold, K. U., V. W. Bowry, et al. (1993). "Autoxidation of lipids and antioxidation by alpha-tocopherol and ubiquinol in homogeneous solution and in aqueous dispersions of lipids: unrecognized consequences of lipid particle size as exemplified by oxidation of human low density lipoprotein." Proc Natl Acad Sci U S A **90**(1): 45-9.

Jialal, I. and C. J. Fuller (1993). "Oxidized LDL and antioxidants." Clin Cardiol **16**(4 Suppl 1): I6-9.

Kanter, M. M., L. A. Nolte, et al. (1993). "Effects of an antioxidant vitamin mixture on lipid peroxidation at rest and postexercise." J Appl Physiol **74**(2): 965-9.

Lavy, A., A. Ben Amotz, et al. (1993). "Preferential inhibition of LDL oxidation by the all-trans isomer of beta-carotene in comparison with 9-cis beta-carotene." Eur J Clin Chem Clin Biochem **31**(2): 83-90.

Lyons, T. J. (1993). "Glycation and oxidation: a role in the pathogenesis of atherosclerosis." Am J Cardiol **71**(6): 26B-31B.

Negre-Salvayre, A., M. T. Pieraggi, et al. (1993). "Protective effect of 17 beta-estradiol against the cytotoxicity of minimally oxidized LDL to cultured bovine aortic endothelial cells." Atherosclerosis **99**(2): 207-17.

Niki, E., S. Minamisawa, et al. (1993). "Membrane damage from lipid oxidation induced by free radicals and cigarette smoke." Ann N Y Acad Sci **686**(1): 29-37.

Ozer, N. K., P. Palozza, et al. (1993). "d-alpha-Tocopherol inhibits low density lipoprotein induced proliferation and protein kinase C activity in vascular smooth muscle cells." Febs Lett **322**(3): 307-10.

Phelps, S. and W. S. Harris (1993). "Garlic supplementation and lipoprotein oxidation susceptibility." Lipids **28**(5): 475-7.

Prasad, K. and J. Kalra (1993). "Oxygen free radicals and hypercholesterolemic atherosclerosis: effect of vitamin E." Am Heart J **125**(4): 958-73.

Rabl, H., G. Khoschsorur, et al. (1993). "A multivitamin infusion prevents lipid peroxidation and improves transplantation performance." Kidney Int **43**(4): 912-7.

Rayssiguier, Y., E. Gueux, et al. (1993). "Dietary magnesium affects susceptibility of lipoproteins and tissues to peroxidation in rats." J Am Coll Nutrt **12**(2): 133-137.

Reaven, P., S. Parthasarathy, et al. (1993). "Effects of oleate-rich and linoleate-rich diets on the susceptibility of low density lipoprotein to oxidative modification in mildly hypercholesterolemic subjects." J Clin Invest **91**(2): 668-76.

Reaven, P. D., A. Khouw, et al. (1993). "Effect of dietary antioxidant combinations in humans. Protection of LDL by vitamin E but not by beta-carotene." Arterioscler Thromb **13**(4): 590-600.

Reaven, P. D. and J. L. Witztum (1993). "Comparison of supplementation of RRR-alpha-tocopherol and racemic alpha-tocopherol in humans. Effects on lipid levels and lipoprotein susceptibility to oxidation." Arterioscler Thromb **13**(4): 601-8.

Retsky, K. L., M. W. Freeman, et al. (1993). "Ascorbic acid oxidation product(s) protect human low density lipoprotein against atherogenic modification. Anti- rather than prooxidant activity of vitamin C in the presence of transition metal ions." J Biol Chem **268**(2): 1304-9.

Sheehy, P. J., P. A. Morrissey, et al. (1993). "Influence of heated vegetable oils and alpha-tocopheryl acetate supplementation on alpha-tocopherol, fatty acids and lipid peroxidation in chicken muscle." Br Poult Sci **34**(2): 367-81.

Shivaswamy, V., C. K. Kurup, et al. (1993). "Ferrous-iron induces lipid peroxidation with little damage to energy transduction in mitochondria." Mol Cell Biochem **120**(2): 141-9.

Smith, D., V. J. O'Leary, et al. (1993). "The role of alpha-tocopherol as a peroxyl radical scavenger in human low density lipoprotein." Biochem Pharmacol **45**(11): 2195-201.

Steinberg, D. (1993). "Modified forms of low-density lipoprotein and atherosclerosis." J Intern Med **233**(3): 227-32.

Walldius, G., J. Regnstrom, et al. (1993). "The role of lipids and antioxidative factors for development of atherosclerosis. The Probucol Quantitative Regression Swedish Trial (PQRST)." Am J Cardiol **71**(6): 15B-19B.

Witztum, J. L. (1993). "Role of oxidised low density lipoprotein in atherogenesis." Br Heart J **69**(1 Suppl): S12-8.

Witztum, J. L. (1993). "Susceptibility of low-density lipoprotein to oxidative modification (Editorial)." AM J Med **94**(4): 347-9.

Abdalla, D. S., A. Campa, et al. (1992). "Low density lipoprotein oxidation by stimulated neutrophils and ferritin." Atherosclerosis **97**(2-3): 149-59.

Aviram, M., G. Dankner, et al. (1992). "Lovastatin inhibits low-density lipoprotein oxidation and alters its fluidity and uptake by macrophages: in vitro and in vivo studies." Metabolism **41**(3): 229-35.

Babiy, A. V., J. M. Gebicki, et al. (1992). "Increased oxidizability of plasma lipoproteins in diabetic patients can be decreased by probucol therapy and is not due to glycation." Biochem Pharmacol **43**(5): 995-1000.

Berliner, J. A., M. Territo, et al. (1992). "Minimally modified lipoproteins in diabetes." Diabetes **41**(1): 74-6.

Bierenbaum, M. L., R. P. Reichstein, et al. (1992). "Relationship between serum lipid peroxidation products in hypercholesterolemic subjects and vitamin E status." Biochem Int **28**(1): 57-66.

Bonanome, A., A. Pagnan, et al. (1992). "Effect of dietary monounsaturated and polyunsaturated fatty acids on the susceptibility of plasma low density lipoproteins to oxidative modification." Arterioscler Thromb **12**(4): 529-33.

Bowry, V. W., K. U. Ingold, et al. (1992). "Vitamin E in human low-density lipoprotein. When and how this antioxidant becomes a pro-oxidant." Biochem J **288**(Pt 2): 341-4.

Chin, J. H., S. Azhar, et al. (1992). "Inactivation of endothelial derived relaxing factor by oxidized lipoproteins." J Clin Invest **89**(1): 10-8.

Chisolm, G. M., K. C. Irwin, et al. (1992). "Lipoprotein oxidation and lipoprotein-induced cell injury in diabetes." Diabetes **41**(1): 61-6.

Cristol, L. S., I. Jialal, et al. (1992). "Effect of low-dose probucol therapy on LDL oxidation and the plasma lipoprotein profile in male volunteers." Atherosclerosis **97**(1): 11-20.

Croft, K. D., S. B. Dimmitt, et al. (1992). "Low density lipoprotein composition and oxidizability in coronary disease—apparent favourable effect of beta blockers." Atherosclerosis **97**(2-3): 123-30.

Dargel, R. (1992). "Lipid peroxidation—a common pathogenetic mechanism?" Exp Toxicol Pathol **44**(4): 169-81.

Darley-Usmar, V. M., N. Hogg, et al. (1992). "The simultaneous generation of superoxide and nitric oxide can initiate lipid peroxidation in human low density lipoprotein." Free Radic Res Commun **17**(1): 9-20.

Dasgupta, A. and T. Zdunek (1992). "In vitro lipid peroxidation of human serum catalyzed by cupric ion: antioxidant rather than prooxidant role of ascorbate." Life Sci **50**(12): 875-82.

Dasgupta, A., T. Zdunek, et al. (1992). "Differential effects of transition metal ions on in vitro lipid peroxidation of human serum and protein precipitated from serum." Clin Physiol Biochem **9**(1): 7-10.

Ernster, L., P. Forsmark, et al. (1992). "The mode of action of lipid-soluble antioxidants in biological membranes. Relationship between the effects of ubiquinol and vitamin E as inhibitors of lipid peroxidation in submitochondrial particles." J Nutr Sci Vitaminol **1**(51): 548-51.

Esterbauer, H., J. Gebicki, et al. (1992). "The role of lipid peroxidation and antioxidants in oxidative modification of LDL." Free Radic Biol Med **13**(4): 341-90.

Esterbauer, H., H. Puhl, et al. (1992). "Vitamin E and atherosclerosis: an overview." J Nutr Sci Vitaminol **1**(82): 177-82.

Esterbauer, H., G. Waeg, et al. (1992). "Inhibition of LDL oxidation by antioxidants." Exs **62**(1): 145-57.

Gonzalez, M. J., J. I. Gray, et al. (1992). "Lipid peroxidation products are elevated in fish oil diets even in the presence of added antioxidants." J Nutr **122**(11): 2190-5.

Haberland, M. E., G. M. Fless, et al. (1992). "Malondialdehyde modification of lipoprotein(a) produces avid uptake by human monocyte-macrophages." J Biol Chem **267**(6): 4143-51.

Hoffman, R., G. J. Brook, et al. (1992). "Hypolipidemic drugs reduce lipoprotein susceptibility to undergo lipid peroxidation: in vitro and ex vivo studies." Atherosclerosis **93**(1-2): 105-13.

Ishikawa, Y., H. Inadera, et al. (1992). "Moderate oxidation of hypertriglyceridemic low-density lipoprotein causes apolipoprotein B epitope change and enhances its uptake by macrophages." Biochim Biophys Acta **1126**(1): 60-4.

Jialal, I. and S. M. Grundy (1992). "Effect of dietary supplementation with alpha-tocopherol on the oxidative modification of low density lipoprotein." J Lipid Res **33**(6): 899-906.

Jialal, I. and S. M. Grundy (1992). "Influence of antioxidant vitamins on LDL oxidation." Ann N Y Acad Sci **669**(1): 237-47.

Kagan, V. E., E. A. Serbinova, et al. (1992). "Recycling of vitamin E in human low density lipoproteins." J Lipid Res **33**(3): 385-97.

Kalyanaraman, B., U. V. Darley, et al. (1992). "Synergistic interaction between the probucol phenoxyl radical and ascorbic acid in inhibiting the oxidation of low density lipoprotein." J Biol Chem **267**(10): 6789-95.

Karlsson, J., B. Diamant, et al. (1992). "Plasma ubiquinone, alpha-tocopherol and cholesterol in man." Int J Vitam Nutr Res **62**(2): 160-4.

Kita, T., M. Yokode, et al. (1992). "The role of oxidized lipoproteins in the pathogenesis of atherosclerosis." Clin Exp Pharmacol Physiol Suppl **20**(1): 37-42.

Kuhn, H., J. Belkner, et al. (1992). "Structure elucidation of oxygenated lipids in human atherosclerotic lesions." Eicosanoids **5**(1): 17-22.

Liu, K. Z., T. E. Cuddy, et al. (1992). "Oxidative status of lipoproteins in coronary disease patients." Am Heart J **123**(2): 285-90.

Mangiapane, H., J. Thomson, et al. (1992). "The inhibition of the oxidation of low density lipoprotein by (+)-catechin, a naturally occurring flavonoid." Biochem Pharmacol **43**(3): 445-50.

Merati, G., P. Pasquali, et al. (1992). "Antioxidant activity of ubiquinone-3 in human low density lipoprotein." Free Radic Res Commun **16**(1): 11-7.

Mohr, D., V. W. Bowry, et al. (1992). "Dietary supplementation with coenzyme Q10 results in increased levels of ubiquinol-10 within circulating lipoproteins and increased resistance of human low-density lipoprotein to the initiation of lipid peroxidation." Biochim Biophys Acta **1126**(3): 247-54.

Musial, J., T. B. Domagala, et al. (1992). "Lipid peroxidation, vitamin E, and cardiovascular disease." J Nutr Sci Vitaminol **1**(3): 200-3.

Naruszewicz, M., E. Selinger, et al. (1992). "Oxidative modification of lipoprotein(a) and the effect of beta-carotene." Metabolism **41**(11): 1215-24.

Negre-Salvayre, A. and R. Salvayre (1992). "Quercetin prevents the cytotoxicity of oxidized LDL on lymphoid cell lines." Free Radic Biol Med **12**(2): 101-6.

Nilsson, J., J. Regnstrom, et al. (1992). "Lipid oxidation and atherosclerosis." Herz **17**(5): 263-9.

Odeleye, O. E., C. D. Eskelson, et al. (1992). "Vitamin E inhibition of lipid peroxidation and ethanol-mediated promotion of esophageal tumorigenesis." Nutr Cancer **17**(3): 223-34.

Parthasarathy, S. (1992). "Evidence for an additional intracellular site of action of probucol in the prevention of oxidative modification of low density lipoprotein. Use of a new water-soluble probucol derivative." J Clin Invest **89**(5): 1618-21.

Parthasarathy, S. (1992). "Role of lipid peroxidation and antioxidants in atherogenesis." J Nutr Sci Vitaminol **1**(6): 183-6.

Parthasarathy, S. and S. M. Rankin (1992). "Role of oxidized low density lipoprotein in atherogenesis." Prog Lipid Res **31**(2): 127-43.

Parthasarathy, S., D. Steinberg, et al. (1992). "The role of oxidized low-density lipoproteins in the pathogenesis of atherosclerosis." Annu Rev Med **43**(1): 219-25.

Princen, H. M., P. G. van, et al. (1992). "Supplementation with vitamin E but not beta-carotene in vivo protects low density lipoprotein from lipid peroxidation in vitro. Effect of cigarette smoking." Arterioscler Thromb **12**(5): 554-62.

Reddy, A. C. and B. R. Lokesh (1992). "Studies on spice principles as antioxidants in the inhibition of lipid peroxidation of rat liver microsomes." Mol Cell Biochem **111**(1-2): 117-24.

Regnstrom, J., J. Nilsson, et al. (1992). "Susceptibility to low-density lipoprotein oxidation and coronary atherosclerosis in man [see comments]." Lancet **339**(8803): 1183-6.

Rifici, V. A. and A. K. Khachadurian (1992). "The inhibition of low-density lipoprotein oxidation by 17-beta estradiol." Metabolism **41**(10): 1110-4.

Salonen, J. T., S. Yla-Herttuala, et al. (1992). "Autoantibody against oxidised LDL and progression of carotid atherosclerosis [see comments]." Lancet **339**(8798): 883-7.

Santiago, L. A., M. Hiramatsu, et al. (1992). "Japanese soybean paste miso scavenges free radicals and inhibits lipid peroxidation." J Nutr Sci Vitaminol **38**(3): 297-304.

Scaccini, C., M. Nardini, et al. (1992). "Effect of dietary oils on lipid peroxidation and on antioxidant parameters of rat plasma and lipoprotein fractions." J Lipid Res **33**(5): 627-33.

Scheffler, E., E. Wiest, et al. (1992). "Smoking influences the atherogenic potential of low-density lipoprotein." Clin Investig **70**(3-4): 263-8.

Schmidt, K., P. Klatt, et al. (1992). "High-density lipoprotein antagonizes the inhibitory effects of oxidized low-density lipoprotein and lysolecithin on soluble guanylyl cyclase." Biochem Biophys Res Commun **182**(1): 302-8.

Sharma, H. M., A. N. Hanna, et al. (1992). "Inhibition of human low-density lipoprotein oxidation in vitro by Maharishi Ayur-Veda herbal mixtures." Pharmacol Biochem Behav **43**(4): 1175-82.

Tihan, T., P. Chiba, et al. (1992). "Serum lipid peroxide levels in the course of coronary by-pass surgery." Eur J Clin Chem Clin Biochem **30**(4): 205-8.

Tribble, D. L., L. G. Holl, et al. (1992). "Variations in oxidative susceptibility among six low density lipoprotein subfractions of differing density and particle size." Atherosclerosis **93**(3): 189-99.

Weisser, B., R. Locher, et al. (1992). "Oxidized low-density lipoproteins in atherogenesis: possible mechanisms of action." J Cardiovasc Pharmacol **19**(1): S4-7.

Weisser, B., R. Locher, et al. (1992). "Oxidation of low density lipoprotein enhances its potential to increase intracellular free calcium concentration in vascular smooth muscle cells." Arterioscler Thromb **12**(2): 231-6.

Yamamoto, Y., K. Wakabayashi, et al. (1992). "Comparison of plasma levels of lipid hydroperoxides and antioxidants in hyperlipidemic Nagase analbuminemic rats, Sprague-Dawley rats, and humans." Biochem Biophys Res Commun **189**(1): 518-23.

Yue, T. L., P. J. McKenna, et al. (1992). "Carvedilol, a new antihypertensive, prevents oxidation of human low density lipoprotein by macrophages and copper." Atherosclerosis **97**(2-3): 209-16.

Aviram, M. (1991). "The contribution of the macrophage receptor for oxidized LDL to its cellular uptake." Biochem Biophys Res Commun **179**(1): 359-65.

Breugnot, C., C. Maziere, et al. (1991). "Calcium antagonists prevent monocyte and endothelial cell-induced modification of low density lipoproteins." Free Radic Res Commun **15**(2): 91-100.

Cathcart, M. K., A. K. McNally, et al. (1991). "Lipoxygenase-mediated transformation of human low density lipoprotein to an oxidized and cytotoxic complex." J Lipid Res **32**(1): 63-70.

Ciavatti, M. and S. Renaud (1991). "Oxidative status and oral contraceptive. Its relevance to platelet abnormalities and cardiovascular risk." Free Radic Biol Med **10**(5): 325-38.

Crawford, D. W. and D. H. Blankenhorn (1991). "Arterial wall oxygenation, oxyradicals, and atherosclerosis." Atherosclerosis **89**(2-3): 97-108.

de Graaf, J., H. L. Hak-Lemmers, et al. (1991). "Enhanced susceptibility to in vitro oxidation of the dense low density lipoprotein subfraction in healthy subjects." Arterioscler Thromb **11**(2): 298-306.

Dieber-Rotheneder, M., H. Puhl, et al. (1991). "Effect of oral supplementation with D-alpha-tocopherol on the vitamin E content of human low density lipoproteins and resistance to oxidation." J Lipid Res **32**(8): 1325-32.

Drake, T. A., K. Hannani, et al. (1991). "Minimally oxidized low-density lipoprotein induces tissue factor expression in cultured human endothelial cells." Am J Pathol **138**(3): 601-7.

Esterbauer, H., M. Dieber-Rotheneder, et al. (1991). "Role of vitamin E in preventing the oxidation of low-density lipoprotein." Am J Clin Nutr **53**(1 Suppl): 314S-321S.

Esterbauer, H., H. Puhl, et al. (1991). "Effect of antioxidants on oxidative modification of LDL." Ann Med **23**(5): 573-81.

Forsmark, P., F. Aberg, et al. (1991). "Inhibition of lipid peroxidation by ubiquinol in submitochondrial particles in the absence of vitamin E." Febs Lett **285**(1): 39-43.

Frei, B. (1991). "Ascorbic acid protects lipids in human plasma and low-density lipoprotein against oxidative damage." Am J Clin Nutr **54**(6 Suppl): 1113S-1118S.

Frei, B., T. M. Forte, et al. (1991). "Gas phase oxidants of cigarette smoke induce lipid peroxidation and changes in lipoprotein properties in human blood plasma. Protective effects of ascorbic acid." Biochem J **277**(Pt 1): 133-8.

Frostegard, J., A. Haegerstrand, et al. (1991). "Biologically modified LDL increases the adhesive properties of endothelial cells." Atherosclerosis **90**(2-3): 119-26.

Galle, J., A. Mulsch, et al. (1991). "Effects of native and oxidized low density lipoproteins on formation and inactivation of endothelium-derived relaxing factor." Arterioscler Thromb **11**(1): 198-203.

Groop, L. C., R. C. Bonadonna, et al. (1991). "Role of free fatty acids and insulin in determining free fatty acid and lipid oxidation in man." J Clin Invest **87**(1): 83-9.

Harats, D., Y. Dabach, et al. (1991). "Fish oil ingestion in smokers and nonsmokers enhances peroxidation of plasma lipoproteins." Atherosclerosis **90**(2-3): 127-39.

Hodis, H. N., D. W. Crawford, et al. (1991). "Cholesterol feeding increases plasma and aortic tissue cholesterol oxide levels in parallel: further evidence for the role of cholesterol oxidation in atherosclerosis." Atherosclerosis **89**(2-3): 117-26.

Hoff, H. F. and J. A. O'Neil (1991). "Oxidation of LDL: role in atherogenesis." Klin Wochenschr **69**(21-23): 1032-8.

Jialal, I., D. A. Freeman, et al. (1991). "Varying susceptibility of different low density lipoproteins to oxidative modification." Arterioscler Thromb **11**(3): 482-8.

Jialal, I. and S. M. Grundy (1991). "Preservation of the endogenous antioxidants in low density lipoprotein by ascorbate but not probucol during oxidative modification." J Clin Invest **87**(2): 597-601.

Jialal, I., E. P. Norkus, et al. (1991). "Beta-Carotene inhibits the oxidative modification of low-density lipoprotein." Biochim Biophys Acta **1086**(1): 134-8.

Kuzuya, M., M. Naito, et al. (1991). "Lipid peroxide and transition metals are required for the toxicity of oxidized low density lipoprotein to cultured endothelial cells." Biochim Biophys Acta **1096**(2): 155-61.

Kuzuya, M., K. Yamada, et al. (1991). "Oxidation of low-density lipoprotein by copper and iron in phosphate buffer." Biochim Biophys Acta **1084**(2): 198-201.

Lavy, A., G. J. Brook, et al. (1991). "Enhanced in vitro oxidation of plasma lipoproteins derived from hypercholesterolemic patients." Metabolism **40**(8): 794-9.

Liu, K. Z., B. Ramjiawan, et al. (1991). "Effects of oxidative modification of cholesterol in isolated low density lipoproteins on cultured smooth muscle cells." Mol Cell Biochem **108**(1): 49-56.

Luc, G. and J. C. Fruchart (1991). "Oxidation of lipoproteins and atherosclerosis." Am J Clin Nutr **53**(1 Suppl): 206S-209S.

Malden, L. T., A. Chait, et al. (1991). "The influence of oxidatively modified low density lipoproteins on expression of platelet-derived growth factor by human monocyte-derived macrophages." J Biol Chem **266**(21): 13901-7.

Masana, L., M. T. Bargallo, et al. (1991). "Effectiveness of probucol in reducing plasma low-density lipoprotein cholesterol oxidation in hypercholesterolemia." Am J Cardiol **68**(9): 863-7.

Maziere, C., M. Auclair, et al. (1991). "Estrogens inhibit copper and cell-mediated modification of low density lipoprotein." Atherosclerosis **89**(2-3): 175-82.

Meydani, M., F. Natiello, et al. (1991). "Effect of long-term fish oil supplementation on vitamin E status and lipid peroxidation in women." J Nutr **121**(4): 484-91.

Niki, E., Y. Yamamoto, et al. (1991). "Membrane damage due to lipid oxidation." Am J Clin Nutr **53**(1 Suppl): 201S-205S.

Panasenko, O. M., T. V. Vol'nova, et al. (1991). "Free-radical generation by monocytes and neutrophils: a possible cause of plasma lipoprotein modification." Biomed Sci **2**(6): 581-9.

Reaven, P., S. Parthasarathy, et al. (1991). "Feasibility of using an oleate-rich diet to reduce the susceptibility of low-density lipoprotein to oxidative modification in humans." Am J Clin Nutr **54**(4): 701-6.

Rosenfeld, M. E., J. C. Khoo, et al. (1991). "Macrophage-derived foam cells freshly isolated from rabbit atherosclerotic lesions degrade modified lipoproteins, promote oxidation of low-density lipoproteins, and contain oxidation-specific lipid-protein adducts." J Clin Invest **87**(1): 90-9.

Sakurai, T., S. Kimura, et al. (1991). "Oxidative modification of glycated low density lipoprotein in the presence of iron." Biochem Biophys Res Commun **177**(1): 433-9.

Steinbrecher, U. P. (1991). "Role of lipoprotein peroxidation in the pathogenesis of atherosclerosis." Clin Cardiol **14**(11): 865-7.

Stocker, R., V. W. Bowry, et al. (1991). "Ubiquinol-10 protects human low density lipoprotein more efficiently against lipid peroxidation than does alpha-tocopherol." Proc Natl Acad Sci U S A **88**(5): 1646-50.

Weisser, B., R. Locher, et al. (1991). "Oxidation of low-density lipoprotein increases vasoconstriction in vitro." J Hypertens Suppl **9**(6): S172-3.

Wiklund, O., L. Mattsson, et al. (1991). "Uptake and degradation of low density lipoproteins in atherosclerotic rabbit aorta: role of local LDL modification." J Lipid Res **32**(1): 55-62.

Witztum, J. L. (1991). "The role of oxidized LDL in atherosclerosis." Adv Exp Med Biol **285**(1): 353-65.

Witztum, J. L. and D. Steinberg (1991). "Role of oxidized low density lipoprotein in atherogenesis." J Clin Invest **88**(6): 1785-92.

Yla-Herttuala, S. (1991). "Macrophages and oxidized low density lipoproteins in the pathogenesis of atherosclerosis." Ann Med **23**(5): 561-7.

Babiy, A. V., J. M. Gebicki, et al. (1990). "Vitamin E content and low density lipoprotein oxidizability induced by free radicals." Atherosclerosis **81**(3): 175-82.

Harats, D., M. Ben-Naim, et al. (1990). "Effect of vitamin C and E supplementation on susceptibility of plasma lipoproteins to peroxidation induced by acute smoking." Atherosclerosis **85**(1): 47-54.

Hoshino, E., R. Shariff, et al. (1990). "Vitamin E suppresses increased lipid peroxidation in cigarette smokers." Jpen J Parenter Enteral Nutr **14**(3): 300-5.

Jialal, I., G. L. Vega, et al. (1990). "Physiologic levels of ascorbate inhibit the oxidative modification of low density lipoprotein." Atherosclerosis **82**(3): 185-91.

Leibovitz, B., M. L. Hu, et al. (1990). "Dietary supplements of vitamin E, beta-carotene, coenzyme Q10 and selenium protect tissues against lipid peroxidation in rat tissue slices." J Nutr **120**(1): 97-104.

Luoma, P. V., J. Stengard, et al. (1990). "Lipid peroxides, glutathione peroxidase, high density lipoprotein subfractions and apolipoproteins in young adults [see comments]." J Intern Med **227**(4): 287-9.

Partial Ileal Bypass Surgery

Buchwald, H., C. T. Campos, et al. (1992). "Women in the POSCH trial. Effects of aggressive cholesterol modification in women with coronary heart disease. The POSCH Group. Program on the Surgical Control of the Hyperlipidemias." Ann Surg **216**(4): 389-98.

Buchwald, H., L. L. Fitch, et al. (1992). "Partial ileal bypass in the treatment of hypercholesterolemia." J Fam Pract **35**(1): 69-76.

Buchwald, H., J. P. Matts, et al. (1992). "Changes in sequential coronary arteriograms and subsequent coronary events. Surgical Control of the Hyperlipidemias (POSCH) Group." Jama **268**(11): 1429-33.

Karnegis, J. N., J. P. Matts, et al. (1992). "Correlation of coronary with peripheral arterial stenosis. The POSCH Group." Atherosclerosis **92**(1): 25-30.

Buchwald, H., R. L. Varco, et al. (1990). "Effect of partial ileal bypass surgery on mortality and morbidity from coronary heart disease in patients with hypercholesterolemia. Report of the Program on the Surgical Control of the Hyperlipidemias (POSCH) [see comments]." N Engl J Med **323**(14): 946-55.

Pathology of Vascular Disease

Chen, Y., M. Zhou, et al. (1993). "Lipoperoxidative damage in experimental rabbits with atherosclerosis." Chin Med J **106**(2): 110-4.

Davies, M. J. and N. Woolf (1993). "Atherosclerosis: what is it and why does it occur?" Br Heart J **69**(1 Suppl): S3-11.

Dzau, V. J., G. H. Gibbons, et al. (1993). "Vascular biology and medicine in the 1990s: scope, concepts, potentials, and perspectives." Circulation **87**(3): 705-19.

Ferns, G. A., M. Konneh, et al. (1993). "Vitamin E: the evidence for an anti-atherogenic role." Artery **20**(2): 61-94.

Freyschuss, A., A. Stiko-Rahm, et al. (1993). "Antioxidant treatment inhibits the development of intimal thickening after balloon injury of the aorta in hypercholesterolemic rabbits." J Clin Invest **91**(4): 1282-8.

Halliwell, B. (1993). "The role of oxygen radicals in human disease, with particular reference to the vascular system." Haemostasis **23**(1): 118-26.

Harrison, D. G. (1993). "Endothelial dysfunction in the coronary microcirculation: a new clinical entity or an experimental finding? [editorial; comment]." J Clin Invest **91**(1): 1-2.

Li, H., M. I. Cybulsky, et al. (1993). "An atherogenic diet rapidly induces VCAM-1, a cytokine-regulatable mononuclear leukocyte adhesion molecule, in rabbit aortic endothelium." Arterioscler Thromb **13**(2): 197-204.

Lyons, T. J. (1993). "Glycation and oxidation: a role in the pathogenesis of atherosclerosis." Am J Cardiol **71**(6): 26B-31B.

Maxwell, S. R. (1993). "Can anti-oxidants prevent ischaemic heart disease?" J Clin Pharm Ther **18**(2): 85-95.

Nakamura, H. and M. Suzukawa (1993). "[Atherosclerosis, with special reference to vitamin E]." Nippon Rinsho **51**(4): 997-1003.

Prasad, K. and J. Kalra (1993). "Oxygen free radicals and hypercholesterolemic atherosclerosis: effect of vitamin E." Am Heart J **125**(4): 958-73.

Ranke, C., H. Hecker, et al. (1993). "Dose-dependent effect of aspirin on carotid atherosclerosis." Circulation **87**(6): 1873-9.

Schwartz, C. J., A. J. Valente, et al. (1993). "A modern view of atherogenesis." Am J Cardiol **71**(6): 9B-14B.

Steinberg, D. (1993). "Modified forms of low-density lipoprotein and atherosclerosis." J Intern Med **233**(3): 227-32.

Sun, Y. P., B. Q. Zhu, et al. (1993). "Aspirin inhibits platelet activity but does not attenuate experimental atherosclerosis." Am Heart J **125**(1): 79-86.

Chobanian, A. V. (1992). "Pathophysiology of atherosclerosis." Am J Cardiol **70**(17): 3G-7G.

Clinton, S. K. and P. Libby (1992). "Cytokines and growth factors in atherogenesis." Arch Pathol Lab Med **116**(12): 1292-300.

Esterbauer, H., H. Puhl, et al. (1992). "Vitamin E and atherosclerosis: an overview." J Nutr Sci Vitaminol **1**(82): 177-82.

Flavahan, N. A. (1992). "Atherosclerosis or lipoprotein-induced endothelial dysfunction. Potential mechanisms underlying reduction in EDRF/nitric oxide activity." Circulation **85**(5): 1927-38.

Fuster, V., J. J. Badimon, et al. (1992). "Clinical-pathological correlations of coronary disease progression and regression." Circulation **86**(6 Suppl): III1-11.

Fuster, V., L. Badimon, et al. (1992). "The pathogenesis of coronary artery disease and the acute coronary syndromes (2)." N Engl J Med **326**(5): 310-8.

Kramsch, D. M. and D. H. Blankenhorn (1992). "Regression of atherosclerosis: which components regress and what influences their reversal." Wien Klin Wochenschr **104**(1): 2-9.

Kuhn, H., J. Belkner, et al. (1992). "Structure elucidation of oxygenated lipids in human atherosclerotic lesions." Eicosanoids **5**(1): 17-22.

Libby, P. (1992). "Do vascular wall cytokines promote atherogenesis?" Hosp Pract **27**(10): 51-8.

Lichtlen, P. R., P. Nikutta, et al. (1992). "Anatomical progression of coronary artery disease in humans as seen by prospective, repeated, quantitated coronary angiography. Relation to clinical events and risk factors. The INTACT Study Group." Circulation **86**(3): 828-38.

Mautner, S. L., G. C. Mautner, et al. (1992). "Comparison of composition of atherosclerotic plaques in saphenous veins used as aortocoronary bypass conduits with plaques in native coronary arteries in the same men." Am J Cardiol **70**(18): 1380-7.

Parthasarathy, S. (1992). "Role of lipid peroxidation and antioxidants in atherogenesis." J Nutr Sci Vitaminol **1**(6): 183-6.

Parthasarathy, S. and S. M. Rankin (1992). "Role of oxidized low density lipoprotein in atherogenesis." Prog Lipid Res **31**(2): 127-43.

Parthasarathy, S., D. Steinberg, et al. (1992). "The role of oxidized low-density lipoproteins in the pathogenesis of atherosclerosis." Annu Rev Med **43**(1): 219-25.

Smith, E. B., W. D. Thompson, et al. (1992). "Fibrinogen/fibrin in atherogenesis." Eur J Epidemiol **8**(1): 83-7.

Stout, R. W. (1992). "Insulin and atherogenesis." Eur J Epidemiol **8**(1): 134-5.

Van Hinsbergh, V. W. (1992). "Arteriosclerosis. Impairment of cellular interactions in the arterial wall." Ann N Y Acad Sci **673**(1): 321-30.

van Hinsbergh, V. W. (1992). "Regulatory functions of the coronary endothelium." Mol Cell Biochem **116**(1-2): 163-9.

Verlangieri, A. J. and M. J. Bush (1992). "Effects of d-alpha-tocopherol supplementation on experimentally induced primate atherosclerosis." J Am Coll Nutr **11**(2): 131-8.

Weisser, B., R. Locher, et al. (1992). "Oxidized low-density lipoproteins in atherogenesis: possible mechanisms of action." J Cardiovasc Pharmacol **19**(1): S4-7.

Williams, R. J., J. M. Motteram, et al. (1992). "Dietary vitamin E and the attenuation of early lesion development in modified Watanabe rabbits." Atherosclerosis **94**(2-3): 153-9.

Wu, K. K. (1992). "Endothelial cells in hemostasis, thrombosis, and inflammation." Hosp Pract **27**(4): 145-50.

Mack, W. J. and D. H. Blankenhorn (1991). "Factors influencing the formation of new human coronary lesions: age, blood pressure, and blood cholesterol." Am J Public Health **81**(9): 1180-4.

Patterson, D. L. and T. Treasure (1991). "The culprit coronary artery lesion [see comments]." Lancet **338**(8779): 1379-80.

Raij, L. (1991). "Hypertension, endothelium, and cardiovascular risk factors." Am J Med **90**(2A): 13S-18S.

Steinbrecher, U. P. (1991). "Role of lipoprotein peroxidation in the pathogenesis of atherosclerosis." Clin Cardiol **14**(11): 865-7.

Stout, R. W. (1991). "Insulin as a mitogenic factor: role in the pathogenesis of cardiovascular disease." Am J Med **90**(2A): 62S-65S.

Wissler, R. W. (1991). "Update on the pathogenesis of atherosclerosis." Am J Med **91**(1B): 3S-9S.

Xu, C. P., S. Glagov, et al. (1991). "Hypertension sustains plaque progression despite reduction of hypercholesterolemia." Hypertension **18**(2): 123-9.

Yla-Herttuala, S. (1991). "Macrophages and oxidized low density lipoproteins in the pathogenesis of atherosclerosis." Ann Med **23**(5): 561-7.

Davies, M. J. (1990). "A macro and micro view of coronary vascular insult in ischemic heart disease." Circulation **82**(3 Suppl): II38-46.

Ip, J. H., V. Fuster, et al. (1990). "Syndromes of accelerated atherosclerosis: role of vascular injury and smooth muscle cell proliferation." J Am Coll Cardiol **15**(7): 1667-87.

Stary, H. C. (1990). "The sequence of cell and matrix changes in atherosclerotic lesions of coronary arteries in the first forty years of life." Eur Heart J **11**(1): 3-19.

Schwartz, C. J., J. L. Kelley, et al. (1989). "Pathophysiology of the atherogenic process." Am J Cardiol **64**(13): 23G-30G.

Peripheral Vascular Disease/Claudication

Donnan, P. T., M. Thomson, et al. (1993). "Diet as a risk factor for peripheral arterial disease in the general population: the Edinburgh Artery Study." Am J Clin Nutr **57**(6): 917-21.

Kiesewetter, H., F. Jung, et al. (1993). "Effects of garlic coated tablets in peripheral arterial occlusive disease." Clin Investig **71**(5): 383-6.

Banerjee, A. K., J. Pearson, et al. (1992). "A six year prospective study of fibrinogen and other risk factors associated with mortality in stable claudicants." Thromb Haemost **68**(3): 261-3.

Coto, V., L. D'Alessandro, et al. (1992). "Evaluation of the therapeutic efficacy and tolerability of levocarnitine propionyl in the treatment of chronic obstructive arteriopathies of the lower extremities: a multicentre controlled study vs. placebo." Drugs Exp Clin Res **18**(1): 29-36.

Criqui, M. H., R. D. Langer, et al. (1992). "Mortality over a period of 10 years in patients with peripheral arterial disease." N Engl J Med **326**(6): 381-6.

Fowkes, F. G., E. Housley, et al. (1992). "Smoking, lipids, glucose intolerance, and blood pressure as risk factors for peripheral atherosclerosis compared with ischemic heart disease in the Edinburgh Artery Study." Am J Epidemiol **135**(4): 331-40.

Goldhaber, S. Z., J. E. Manson, et al. (1992). "Low-dose aspirin and subsequent peripheral arterial surgery in the Physicians' Health Study." Lancet **340**(8812): 143-5.

Karnegis, J. N., J. P. Matts, et al. (1992). "Correlation of coronary with peripheral arterial stenosis. The POSCH Group." Atherosclerosis **92**(1): 25-30.

Molgaard, J., M. R. Malinow, et al. (1992). "Hyperhomocyst(e)inaemia: an independent risk factor for intermittent claudication." J Intern Med **231**(3): 273-9.

Olin, J. W., M. D. Cressman, et al. (1992). "Lipid and lipoprotein abnormalities in lower-extremity arteriosclerosis obliterans." Cleve Clin J Med **59**(5): 491-7.

Tyrrell, J., T. Cooke, et al. (1992). "Lipoprotein [Lp(a)] and peripheral vascular disease." J Intern Med **232**(4): 349-52.

Vogt, M. T., S. K. Wolfson, et al. (1992). "Lower extremity arterial disease and the aging process: a review." J Clin Epidemiol **45**(5): 529-42.

Ernst, E. (1991). "Peripheral vascular disease. Benefits of exercise." Sports Med **12**(3): 149-51.

Katsouyanni, K., Y. Skalkidis, et al. (1991). "Diet and peripheral arterial occlusive disease: the role of poly-, mono-, and saturated fatty acids." Am J Epidemiol **133**(1): 24-31.

Krupski, W. C. (1991). "The peripheral vascular consequences of smoking." Ann Vasc Surg **5**(3): 291-304.

Lassila, R., M. Lepantalo, et al. (1991). "The effect of acetylsalicylic acid on the outcome after lower limb arterial surgery with special reference to cigarette smoking." World J Surg **15**(3): 378-82.

Lind, J., M. Kramhoft, et al. (1991). "The influence of smoking on complications after primary amputations of the lower extremity." Clin Orthop **267**: 211-7.

Plaque Fissures

Brown, B. G., X. Q. Zhao, et al. (1993). "Arteriographic view of treatment to achieve regression of coronary atherosclerosis and to prevent plaque disruption and clinical cardiovascular events." Br Heart J **69**(1 Suppl): S48-53.

Brown, B. G., X. Q. Zhao, et al. (1993). "Atherosclerosis regression, plaque disruption, and cardiovascular events: a rationale for lipid lowering in coronary artery disease." Annu Rev Med **44**(1): 365-76.

Brown, B. G., X. Q. Zhao, et al. (1993). "Lipid lowering and plaque regression. New insights into prevention of plaque disruption and clinical events in coronary disease." Circulation **87**(6): 1781-91.

Cheng, G. C., et al (1993). "Distribution of circumferential stress in ruptured and stable atherosclerotic lesions." Circulation **87**(4): 1179-1187.

Ambrose, J. A. (1992). "Plaque disruption and the acute coronary syndromes of unstable angina and myocardial infarction: if the substrate is similar, why is the clinical presentation different? [editorial]." J Am Coll Cardiol **19**(7): 1653-8.

Badimon, L., J. H. Chesebro, et al. (1992). "Thrombus formation on ruptured atherosclerotic plaques and rethrombosis on evolving thrombi." Circulation **86**(6 Suppl): III74-85.

Falk, E. (1992). "Why do plaques rupture?" Circulation **86**(6 Suppl): III30-42.

Vanhoutte, P. M. (1992). "Platelets, endothelium-derived vasoactive factors, and coronary disease [editorial]." Cardiologia **37**(2): 89-93.

Chesebro, J. H., P. Zoldhelyi, et al. (1991). "Plaque disruption and thrombosis in unstable angina pectoris." Am J Cardiol **68**(12): 9C-15C.

Lendon, C. L., M. J. Davies, et al. (1991). "Atherosclerotic plaque caps are locally weakened when macrophages density is increased." Atherosclerosis **87**(1): 87-90.

Qiao, J. H., A. E. Walts, et al. (1991). "The severity of atherosclerosis at sites of plaque rupture with occlusive thrombosis in saphenous vein coronary artery bypass grafts." Am Heart J **122**(4 Pt 1): 955-8.

Fuster, V., B. Stein, et al. (1990). "Atherosclerotic plaque rupture and thrombosis. Evolving concepts." Circulation **82**(3 Suppl): II47-59.

Davies, M. J. and A. C. Thomas (1985). "Plaque fissuring—the cause of acute myocardial infarction, sudden ischaemic death, and crescendo angina." Br Heart J **53**(4): 363-73.

Platelets

Becker, R. C. (1993). "Antiplatelet therapy in coronary heart disease. Emerging strategies for the treatment and prevention of acute myocardial infarction." Arch Pathol Lab Med **117**(1): 89-96.

Budd, J. S., K. Allen, et al. (1993). "The effectiveness of low dose slow release aspirin as an antiplatelet agent." J R Soc Med **86**(5): 261-3.

Glassman, A. B. (1993). "Platelet abnormalities in diabetes mellitus." Ann Clin Lab Sci **23**(1): 47-50.

Hwang, D. L., C. F. Yen, et al. (1993). "Insulin increases intracellular magnesium transport in human platelets." J Clin Endocrinol Metab **76**(3): 549-53.

Karlberg, K. E., J. Ahlner, et al. (1993). "Effects of nitroglycerin on platelet aggregation beyond the effects of acetylsalicylic acid in healthy subjects." Am J Cardiol **71**(4): 361-4.

Legnani, C., M. Frascaro, et al. (1993). "Effects of a dried garlic preparation on fibrinolysis and platelet aggregation in healthy subjects." Arzneimittelforschung **43**(2): 119-22.

Mohri, H. and T. Ohkubo (1993). "Single-dose effect of enteric-coated aspirin on platelet function and thromboxane generation in middle-aged men." Ann Pharmacother **27**(4): 405-10.

Steiner, M. (1993). "Vitamin E: more than an antioxidant." Clin Cardiol **16**(4 Suppl 1): I16-8.

Sun, Y. P., B. Q. Zhu, et al. (1993). "Aspirin inhibits platelet activity but does not attenuate experimental atherosclerosis." Am Heart J **125**(1): 79-86.

Ware, J. A. and D. D. Heistad (1993). "Seminars in medicine of the Beth Israel Hospital, Boston. Platelet-endothelium interactions." N Engl J Med **328**(9): 628-35.

Apitz-Castro, R., J. J. Badimon, et al. (1992). "Effect of ajoene, the major antiplatelet compound from garlic, on platelet thrombus formation." Thromb Res **68**(2): 145-55.

Blache, D., D. Bouthillier, et al. (1992). "Acute influence of smoking on platelet behaviour, endothelium and plasma lipids and normalization by aspirin." Atherosclerosis **93**(3): 179-88.

Chirkov, Y. Y., J. I. Naujalis, et al. (1992). "Reversal of human platelet aggregation by low concentrations of nitroglycerin in vitro in normal subjects." Am J Cardiol **70**(7): 802-6.

Colwell, J. A. (1992). "Antiplatelet drugs and prevention of macrovascular disease in diabetes mellitus." Metabolism **41**(5 Suppl 1): 7-10.

Ferroni, P. and P. P. Gazzaniga (1992). "Evaluation of the clinical utility of platelet aggregation studies in the long-term follow-up of patients with atherosclerotic vascular disease." J Clin Lab Anal **6**(5): 257-63.

Green, M. S., I. Peled, et al. (1992). "Gender differences in platelet count and its association with cigarette smoking in a large cohort in Israel." J Clin Epidemiol **45**(1): 77-84.

Grignani, G., L. Pacchiarini, et al. (1992). "Effect of mental stress on platelet function in normal subjects and in patients with coronary artery disease." Haemostasis **22**(3): 138-46.

Grines, C. L. (1992). "Thrombolytic, antiplatelet, and antithrombotic agents." Am J Cardiol **70**(21): 18I-26I.

Hwang, D. L., C. F. Yen, et al. (1992). "Effect of extracellular magnesium on platelet activation and intracellular calcium mobilization." Am J Hypertens **5**(10): 700-6.

Jafri, S. M., M. Van Rollins, et al. (1992). "Circadian variation in platelet function in healthy volunteers." Am J Cardiol **69**(9): 951-4.

Jimenez, A. H., M. E. Stubbs, et al. (1992). "Rapidity and duration of platelet suppression by enteric-coated aspirin in healthy young men." Am J Cardiol **69**(3): 258-62.

Kario, K., T. Matsuo, et al. (1992). "Cigarette smoking increases the mean platelet volume in elderly patients with risk factors for atherosclerosis." Clin Lab Haematol **14**(4): 281-7.

Lam, J. Y., J. J. Badimon, et al. (1992). "Cod liver oil alters platelet-arterial wall response to injury in pigs." Circ Res **71**(4): 769-75.

Lassila, R. and K. E. Laustiola (1992). "Cigarette smoking and platelet-vessel wall interactions." Prostaglandins Leukot Essent Fatty Acids **46**(2): 81-6.

Lawson, L. D., D. K. Ransom, et al. (1992). "Inhibition of whole blood platelet-aggregation by compounds in garlic clove extracts and commercial garlic products." Thromb Res **65**(2): 141-56.

Loscalzo, J. (1992). "Antiplatelet and antithrombotic effects of organic nitrates." Am J Cardiol **70**(8): 18B-22B.

Meydani, M. (1992). "Modulation of the platelet thromboxane A2 and aortic prostacyclin synthesis by dietary selenium and vitamin E." Biol Trace Elem Res **33**(1): 79-86.

Mori, T. A., R. Vandongen, et al. (1992). "Differential effect of aspirin on platelet aggregation in IDDM." Diabetes **41**(3): 261-6.

Mori, T. A., R. Vandongen, et al. (1992). "Plasma lipid levels and platelet and neutrophil function in patients with vascular disease following fish oil and olive oil supplementation." Metabolism **41**(10): 1059-67.

Mutanen, M., R. Freese, et al. (1992). "Rapeseed oil and sunflower oil diets enhance platelet in vitro aggregation and thromboxane production in healthy men when compared with milk fat or habitual diets." Thromb Haemost **67**(3): 352-6.

Nadler, J. L., S. Malayan, et al. (1992). "Intracellular free magnesium deficiency plays a key role in increased platelet reactivity in type II diabetes mellitus." Diabetes Care **15**(7): 835-41.

Notarbartolo, A., I. Catalano, et al. (1992). "Platelets, eicosanoids and aging." Aging **4**(1): 13-20.

Ozdemir, O., Y. Karaaslan, et al. (1992). "The acute effect of smoking on platelet and endothelial release reaction is suppressed in chronic smokers." Thromb Res **65**(2): 263-74.

Prescott, S. M. (1992). "What are the effects of dietary fatty acid modification on platelet eicosanoid metabolism, platelet-activating factor, and platelet function? How might these metabolic alterations influence thrombosis?" Am J Clin Nutr **56**(4 Suppl): 801S-802S.

Rand, M. L., P. L. Gross, et al. (1992). "Acute in vitro effects of ethanol on responses of platelets from cholesterol-fed and Watanabe heritable hyperlipidemic rabbits." Arterioscler Thromb **12**(4): 437-45.

Ratnatunga, C. P., S. F. Edmondson, et al. (1992). "High-dose aspirin inhibits shear-induced platelet reaction involving thrombin generation." Circulation **85**(3): 1077-82.

Renaud, S. and M. de Lorgeril (1992). "Wine, alcohol, platelets, and the French paradox for coronary heart disease." Lancet **339**(8808): 1523-6.

Renaud, S. C., A. D. Beswick, et al. (1992). "Alcohol and platelet aggregation: the Caerphilly Prospective Heart Disease Study." Am J Clin Nutr **55**(5): 1012-7.

Sivenius, J., M. Laakso, et al. (1992). "European stroke prevention study: effectiveness of antiplatelet therapy in diabetic patients in secondary prevention of stroke." Stroke **23**(6): 851-4.

Steiner, M. (1992). "Alpha-tocopherol: a potent inhibitor of platelet adhesion." J Nutr Sci Vitaminol **1**(5): 191-5.

Terres, W., C. W. Hamm, et al. (1992). "Residual platelet function under acetylsalicylic acid and the risk of restenosis after coronary angioplasty." J Cardiovasc Pharmacol **19**(2): 190-3.

Tohgi, H., S. Konno, et al. (1992). "Effects of low-to-high doses of aspirin on platelet aggregability and metabolites of thromboxane A2 and prostacyclin." Stroke **23**(10): 1400-3.

Vericel, E., C. Rey, et al. (1992). "Age-related changes in arachidonic acid peroxidation and glutathione-peroxidase activity in human platelets." Prostaglandins **43**(1): 75-85.

Winther, K., W. Hillegass, et al. (1992). "Effects on platelet aggregation and fibrinolytic activity during upright posture and exercise in healthy men." Am J Cardiol **70**(11): 1051-5.

Wu, H. P., T. Y. Tai, et al. (1992). "Effect of tocopherol on platelet aggregation in non-insulin-dependent diabetes mellitus: ex vivo and in vitro studies." Taiwan I Hsueh Hui Tsa Chih **91**(3): 270-5.

Becker, R. C. (1991). "Seminars in thrombosis, thrombolysis and vascular biology. 3. Platelet activity in cardiovascular disease." Cardiology **79**(1): 49-63.

Berglund, U. and L. Wallentin (1991). "Persistent inhibition of platelet function during long-term treatment with 75 mg acetylsalicylic acid daily in men with unstable coronary artery disease." Eur Heart J **12**(3): 428-33.

Beswick, A. D., A. M. Fehily, et al. (1991). "Long-term diet modification and platelet activity." J Intern Med **229**(6): 511-5.

Burri, B. J., R. M. Dougherty, et al. (1991). "Platelet aggregation in humans is affected by replacement of dietary linoleic acid with oleic acid." Am J Clin Nutr **54**(2): 359-62.

Chan, A. C., K. Tran, et al. (1991). "Regeneration of vitamin E in human platelets." J Biol Chem **266**(26): 17290-5.

Ciavatti, M. and S. Renaud (1991). "Oxidative status and oral contraceptive. Its relevance to platelet abnormalities and cardiovascular risk." Free Radic Biol Med **10**(5): 325-38.

Elwood, P. C., S. Renaud, et al. (1991). "Ischemic heart disease and platelet aggregation. The Caerphilly Collaborative Heart Disease Study." Circulation **83**(1): 38-44.

Kerins, D. M. and G. A. Fitz Gerald (1991). "The current role of platelet-active drugs in ischaemic heart disease." Drugs **41**(5): 665-71.

Kiesewetter, H., F. Jung, et al. (1991). "Effect of garlic on thrombocyte aggregation, microcirculation, and other risk factors." Int J Clin Pharmacol Ther Toxicol **29**(4): 151-5.

Kwon, J. S., J. T. Snook, et al. (1991). "Effects of diets high in saturated fatty acids, canola oil, or safflower oil on platelet function, thromboxane B2 formation, and fatty acid composition of platelet phospholipids." Am J Clin Nutr **54**(2): 351-8.

Malle, E., W. Sattler, et al. (1991). "Effects of dietary fish oil supplementation on platelet aggregability and platelet membrane fluidity in normolipemic subjects with and without high plasma Lp(a) concentrations." Atherosclerosis **88**(2-3): 193-201.

McCall, N. T., G. H. Tofler, et al. (1991). "The effect of enteric-coated aspirin on the morning increase in platelet activity." Am Heart J **121**(5): 1382-8.

Mori, T. A., R. Vandongen, et al. (1991). "The effect of fish oil on plasma lipids, platelet and neutrophil function in patients with vascular disease." Adv Prostaglandin Thromboxane Leukot Res **1**: 229-32.

Nelson, G. J., P. C. Schmidt, et al. (1991). "The effect of a salmon diet on blood clotting, platelet aggregation and fatty acids in normal adult men." Lipids **26**(2): 87-96.

Numminen, H., M. Hillbom, et al. (1991). "Effects of exercise and ethanol ingestion on platelet thromboxane release in healthy men." Metabolism **40**(7): 695-701.

Rabinovici, R., T. L. Yue, et al. (1991). "Platelet-activating factor in cardiovascular stress situations." Lipids **26**(12): 1257-63.

Ridker, P. M., J. E. Manson, et al. (1991). "Clinical characteristics of nonfatal myocardial infarction among individuals on prophylactic low-dose aspirin therapy." Circulation **84**(2): 708-11.

Ridker, P. M., J. E. Manson, et al. (1991). "The effect of chronic platelet inhibition with low-dose aspirin on atherosclerotic progression and acute thrombosis: clinical evidence from the Physicians' Health Study." Am Heart J **122**(6): 1588-92.

Ridker, P. M., J. E. Manson, et al. (1991). "Low-dose aspirin therapy for chronic stable angina. A randomized, placebo-controlled clinical trial." Ann Intern Med **114**(10): 835-9.

Ridker, P. M., S. N. Willich, et al. (1991). "Aspirin, platelet aggregation, and the circadian variation of acute thrombotic events." Chronobiol Int **8**(5): 327-35.

Salonen, J. T., R. Salonen, et al. (1991). "Effects of antioxidant supplementation on platelet function: a randomized pair-matched, placebo-controlled, double-blind trial in men with low antioxidant status [see comments]." Am J Clin Nutr **53**(5): 1222-9.

Steiner, M. (1991). "Influence of vitamin E on platelet function in humans." J Am Coll Nutr **10**(5): 466-73.

Polyunsaturated Fatty Acid (PUFA)

Bonanome, A., A. Pagnan, et al. (1992). "Effect of dietary monounsaturated and polyunsaturated fatty acids on the susceptibility of plasma low density lipoproteins to oxidative modification." Arterioscler Thromb **12**(4): 529-33.

Dolecek, T. A. (1992). "Epidemiological evidence of relationships between dietary polyunsaturated fatty acids and mortality in the multiple risk factor intervention trial." Proc Soc Exp Biol Med **200**(2): 177-82.

Foley, M., M. Ball, et al. (1992). "Should mono- or poly-unsaturated fats replace saturated fat in the diet?" Eur J Clin Nutr **46**(6): 429-36.

Gustafsson, I. B., B. Vessby, et al. (1992). "Effects of lipid-lowering diets enriched with monounsaturated and polyunsaturated fatty acids on serum lipoprotein composition in patients with hyperlipoproteinaemia." Atherosclerosis **96**(2-3): 109-18.

Khosla, P. and K. C. Hayes (1992). "Comparison between the effects of dietary saturated (16:0), monounsaturated (18:1), and polyunsaturated (18:2) fatty acids on plasma lipoprotein metabolism in cebus and rhesus monkeys fed cholesterol-free diets." Am J Clin Nutr **55**(1): 51-62.

Mata, P., L. A. Alvarez-Sala, et al. (1992). "Effects of long-term monounsaturated- vs polyunsaturated-enriched diets on lipoproteins in healthy men and women." Am J Clin Nutr **55**(4): 846-50.

Mutanen, M., P. Kleemola, et al. (1992). "Lack of effect on blood pressure by polyunsaturated and monounsaturated fat diets." Eur J Clin Nutr **46**(1): 1-6.

Valsta, L. M., M. Jauhiainen, et al. (1992). "Effects of a monounsaturated rapeseed oil and a polyunsaturated sunflower oil diet on lipoprotein levels in humans." Arterioscler Thromb **12**(1): 50-7.

Berry, E. M., S. Eisenberg, et al. (1991). "Effects of diets rich in monounsaturated fatty acids on plasma lipoproteins—the Jerusalem Nutrition Study: high MUFAs vs high PUFAs." Am J Clin Nutr **53**(4): 899-907.

Fumeron, F., L. Brigant, et al. (1991). "Lowering of HDL2-cholesterol and lipoprotein A-I particle levels by increasing the ratio of polyunsaturated to saturated fatty acids." Am J Clin Nutr **53**(3): 655-9.

Kok, F. J., G. van Poppel, et al. (1991). "Do antioxidants and polyunsaturated fatty acids have a combined association with coronary atherosclerosis?" Atherosclerosis **86**(1): 85-90.

Wardlaw, G. M., J. T. Snook, et al. (1991). "Serum lipid and apolipoprotein concentrations in healthy men on diets enriched in either canola oil or safflower oil." Am J Clin Nutr **54**(1): 104-10.

Mensink, R. P. and M. B. Katan (1989). "Effect of a diet enriched with monounsaturated or polyunsaturated fatty acids on levels of low-density and high-density lipoprotein cholesterol in healthy women and men [see comments]." N Engl J Med **321**(7): 436-41.

Potassium

Gettes, L. S. (1992). "Electrolyte abnormalities underlying lethal and ventricular arrhythmias." Circulation **85**(1 Suppl): I70-6.

Mervaala, E. M., J. J. Himberg, et al. (1992). "Beneficial effects of a potassium- and magnesium-enriched salt alternative." Hypertension **19**(6 Pt 1): 535-40.

Siegel, D., S. B. Hulley, et al. (1992). "Diuretics, serum and intracellular electrolyte levels, and ventricular arrhythmias in hypertensive men." Jama **267**(8): 1083-9.

Whang, R., D. D. Whang, et al. (1992). "Refractory potassium repletion. A consequence of magnesium deficiency." Arch Intern Med **152**(1): 40-5.

Andersson, O. K., T. Gudbrandsson, et al. (1991). "Metabolic adverse effects of thiazide diuretics: the importance of normokalaemia." J Intern Med Suppl **735**(1): 89-96.

Cappuccio, F. P. and G. A. Mac Gregor (1991). "Does potassium supplementation lower blood pressure? A meta-analysis of published trials." J Hypertens **9**(5): 465-73.

Friedensohn, A., H. E. Faibel, et al. (1991). "Malignant arrhythmias in relation to values of serum potassium in patients with acute myocardial infarction." Int J Cardiol **32**(3): 331-8.

Krishna, G. G. and S. C. Kapoor (1991). "Potassium depletion exacerbates essential hypertension." Ann Intern Med **115**(2): 77-83.

Langford, H. G. (1991). "Sodium-potassium interaction in hypertension and hypertensive cardiovascular disease." Hypertension **17**(1 Suppl): I155-7.

Overlack, A., H. Conrad, et al. (1991). "The influence of oral potassium citrate/bicarbonate on blood pressure in essential hypertension during unrestricted salt intake (no effect)." Klin Wochenschr **69**(1): 79-83.

Siani, A., P. Strazzullo, et al. (1991). "Increasing the dietary potassium intake reduces the need for antihypertensive medication." Ann Intern Med **115**(10): 753-9.

Khaw, K. T. and E. Barrett-Connor (1987). "Dietary potassium and stroke-associated mortality. A 12-year prospective population study." N Engl J Med **316**(5): 235-40.

Primary Prevention of Coronary Heart Disease

Maxwell, S. R. (1993). "Can anti-oxidants prevent ischaemic heart disease?" J Clin Pharm Ther **18**(2): 85-95.

Gunby, P. (1992). "Forum offers hints of future therapy, prevention programs for combating cardiovascular problems [news] [published errata appear in JAMA 1992 Apr 15; 267(15):2039 and 1992 Jul 22-29; 268(4):475]." Jama **267**(7): 905-6.

Harris, W. S. (1992). "The prevention of atherosclerosis with antioxidants." Clin Cardiol **15**(9): 636-40.

Johnson, K. and E. W. Kligman (1992). "Preventive nutrition: disease-specific dietary interventions for older adults." Geriatrics **47**(11): 39-40.

Juul-Moller, S., N. Edvardsson, et al. (1992). "Double-blind trial of aspirin in primary prevention of myocardial infarction in patients with stable chronic angina pectoris. The Swedish Angina Pectoris Aspirin Trial (SAPAT) Group." Lancet **340**(8833): 1421-5.

Kaplan, N. M. (1992). "Lipid intervention trials in primary prevention: a critical review." Clin Exp Hypertens [a] **14**(1-2): 109-18.

Kaplan, N. M. (1992). "A new era in hypertension therapy. Protecting patients from premature cardiovascular disease." Postgrad Med **91**(8): 225-6.

Kavey, R. E. (1992). "Preventive cardiology for the pediatrician." Curr Probl Pediatr **22**(6): 258-81.

Lush, D. T. (1992). "Coronary artery disease. The latest on prevention." Postgrad Med **91**(3): 179-85.

Manson, J. E., H. Tosteson, et al. (1992). "The primary prevention of myocardial infarction." N Engl J Med **326**(21): 1406-16.

Miettinen, T. A. and T. E. Strandberg (1992). "Implications of recent results of long term multifactorial primary prevention of cardiovascular diseases." Ann Med **24**(2): 85-9.

Mogelvang, B. (1992). "[Can arteriosclerosis be prevented by antioxidants?]." Nord Med **107**(2): 53-6.

Rothenberg, R., E. S. Ford, et al. (1992). "Ischemic heart disease prevention: estimating the impact of interventions [see comments]." J Clin Epidemiol **45**(1): 21-9.

Grundy, S. M. (1991). "George Lyman Duff Memorial Lecture. Multifactorial etiology of hypercholesterolemia. Implications for prevention of coronary heart disease." Arterioscler Thromb **11**(6): 1619-35.

Gurr, M. I. (1991). "Diet, nutrition and the prevention of chronic diseases (WHO, 1990) [letter]." Eur J Clin Nutr **45**(12): 619-23.

Lawrence, M., M. Arbeit, et al. (1991). "Prevention of adult heart disease beginning in childhood: intervention programs." Cardiovasc Clin **21**(3): 249-62.

Manson, J. E., M. J. Stampfer, et al. (1991). "A prospective study of aspirin use and primary prevention of cardiovascular disease in women [see comments]." Jama **266**(4): 521-7.

Probstfield, J. L. and B. M. Rifkind (1991). "The Lipid Research Clinics Coronary Primary Prevention Trial: design, results, and implications." Eur J Clin Pharmacol **40**(1): S69-75.

Scrogin, K. E., D. C. Hatton, et al. (1991). "The interactive effects of dietary sodium chloride and calcium on cardiovascular stress responses." Am J Physiol **261**(4 Pt 2): R945-9.

Strong, W. B. (1991). "Cholesterol screening as a component of pediatric preventive cardiology. The office setting in hyperlipidemia in children." Ann N Y Acad Sci **623**(1): 214-21.

Pritikin

Barnard, R. J. (1991). "Effects of life-style modification on serum lipids [see comments]." Arch Intern Med **151**(7): 1389-94.

Martin, W. (1991). "Nathan Pritikin and atheroma." Med Hypotheses **36**(3): 181-2.

Probucol

Kuzuya, M. and F. Kuzuya (1993). "Probucol as an antioxidant and antiatherogenic drug." Free Radic Biol Med **14**(1): 67-77.

Walldius, G., J. Regnstrom, et al. (1993). "The role of lipids and antioxidative factors for development of atherosclerosis. The Probucol Quantitative Regression Swedish Trial (PQRST)." Am J Cardiol **71**(6): 15B-19B.

Babiy, A. V., J. M. Gebicki, et al. (1992). "Increased oxidizability of plasma lipoproteins in diabetic patients can be decreased by probucol therapy and is not due to glycation." Biochem Pharmacol **43**(5): 995-1000.

Baumstark, M. W., R. Aristegui, et al. (1992). "Probucol, incorporated into LDL particles in vivo, inhibits generation of lipid peroxides more effectively than endogenous antioxidants alone." Clin Biochem **25**(5): 395-7.

Cristol, L. S., I. Jialal, et al. (1992). "Effect of low-dose probucol therapy on LDL oxidation and the plasma lipoprotein profile in male volunteers." Atherosclerosis **97**(1): 11-20.

Gotoh, N., K. Shimizu, et al. (1992). "Antioxidant activities of probucol against lipid peroxidations." Biochim Biophys Acta **1128**(2-3): 147-54.

Kalyanaraman, B., U. V. Darley, et al. (1992). "Synergistic interaction between the probucol phenoxyl radical and ascorbic acid in inhibiting the oxidation of low density lipoprotein." J Biol Chem **267**(10): 6789-95.

Kita, T., M. Yokode, et al. (1992). "The role of oxidized lipoproteins in the pathogenesis of atherosclerosis." Clin Exp Pharmacol Physiol Suppl **20**(1): 37-42.

Naruszewicz, M., E. Selinger, et al. (1992). "Probucol protects lipoprotein (a) against oxidative modification." Metabolism **41**(11): 1225-8.

Parthasarathy, S. (1992). "Evidence for an additional intracellular site of action of probucol in the prevention of oxidative modification of low density lipoprotein. Use of a new water-soluble probucol derivative." J Clin Invest **89**(5): 1618-21.

Paterson, J. R., A. G. Rumley, et al. (1992). "Probucol reduces plasma lipid peroxides in man." Atherosclerosis **97**(1): 63-6.

Reaven, P. D., S. Parthasarathy, et al. (1992). "Effect of probucol dosage on plasma lipid and lipoprotein levels and on protection of low density lipoprotein against in vitro oxidation in humans." Arterioscler Thromb **12**(3): 318-24.

Bridges, A. B., N. A. Scott, et al. (1991). "Probucol, a superoxide free radical scavenger in vitro." Atherosclerosis **89**(2-3): 263-5.

Kuzuya, M., M. Naito, et al. (1991). "Probucol prevents oxidative injury to endothelial cells." J Lipid Res **32**(2): 197-204.

Mao, S. J., M. T. Yates, et al. (1991). "Antioxidant activity of probucol and its analogues in hypercholesterolemic Watanabe rabbits." J Med Chem **34**(1): 298-302.

Masana, L., M. T. Bargallo, et al. (1991). "Effectiveness of probucol in reducing plasma low-density lipoprotein cholesterol oxidation in hypercholesterolemia." Am J Cardiol **68**(9): 863-7.

Psychological Factors and Stress

Fleury, J. (1993). "An exploration of the role of social networks in cardiovascular risk reduction." Heart Lung **22**(2): 134-44.

Gorkin, L., E. B. Schron, et al. (1993). "Psychosocial predictors of mortality in the Cardiac Arrhythmia Suppression Trial-1 (CAST-1)." Am J Cardiol **71**(4): 263-7.

Morgan, R. E., L. A. Palinkas, et al. (1993). "Plasma cholesterol and depressive symptoms in older men." Lancet **341**(8837): 75-9.

Netterstrom, B. and P. Suadicani (1993). "Self-assessed job satisfaction and ischaemic heart disease mortality: a 10-year follow-up of urban bus drivers." Int J Epidemiol **22**(1): 51-6.

Orth-Gomer, K., A. Rosengren, et al. (1993). "Lack of social support and incidence of coronary heart disease in middle-aged Swedish men." Psychosom Med **55**(1): 37-43.

Schonwetter, D. J., J. M. Gerrard, et al. (1993). "Type A behavior and alcohol consumption: effects on resting and post-exercise bleeding time thromboxane and prostacyclin metabolites." Prostaglandins Leukot Essent Fatty Acids **48**(2): 143-8.

Schonwetter, D. J., J. M. Gerrard, et al. (1993). "Type A behavior and alcohol consumption: effects on resting and post-exercise bleeding time thromboxane and prostacyclin metabolites." Prostaglandins Leukot Essent Fatty Acids **48**(2): 143-8.

Anderson, W. P., C. M. Reid, et al. (1992). "Pet ownership and risk factors for cardiovascular disease." Med J Aust **157**(5): 298-301.

Berkman, L. F., L. Leo-Summers, et al. (1992). "Emotional support and survival after myocardial infarction. A prospective, population-based study of the elderly." Ann Intern Med **117**(12): 1003-9.

Brill, P. A., H. W. Kohl, et al. (1992). "Anxiety, depression, physical fitness, and all-cause mortality in men." J Psychosom Res **36**(3): 267-73.

Brown, P. C. and T. W. Smith (1992). "Social influence, marriage, and the heart: cardiovascular consequences of interpersonal control in husbands and wives." Health Psychol **11**(2): 88-96.

Case, R. B., A. J. Moss, et al. (1992). "Living alone after myocardial infarction. Impact on prognosis [see comments]." Jama **267**(4): 515-9.

Conduit, E. H. (1992). "If (Type) A-B does not predict heart disease, why bother with it? A clinician's view." Br J Med Psychol **65**(Pt 3): 289-96.

Denollet, J. and B. De Potter (1992). "Coping subtypes for men with coronary heart disease: relationship to well-being, stress and Type-A behaviour." Psychol Med **22**(3): 667-84.

Eaker, E. D., J. Pinsky, et al. (1992). "Myocardial infarction and coronary death among women: psychosocial predictors from a 20-year follow-up of women in the Framingham Study." Am J Epidemiol **135**(8): 854-64.

Eliot, R. S. (1992). "Stress and the heart. Mechanisms, measurement, and management." Postgrad Med **92**(5): 237-42.

Eysenck, H. J. (1992). "Psychosocial factors, cancer, and ischaemic heart disease." Bmj **305**(6851): 457-9.

Fava, M., A. Littman, et al. (1992). "Psychological, behavioral and biochemical risk factors for coronary artery disease among American and Italian male corporate managers." Am J Cardiol **70**(18): 1412-6.

Frasure-Smith, N., F. Lesperance, et al. (1992). "Differential long-term impact of in-hospital symptoms of psychological stress after non-Q-wave and Q-wave acute myocardial infarction." Am J Cardiol **69**(14): 1128-34.

Freedland, K. E., R. M. Carney, et al. (1992). "Major depression in coronary artery disease patients with vs. without a prior history of depression." Psychosom Med **54**(4): 416-21.

Freedland, K. E., P. J. Lustman, et al. (1992). "Underdiagnosis of depression in patients with coronary artery disease: the role of nonspecific symptoms." Int J Psychiatry Med **22**(3): 221-9.

Grignani, G., L. Pacchiarini, et al. (1992). "Effect of mental stress on platelet function in normal subjects and in patients with coronary artery disease." Haemostasis **22**(3): 138-46.

Houston, B. K., M. A. Chesney, et al. (1992). "Behavioral clusters and coronary heart disease risk." Psychosom Med **54**(4): 447-61.

Ironson, G., C. B. Taylor, et al. (1992). "Effects of anger on left ventricular ejection fraction in coronary artery disease." Am J Cardiol **70**(3): 281-5.

Lewin, B., I. H. Robertson, et al. (1992). "Effects of self-help post-myocardial-infarction rehabilitation on psychological adjustment and use of health services." Lancet **339**(8800): 1036-40.

Mark, D. B., L. C. Lam, et al. (1992). "Identification of patients with coronary disease at high risk for loss of employment. A prospective validation study." Circulation **86**(5): 1485-94.

Mitsibounas, D. N., E. D. Tsouna-Hadjis, et al. (1992). "Effects of group psychosocial intervention on coronary risk factors." Psychother Psychosom **58**(2): 97-102.

Niaura, R., P. N. Herbert, et al. (1992). "Repressive coping and blood lipids in men and women." Psychosom Med **54**(6): 698-706.

Niaura, R., C. M. Stoney, et al. (1992). "Lipids in psychological research: the last decade." Biol Psychol **34**(1): 1-43.

Palm, T. and A. Ohman (1992). "Social interaction, cardiovascular activation and the Type A behavior pattern." Int J Psychophysiol **13**(2): 101-10.

Rejeski, W. J., A. Thompson, et al. (1992). "Acute exercise: buffering psychosocial stress responses in women." Health Psychol **11**(6): 355-62.

Rost, K. and G. R. Smith (1992). "Return to work after an initial myocardial infarction and subsequent emotional distress." Arch Intern Med **152**(2): 381-5.

Ruberman, W. (1992). "Psychosocial influences on mortality of patients with coronary heart disease [editorial; comment]." Jama **267**(4): 559-60.

Schnall, P. L., J. E. Schwartz, et al. (1992). "Relation between job strain, alcohol, and ambulatory blood pressure." Hypertension **19**(5): 488-94.

Siegler, I. C., B. L. Peterson, et al. (1992). "Hostility during late adolescence predicts coronary risk factors at mid-life." Am J Epidemiol **136**(2): 146-54.

Sykes, D. H., U. Haertel, et al. (1992). "The Framingham Type A behaviour pattern and coronary heart disease in three countries: a cross-cultural comparison." Int J Epidemiol **21**(6): 1081-9.

Weidner, G., S. L. Connor, et al. (1992). "Improvements in hostility and depression in relation to dietary change and cholesterol lowering. The Family Heart Study." Ann Intern Med **117**(10): 820-3.

Williams, R. B., J. C. Barefoot, et al. (1992). "Prognostic importance of social and economic resources among medically treated patients with angiographically documented coronary artery disease [see comments]." Jama **267**(4): 520-4.

Freedland, K. E., P. J. Lustman, et al. (1992). "Underdiagnosis of depression in patients with coronary artery disease: the role of nonspecific symptoms." Int J Psychiatry Med **22**(3): 221-9.

Grignani, G., L. Pacchiarini, et al. (1992). "Effect of mental stress on platelet function in normal subjects and in patients with coronary artery disease." Haemostasis **22**(3): 138-46.

Houston, B. K., M. A. Chesney, et al. (1992). "Behavioral clusters and coronary heart disease risk." Psychosom Med **54**(4): 447-61.

Ironson, G., C. B. Taylor, et al. (1992). "Effects of anger on left ventricular ejection fraction in coronary artery disease." Am J Cardiol **70**(3): 281-5.

Lewin, B., I. H. Robertson, et al. (1992). "Effects of self-help post-myocardial-infarction rehabilitation on psychological adjustment and use of health services." Lancet **339**(8800): 1036-40.

Mark, D. B., L. C. Lam, et al. (1992). "Identification of patients with coronary disease at high risk for loss of employment. A prospective validation study." Circulation **86**(5): 1485-94.

Mitsibounas, D. N., E. D. Tsouna-Hadjis, et al. (1992). "Effects of group psychosocial intervention on coronary risk factors." Psychother Psychosom **58**(2): 97-102.

Niaura, R., P. N. Herbert, et al. (1992). "Repressive coping and blood lipids in men and women." Psychosom Med **54**(6): 698-706.

Niaura, R., C. M. Stoney, et al. (1992). "Lipids in psychological research: the last decade." Biol Psychol **34**(1): 1-43.

Palm, T. and A. Ohman (1992). "Social interaction, cardiovascular activation and the Type A behavior pattern." Int J Psychophysiol **13**(2): 101-10.

Rejeski, W. J., A. Thompson, et al. (1992). "Acute exercise: buffering psychosocial stress responses in women." Health Psychol **11**(6): 355-62.

Rost, K. and G. R. Smith (1992). "Return to work after an initial myocardial infarction and subsequent emotional distress." Arch Intern Med **152**(2): 381-5.

Ruberman, W. (1992). "Psychosocial influences on mortality of patients with coronary heart disease [editorial; comment]." Jama **267**(4): 559-60.

Schnall, P. L., J. E. Schwartz, et al. (1992). "Relation between job strain, alcohol, and ambulatory blood pressure." Hypertension **19**(5): 488-94.

Siegler, I. C., B. L. Peterson, et al. (1992). "Hostility during late adolescence predicts coronary risk factors at mid-life." Am J Epidemiol **136**(2): 146-54.

Sykes, D. H., U. Haertel, et al. (1992). "The Framingham Type A behaviour pattern and coronary heart disease in three countries: a cross-cultural comparison." Int J Epidemiol **21**(6): 1081-9.

Weidner, G., S. L. Connor, et al. (1992). "Improvements in hostility and depression in relation to dietary change and cholesterol lowering. The Family Heart Study." Ann Intern Med **117**(10): 820-3.

Williams, R. B., J. C. Barefoot, et al. (1992). "Prognostic importance of social and economic resources among medically treated patients with angiographically documented coronary artery disease [see comments]." Jama **267**(4): 520-4.

Red Meat

(1991). "Meat—can we live without it?" World Health Forum **12**(3): 251-60.

Bodenmann, A., U. Ackermann-Liebrich, et al. (1991). "[Meat consumption and serum cholesterol concentration]." Dtsch Med Wochenschr **116**(28-29): 1089-94.

Denke, M. A. and S. M. Grundy (1991). "Effects of fats high in stearic acid on lipid and lipoprotein concentrations in men." Am J Clin Nutr **54**(6): 1036-40.

Red Wine

Frankel, E. N., J. Kanner, et al. (1993). "Inhibition of oxidation of human low-density lipoprotein by phenolic substances in red wine." Lancet **341**(8843): 454-7.

Klatsky, A. L. and M. A. Armstrong (1993). "Alcoholic beverage choice and risk of coronary artery disease mortality: do red wine drinkers fare best?" Am J Cardiol **71**(5): 467-9.

Regression and Reversal of Heart Disease

Brown, B. G., L. A. Hillger, et al. (1993). "A maximum confidence approach for measuring progression and regression of coronary artery disease in clinical trials." Circulation **87**(3 Suppl): II66-73.

Brown, B. G., X. Q. Zhao, et al. (1993). "Arteriographic view of treatment to achieve regression of coronary atherosclerosis and to prevent plaque disruption and clinical cardiovascular events." Br Heart J **69**(1 Suppl): S48-53.

Brown, B. G., X. Q. Zhao, et al. (1993). "Atherosclerosis regression, plaque disruption, and cardiovascular events: a rationale for lipid lowering in coronary artery disease." Annu Rev Med **44**(1): 365-76.

Brown, B. G., X. Q. Zhao, et al. (1993). "Lipid lowering and plaque regression. New insights into prevention of plaque disruption and clinical events in coronary disease." Circulation **87**(6): 1781-91.

Stone, P. H., C. M. Gibson, et al. (1993). "Natural history of coronary atherosclerosis using quantitative angiography in men, and implications for clinical trials of coronary regression. The Harvard Atherosclerosis Reversibility Project Study Group." Am J Cardiol **71**(10): 766-72.

(1992). "Progression-Regression of Atherogenesis: Molecular, Cellular, and Clinical Bases. Symposium proceedings. Scottsdale, Arizona, April 5-7, 1991." Circulation **86**(6 Suppl): III1-123.

Badimon, J. J., V. Fuster, et al. (1992). "Role of high density lipoproteins in the regression of atherosclerosis." Circulation **86**(6 Suppl): III86-94.

Barth, J. D. (1992). "Regression of atherosclerosis [editorial]." Can J Cardiol **8**(9): 911-2.

Brown, B. G. (1992). "Effect of lovastatin or niacin combined with colestipol and regression of coronary atherosclerosis." Eur Heart J **13**(1): 17-20.

Fuster, V., J. J. Badimon, et al. (1992). "Clinical-pathological correlations of coronary disease progression and regression." Circulation **86**(6 Suppl): III1-11.

Gohlke, H. (1992). "[Effect of the LDL-/HDL-cholesterol quotient on progression and regression of arteriosclerotic lesions. An analysis of controlled angiographic intervention studies]." Wien Klin Wochenschr **104**(11): 309-13.

Gould, K. L., D. Ornish, et al. (1992). "Improved stenosis geometry by quantitative coronary arteriography after vigorous risk factor modification." Am J Cardiol **69**(9): 845-53.

Kramsch, D. M. and D. H. Blankenhorn (1992). "Regression of atherosclerosis: which components regress and what influences their reversal." Wien Klin Wochenschr **104**(1): 2-9.

La Rosa, J. C. and J. I. Cleeman (1992). "Cholesterol lowering as a treatment for established coronary heart disease." Circulation **85**(3): 1229-35.

Schuler, G., R. Hambrecht, et al. (1992). "Myocardial perfusion and regression of coronary artery disease in patients on a regimen of intensive physical exercise and low fat diet." J Am Coll Cardiol **19**(1): 34-42.

Schuler, G., R. Hambrecht, et al. (1992). "Regular physical exercise and low-fat diet. Effects on progression of coronary artery disease." Circulation **86**(1): 1-11.

Schwartz, C. J., A. J. Valente, et al. (1992). "Atherosclerosis. Potential targets for stabilization and regression." Circulation **86**(6 Suppl): III117-23.

Tatami, R., N. Inoue, et al. (1992). "Regression of coronary atherosclerosis by combined LDL-apheresis and lipid-lowering drug therapy in patients with familial hypercholesterolemia: a multicenter study. The LARS Investigators." Atherosclerosis **95**(1): 1-13.

(1991). "The lifestyle heart trial: regression of coronary artery blockage." Nutr Rev **49**(8): 250-2.

Arntzenius, A. C. (1991). "Regression of atherosclerosis. Benefit can be expected from low LDL-C and high HDL-C levels [editorial]." Acta Cardiol **46**(4): 431-8.

Barth, J. D. and A. C. Arntzenius (1991). "Progression and regression of atherosclerosis, what roles for LDL-cholesterol and HDL-cholesterol: a perspective." Eur Heart J **12**(8): 952-7.

Blankenhorn, D. H. (1991). "Regression of atherosclerosis: what does it mean?" Am J Med **90**(2A): 42S-47S.

Blankenhorn, D. H., S. P. Azen, et al. (1991). "Effects of colestipol-niacin therapy on human femoral atherosclerosis [see comments]." Circulation **83**(2): 438-47.

Blankenhorn, D. H. and H. N. Hodis (1991). "Treating serum lipid abnormalities in high-priority patients." Postgrad Med **89**(1): 81-2.

Brown, B. G. (1991). "Workshop VI—Regression of atherosclerosis: what does it mean?" Am J Med **90**(2A): 53S-55S.

Gotto, A., Jr. (1991). "Rationale for treatment." Am J Med **91**(1B): 31S-36S.

Hahmann, H. W., T. Bunte, et al. (1991). "Progression and regression of minor coronary arterial narrowings by quantitative angiography after fenofibrate therapy." Am J Cardiol **67**(11): 957-61.

Koga, N. and Y. Iwata (1991). "Pathological and angiographic regression of coronary atherosclerosis by LDL-apheresis in a patient with familial hypercholesterolemia." Atherosclerosis **90**(1): 9-21.

Superko, H. R. (1991). "Prevention and regression of atherosclerosis with drug therapy." Clin Cardiol **14**(2 Suppl 1): I40-7.

Waters, D. and J. Lesperance (1991). "Regression of coronary atherosclerosis: an achievable goal? Review of results from recent clinical trials." Am J Med **91**(1B): 10S-17S.

Yamamoto, A. (1991). "Regression of atherosclerosis in humans by lowering serum cholesterol." Atherosclerosis **89**(1): 1-10.

Blankenhorn, D. H. (1990). "Can atherosclerotic lesions regress? Angiographic evidence in humans." Am J Cardiol **65**(12): 41F-43F.

Blankenhorn, D. H., P. Alaupovic, et al. (1990). "Prediction of angiographic change in native human coronary arteries and aortocoronary bypass grafts. Lipid and nonlipid factors [see comments]." Circulation **81**(2): 470-6.

Blankenhorn, D. H., R. L. Johnson, et al. (1990). "The influence of diet on the appearance of new lesions in human coronary arteries [see comments]." Jama **263**(12): 1646-52.

Brown, G., J. J. Albers, et al. (1990). "Regression of coronary artery disease as a result of intensive lipid-lowering therapy in men with high levels of apolipoprotein B [see comments]." N Engl J Med **323**(19): 1289-98.

Cashin-Hemphill, L., W. J. Mack, et al. (1990). "Beneficial effects of colestipol-niacin on coronary atherosclerosis. A 4-year follow-up [see comments]." Jama **264**(23): 3013-7.

Kane, J. P., M. J. Malloy, et al. (1990). "Regression of coronary atherosclerosis during treatment of familial hypercholesterolemia with combined drug regimens [see comments]." Jama **264**(23): 3007-12.

Loscalzo, J. (1990). "Regression of coronary atherosclerosis [editorial; comment]." N Engl J Med **323**(19): 1337-9.

Ornish, D., S. E. Brown, et al. (1990). "Can lifestyle changes reverse coronary heart disease? The Lifestyle Heart Trial [see comments]." Lancet **336** (8708): 129-33.

Blankenhorn, D. H. (1989). "Prevention or reversal of atherosclerosis: review of current evidence." Am J Cardiol **63**(16): 38H-41H.

Blankenhorn, D. H. and D. M. Kramsch (1989). "Reversal of atherosis and sclerosis. The two components of atherosclerosis." Circulation **79**(1): 1-7.

Blankenhorn, D. H., S. A. Nessim, et al. (1987). "Beneficial effects of combined colestipol-niacin therapy on coronary atherosclerosis and coronary venous bypass grafts [published erratum appears in JAMA 1988 May 13; 259(18):2698]." Jama **257**(23): 3233-40.

Rice Bran Oil

Kahlon, T. S., F. I. Chow, et al. (1992). "Cholesterol-lowering in hamsters fed rice bran at various levels, defatted rice bran and rice bran oil." J Nutr **122**(3): 513-9.

Nicolosi, R. J., L. M. Ausman, et al. (1991). "Rice bran oil lowers serum total and low density lipoprotein cholesterol and apo B levels in nonhuman primates." Atherosclerosis **88**(2-3): 133-42.

Rukmini, C. and T. C. Raghuram (1991). "Nutritional and biochemical aspects of the hypolipidemic action of rice bran oil: a review." J Am Coll Nutr **10**(6): 593-601.

Risk Factors

Gey, K. F., U. K. Moser, et al. (1993). "Increased risk of cardiovascular disease at suboptimal plasma concentrations of essential antioxidants: an epidemiological update with special attention to carotene and vitamin C." Am J Clin Nutr **57**(5 Suppl): 787S-797S.

Haffner, S. M., P. A. Morales, et al. (1993). "Cardiovascular risk factors in non-insulin-dependent diabetic subjects with microalbuminuria." Arterioscler Thromb **13**(2): 205-10.

Stamler, J., O. Vaccaro, et al. (1993). "Diabetes, other risk factors, and 12-yr cardiovascular mortality for men screened in the Multiple Risk Factor Intervention Trial." Diabetes Care **16**(2): 434-44.

Willett, W. C., M. J. Stampfer, et al. (1993). "Intake of trans fatty acids and risk of coronary heart disease among women." Lancet **341**(8845): 581-5.

Ballor, D. L. and E. T. Poehlman (1992). "Resting metabolic rate and coronary-heart-disease risk factors in aerobically and resistance-trained women." Am J Clin Nutr **56**(6): 968-74.

Barnard, R. J., E. J. Ugianskis, et al. (1992). "Role of diet and exercise in the management of hyperinsulinemia and associated atherosclerotic risk factors." Am J Cardiol **69**(5): 440-4.

Benotti, P. N., B. Bistrain, et al. (1992). "Heart disease and hypertension in severe obesity: the benefits of weight reduction." Am J Clin Nutr **55**(2 Suppl): 586S-590S.

Berenson, G. S., W. A. Wattigney, et al. (1992). "Atherosclerosis of the aorta and coronary arteries and cardiovascular risk factors in persons aged 6 to 30 years and studied at necropsy (The Bogalusa Heart Study)." Am J Cardiol **70**(9): 851-8.

Ding, Y. A. (1992). "Plasma triglycerides: a cardiovascular risk factor?" Chung Hua I Hsueh Tsa Chih **49**(5): 297-302.

Fraser, G. E., T. M. Strahan, et al. (1992). "Effects of traditional coronary risk factors on rates of incident coronary events in a low-risk population. The Adventist Health Study." Circulation **86**(2): 406-13.

Fulcher, G. (1992). "Lipoprotein(a): a new independent risk factor for atherosclerosis [editorial; comment]." Aust N Z J Med **22**(4): 326-8.

Genest, J., Jr., J. R. McNamara, et al. (1992). "Lipoprotein cholesterol, apolipoprotein A-I and B and lipoprotein (a) abnormalities in men with premature coronary artery disease." J Am Coll Cardiol **19**(4): 792-802.

Greenlee, P., C. H. Castle, et al. (1992). "Successful modification of medical students' cardiovascular risk factors." Am J Prev Med **8**(1): 43-52.

Hebert, P. R., J. E. Buring, et al. (1992). "Occupation and risk of nonfatal myocardial infarction." Arch Intern Med **152**(11): 2253-7.

Hostmark, A. T., J. Berg, et al. (1992). "Coronary risk factors in middle-aged men as related to smoking, coffee intake and physical activity." Scand J Soc Med **20**(4): 196-203.

Kalandidi, A., A. Tzonou, et al. (1992). "A case-control study of coronary heart disease in Athens, Greece." Int J Epidemiol **21**(6): 1074-80.

Kannel, W. B. (1992). "Epidemiology of cardiovascular disease in the elderly: an assessment of risk factors." Cardiovasc Clin **22**(2): 9-22.

Lindholm, L. H., A. D. Koutis, et al. (1992). "Risk factors for ischaemic heart disease in a Greek population. A cross-sectional study of men and women living in the village of Spili in Crete." Eur Heart J **13**(3): 291-8.

Michel, U. and B. Riechers (1992). "Cardiovascular risk factors in schoolchildren." J Am Coll Nutr **11**(1): 36S-40S.

Mitsibounas, D. N., E. D. Tsouna-Hadjis, et al. (1992). "Effects of group psychosocial intervention on coronary risk factors." Psychother Psychosom **58**(2): 97-102.

Neaton, J. D. and D. Wentworth (1992). "Serum cholesterol, blood pressure, cigarette smoking, and death from coronary heart disease. Overall findings and differences by age for 316,099 white men. Multiple Risk Factor Intervention Trial Research Group." Arch Intern Med **152**(1): 56-64.

Rocchini, A. P. (1992). "Adolescent obesity and cardiovascular risk." Pediatr Ann **21**(4): 235-40.

Rosengren, A., L. Wilhelmsen, et al. (1992). "Coronary heart disease, cancer and mortality in male middle-aged light smokers." J Intern Med **231**(4): 357-62.

Schoenberger, J. A. (1992). "Effects of antihypertensive agents on coronary artery disease risk factors." Am J Cardiol **69**(10): 33C-39C.

Simons, L. A. (1992). "Triglyceride levels and the risk of coronary artery disease: a view from Australia." Am J Cardiol **70**(19): 14H-18H.

(1991). "National Education Programs Working Group report on the management of patients with hypertension and high blood cholesterol." Ann Intern Med **114**(3): 224-37.

Altura, B. M. and B. T. Altura (1991). "Cardiovascular risk factors and magnesium: relationships to atherosclerosis, ischemic heart disease and hypertension." Magnes Trace Elem **10**(2-4): 182-92.

Risk Factors—Nontraditional

Gey, K. F., U. K. Moser, et al. (1993). "Increased risk of cardiovascular disease at suboptimal plasma concentrations of essential antioxidants: an epidemiological update with special attention to carotene and vitamin C." Am J Clin Nutr **57**(5 Suppl): 787S-797S.

Rimm, E. B., A. Ascherio, et al. (1993). "Dietary iron intake and risk of coronary disease among men. (abstract)." Circulation **87**(2): 692.

Rimm, E. B., M. J. Stampfer, et al. (1993). "Vitamin E consumption and the risk of coronary heart disease in men [see comments]." N Engl J Med **328**(20): 1450-6.

Beilin, L. J. (1992). "Dietary salt and risk factors for cardiovascular disease." Kidney Int Suppl **37**(1): S90-6.

Bonora, E., M. Zenere, et al. (1992). "Influence of body fat and its regional localization on risk factors for atherosclerosis in young men." Am J Epidemiol **135**(11): 1271-8.

Gliksman, M. and A. Wilson (1992). "Are hemostatic factors responsible for the paradoxical risk factors for coronary heart disease and stroke?" Stroke **23**(4): 607-10.

Jackson, R., R. Scragg, et al. (1992). "Does recent alcohol consumption reduce the risk of acute myocardial infarction and coronary death in regular drinkers?" Am J Epidemiol **136**(7): 819-24.

Kannel, W. B., et al (1992). "Update on fibrinogen as a cardiovascular risk factor." Ann Epidem **2**: 457-466.

Kovacs, I. B., C. P. Ratnatunga, et al. (1992). "Significance of plasma fibrinogen in coronary arterial disease: marker or causative risk factor for arterial thrombosis?" Int J Cardiol **35**(1): 57-64.

Resch, K. L., E. Ernst, et al. (1992). "Fibrinogen and viscosity as risk factors for subsequent cardiovascular events in stroke survivors." Ann Intern Med **117**(5): 371-5.

Salonen, J. T., K. Nyyssonen, et al. (1992). "High stored iron levels are associated with excess risk of myocardial infarction in eastern Finnish men [see comments]." Circulation **86**(3): 803-11.

Seidelin, K. N., B. Myrup, et al. (1992). "n-3 fatty acids in adipose tissue and coronary artery disease are inversely related." Am J Clin Nutr **55**(6): 1117-9.

Suadicani, P., H. O. Hein, et al. (1992). "Serum selenium concentration and risk of ischaemic heart disease in a prospective cohort study of 3000 males." Atherosclerosis **96**(1): 33-42.

Altura, B. M. and B. T. Altura (1991). "Cardiovascular risk factors and magnesium: relationships to atherosclerosis, ischemic heart disease and hypertension." Magnes Trace Elem **10**(2-4): 182-92.

Ciavatti, M. and S. Renaud (1991). "Oxidative status and oral contraceptive. Its relevance to platelet abnormalities and cardiovascular risk." Free Radic Biol Med **10**(5): 325-38.

Dobson, A. J., H. M. Alexander, et al. (1991). "Passive smoking and the risk of heart attack or coronary death." Med J Aust **154**(12): 793-7.

Elliott, W. J. and T. Karrison (1991). "Increased all-cause and cardiac morbidity and mortality associated with the diagonal earlobe crease: a prospective cohort study." Am J Med **91**(3): 247-54.

Folsom, A. R., K. K. Wu, et al. (1991). "Population correlates of plasma fibrinogen and factor VII, putative cardiovascular risk factors." Atherosclerosis **91**(3): 191-205.

Gey, K. F., P. Puska, et al. (1991). "Inverse correlation between plasma vitamin E and mortality from ischemic heart disease in cross-cultural epidemiology." Am J Clin Nutr **53**(1 Suppl): 326S-334S.

Jackson, R., R. Scragg, et al. (1991). "Alcohol consumption and risk of coronary heart disease [see comments]." Bmj **303**(6796): 211-6.

McCord, J. M. (1991). "Is iron sufficiency a risk factor in ischemic heart disease? [editorial; comment]." Circulation **83**(3): 1112-4.

Rimm, E. B., E. L. Giovannucci, et al. (1991). "Prospective study of alcohol consumption and risk of coronary disease in men [see comments]." Lancet **338**(8765): 464-8.

Thompson, C. J., J. E. Ryu, et al. (1991). "Central adipose distribution is related to coronary atherosclerosis." Arterioscler Thromb **11**(2): 327-33.

Yarnell, J. W., I. A. Baker, et al. (1991). "Fibrinogen, viscosity, and white blood cell count are major risk factors for ischemic heart disease. The Caerphilly and Speedwell collaborative heart disease studies [see comments]." Circulation **83**(3): 836-44.

Salt

Lind, L., H. Lithell, et al. (1993). "Calcium metabolism and sodium sensitivity in hypertensive subjects." J Hum Hypertens **7**(1): 53-7.

Beilin, L. J. (1992). "Dietary salt and risk factors for cardiovascular disease." Kidney Int Suppl **37**(1): S90-6.

Cobiac, L., P. J. Nestel, et al. (1992). "A low-sodium diet supplemented with fish oil lowers blood pressure in the elderly." J Hypertens **10**(1): 87-92.

Correa, P. (1992). "Diet modification and gastric cancer prevention." Monogr Natl Cancer Inst **12**: 75-8.

Feldman, R. D. (1992). "A low-sodium diet corrects the defect in beta-adrenergic response in older subjects." Circulation **85**(2): 612-8.

Hamet, P., M. Daignault-Gelinas, et al. (1992). "Epidemiological evidence of an interaction between calcium and sodium intake impacting on blood pressure. A Montreal study." Am J Hypertens **5**(6 Pt 1): 378-85.

Lind, L., H. Lithell, et al. (1992). "Metabolic cardiovascular risk factors and sodium sensitivity in hypertensive subjects." Am J Hypertens **5**(8): 502-5.

Cappuccio, F. P., N. D. Markandu, et al. (1991). "Dietary salt intake and hypertension." Klin Wochenschr **69**(1): 17-25.

Drueke, T. B. and M. Muntzel (1991). "Heterogeneity of blood pressure responses to salt restriction and salt appetite in rats." Klin Wochenschr **69**(1): 73-8.

Dustan, H. P. (1991). "A perspective on the salt-blood pressure relation." Hypertension **17**(1 Suppl): I166-9.

Elmer, P. J., R. Grimm Jr., et al. (1991). "Dietary sodium reduction for hypertension prevention and treatment." Hypertension **17**(1 Suppl): I182-9.

Hamet, P., E. Mongeau, et al. (1991). "Interactions among calcium, sodium, and alcohol intake as determinants of blood pressure." Hypertension **17**(1 Suppl): I150-4.

He, J., G. S. Tell, et al. (1991). "Relation of electrolytes to blood pressure in men. The Yi people study." Hypertension **17**(3): 378-85.

Heagerty, A. M. (1991). "Salt restriction, a sceptic's viewpoint." Klin Wochenschr **69**(1): 26-9.

Hegsted, D. M. (1991). "A perspective on reducing salt intake." Hypertension **17**(1 Suppl): I201-4.

Krakoff, L. R. (1991). "Is reduction of dietary salt a treatment for hypertension? [editorial] [published erratum appears in Am J Hypertens 1991 Jul; 4(7 Pt 1):644] [comment]." Am J Hypertens **4**(5 Pt 1): 481-2.

Kuller, L. H. (1991). "Research and policy directions. Salt and blood pressure." Hypertension **17**(1 Suppl): I211-5.

Langford, H. G. (1991). "Sodium-potassium interaction in hypertension and hypertensive cardiovascular disease." Hypertension **17**(1 Suppl): I155-7.

Reusch, H. P. and F. C. Luft (1991). "[The role of chlorides in sodium-induced "salt-sensitive" hypertension]." Klin Wochenschr **69**(1): 90-6.

Ruppert, M., J. Diehl, et al. (1991). "Short-term dietary sodium restriction increases serum lipids and insulin in salt-sensitive and salt-resistant normotensive adults." Klin Wochenschr **69**(1): 51-7.

Scrogin, K. E., D. C. Hatton, et al. (1991). "The interactive effects of dietary sodium chloride and calcium on cardiovascular stress responses." Am J Physiol **261**(4 Pt 2): R945-9.

Sowers, J. R., M. B. Zemel, et al. (1991). "Calcium metabolism and dietary calcium in salt sensitive hypertension." Am J Hypertens **4**(6): 557-63.

Weder, A. B. and B. M. Egan (1991). "Potential deleterious impact of dietary salt restriction on cardiovascular risk factors." Klin Wochenschr **69**(1): 45-50.

Saturated Fats (SFA)

Lichtenstein, A. H., L. M. Ausman, et al. (1993). "Hydrogenation impairs the hypolipidemic effect of corn oil in humans. Hydrogenation, trans fatty acids, and plasma lipids." Arterioscler Thromb **13**(2): 154-61.

Barr, S. L., R. Ramakrishnan, et al. (1992). "Reducing total dietary fat without reducing saturated fatty acids does not significantly lower total plasma cholesterol concentrations in normal males." Am J Clin Nutr **55**(3): 675-81.

Foley, M., M. Ball, et al. (1992). "Should mono- or poly-unsaturated fats replace saturated fat in the diet?" Eur J Clin Nutr **46**(6): 429-36.

Khosla, P. and K. C. Hayes (1992). "Comparison between the effects of dietary saturated (16:0), monounsaturated (18:1), and polyunsaturated (18:2) fatty acids on plasma lipoprotein metabolism in cebus and rhesus monkeys fed cholesterol-free diets." Am J Clin Nutr **55**(1): 51-62.

Mott, G. E., E. M. Jackson, et al. (1992). "Dietary cholesterol and type of fat differentially affect cholesterol metabolism and atherosclerosis in baboons." J Nutr **122**(7): 1397-406.

Sundram, K., G. Hornstra, et al. (1992). "Replacement of dietary fat with palm oil: effect on human serum lipids, lipoproteins and apolipoproteins." Br J Nutr **68**(3): 677-92.

Dupont, J., P. J. White, et al. (1991). "Saturated and hydrogenated fats in food in relation to health [see comments]." J Am Coll Nutr **10**(6): 577-92.

Kwon, J. S., J. T. Snook, et al. (1991). "Effects of diets high in saturated fatty acids, canola oil, or safflower oil on platelet function, thromboxane B2 formation, and fatty acid composition of platelet phospholipids." Am J Clin Nutr **54**(2): 351-8.

Maron, D. J., J. M. Fair, et al. (1991). "Saturated fat intake and insulin resistance in men with coronary artery disease. The Stanford Coronary Risk Intervention Project Investigators and Staff." Circulation **84**(5): 2020-7.

Connor, S. L., J. R. Gustafson, et al. (1986). "The cholesterol/saturated-fat index: an indication of the hypercholesterolaemic and atherogenic potential of food." Lancet **1**(8492): 1229-32.

Secondary Prevention of Coronary Heart Disease

Bissett, J. K., R. P. Wyeth, et al. (1993). "Plasma lipid concentrations and subsequent coronary occlusion after a first myocardial infarction. The POSCH Group." Am J Med Sci **305**(3): 139-44.

Cupples, L. A., D. R. Gagnon, et al. (1993). "Preexisting cardiovascular conditions and long-term prognosis after initial myocardial infarction: the Framingham Study." Am Heart J **125**(3): 863-72.

Deedwania, P. C. and E. V. Carbajal (1993). "Secondary prevention after myocardial infarction. Too many choices, which ones work? [editorial; comment]." Arch Intern Med **153**(3): 285-8.

Burr, M. L., R. M. Holliday, et al. (1992). "Haematological prognostic indices after myocardial infarction: evidence from the diet and reinfarction trial (DART)." Eur Heart J **13**(2): 166-70.

Friedensohn, A. and Z. Schlesinger (1992). "Pharmacological aspects in secondary prevention of coronary artery disease." Ann Acad Med Singapore **21**(1): 73-7.

Sleight, P. (1992). "The secondary prevention of myocardial infarction by drug treatment; excluding lipid lowering agents." Clin Exp Hypertens [a] **14**(1-2): 239-50.

Criqui, M. H. (1991). "Cholesterol, primary and secondary prevention, and all-cause mortality." Ann Intern Med **115**(12): 973-6.

Lewis, B. (1991). "On lowering lipids in the post-infarction patient." J Intern Med **229**(6): 483-8.

Selenium

Clark, L. C., L. J. Hixson, et al. (1993). "Plasma selenium concentration predicts the prevalence of colorectal adenomatous polyps." Cancer Epidemiol Biomarkers Prev **2**(1): 41-6.

Vadhanavikit, S. and H. E. Ganther (1993). "Decreased ubiquinone levels in tissues of rats deficient in selenium." Biochem Biophys Res Commun **190**(3): 921-6.

Comstock, G. W., T. L. Bush, et al. (1992). "Serum retinol, beta-carotene, vitamin E, and selenium as related to subsequent cancer of specific sites." Am J Epidemiol **135**(2): 115-21.

Meydani, M. (1992). "Modulation of the platelet thromboxane A2 and aortic prostacyclin synthesis by dietary selenium and vitamin E." Biol Trace Elem Res **33**(1): 79-86.

Suadicani, P., H. O. Hein, et al. (1992). "Serum selenium concentration and risk of ischaemic heart disease in a prospective cohort study of 3000 males." Atherosclerosis **96**(1): 33-42.

Tominaga, K., Y. Saito, et al. (1992). "An evaluation of serum microelement concentrations in lung cancer and matched non-cancer patients to determine the risk of developing lung cancer: a preliminary study." Jpn J Clin Oncol **22**(2): 96-101.

Van Dokkum, W., H. W. Van der Torre, et al. (1992). "Supplementation with selenium-rich bread does not influence platelet aggregation in healthy volunteers." Eur J Clin Nutr **46**(6): 445-50.

Van Vleet, J. F. and V. J. Ferrans (1992). "Etiologic factors and pathologic alterations in selenium-vitamin E deficiency and excess in animals and humans." Biol Trace Elem Res **33**(1): 1-21.

Veera Reddy, K., T. Charles Kumar, et al. (1992). "Exercise-induced oxidant stress in the lung tissue: role of dietary supplementation of vitamin E and selenium." Biochem Int **26**(5): 863-71.

Clark, L. C., K. P. Cantor, et al. (1991). "Selenium in forage crops and cancer mortality in U.S. counties." Arch Environ Health **46**(1): 37-42.

Clausen, J. (1991). "The influence of selenium and vitamin E on the enhanced respiratory burst reaction in smokers." Biol Trace Elem Res **31**(3): 281-91.

Jossa, F., M. Trevisan, et al. (1991). "Serum selenium and coronary heart disease risk factors in southern Italian men." Atherosclerosis **87**(2-3): 129-34.

Pawlowicz, Z., B. A. Zachara, et al. (1991). "Blood selenium concentrations and glutathione peroxidase activities in patients with breast cancer and with advanced gastrointestinal cancer." J Trace Elem Electrolytes Health Dis **5**(4): 275-7.

Rozewicka, L., W. B. Barcew, et al. (1991). "Protective effect of selenium and vitamin E against changes induced in heart vessels of rabbits fed chronically on a high-fat diet." Kitasato Arch Exp Med **64**(4): 183-92.

Salonen, J. T., R. Salonen, et al. (1991). "Interactions of serum copper, selenium, and low density lipoprotein cholesterol in atherogenesis." Bmj **302**(6779): 756-60.

Siegel, B. Z., S. M. Siegel, et al. (1991). "The protection of invertebrates, fish, and vascular plants against inorganic mercury poisoning by sulfur and selenium derivatives." Arch Environ Contam Toxicol **20**(2): 241-6.

Wojcicki, J., L. Rozewicka, et al. (1991). "Effect of selenium and vitamin E on the development of experimental atherosclerosis in rabbits." Atherosclerosis **87**(1): 9-16.

Zamora, R., F. J. Hidalgo, et al. (1991). "Comparative antioxidant effectiveness of dietary beta-carotene, vitamin E, selenium and coenzyme Q10 in rat erythrocytes and plasma." J Nutr **121**(1): 50-6.

Bukkens, S. G., N. de Vos, et al. (1990). "Selenium status and cardiovascular risk factors in healthy Dutch subjects." J Am Coll Nutr **9**(2): 128-35.

Knekt, P., A. Aromaa, et al. (1990). "Serum selenium and subsequent risk of cancer among Finnish men and women." J Natl Cancer Inst **82**(10): 864-8.

Leibovitz, B., M. L. Hu, et al. (1990). "Dietary supplements of vitamin E, beta-carotene, coenzyme Q10 and selenium protect tissues against lipid peroxidation in rat tissue slices." J Nutr **120**(1): 97-104.

Riemersma, R. A., M. Oliver, et al. (1990). "Plasma antioxidants and coronary heart disease: vitamins C and E, and selenium." Eur J Clin Nutr **44**(2): 143-50.

Swanson, C. A., M. P. Longnecker, et al. (1990). "Selenium intake, age, gender, and smoking in relation to indices of selenium status of adults residing in a seleniferous area." Am J Clin Nutr **52**(5): 858-62.

Yang, G., S. Yin, et al. (1989). "Studies of safe maximal daily dietary Se-intake in a seleniferous area in China. Part II: Relation between Se-intake and the manifestation of clinical signs and certain biochemical alterations in blood and urine." J Trace Elem Electrolytes Health Dis **3**(3): 123-30.

Salonen, J. T., R. Salonen, et al. (1988). "Relationship of serum selenium and antioxidants to plasma lipoproteins, platelet aggregability and prevalent ischaemic heart disease in Eastern Finnish men." Atherosclerosis **70**(1-2): 155-60.

Salonen, J. T., R. Salonen, et al. (1985). "Serum fatty acids, apolipoproteins, selenium and vitamin antioxidants and the risk of death from coronary artery disease." Am J Cardiol **56**(4): 226-31.

Smoking

Barbash, G. I., H. D. White, et al. (1993). "Significance of smoking in patients receiving thrombolytic therapy for acute myocardial infarction. Experience gleaned from the International Tissue Plasminogen Activator/Streptokinase Mortality Trial [see comments]." Circulation **87**(1): 53-8.

Chow, C. K. (1993). "Cigarette smoking and oxidative damage in the lung." Ann N Y Acad Sci **686**(1): 289-98.

Chung, F. L., M. A. Morse, et al. (1993). "Inhibition of tobacco-specific nitrosamine-induced lung tumorigenesis by compounds derived from cruciferous vegetables and green tea." Ann N Y Acad Sci **686**(1): 186-201.

Cross, C. E., C. A. O'Neill, et al. (1993). "Cigarette smoke oxidation of human plasma constituents." Ann N Y Acad Sci **686**(1): 72-89.

Duthie, G. G., J. R. Arthur, et al. (1993). "Cigarette smoking, antioxidants, lipid peroxidation, and coronary heart disease." Ann N Y Acad Sci **686**(1): 120-9.

Hoffmann, D., A. Rivenson, et al. (1993). "Potential inhibitors of tobacco carcinogenesis." Ann N Y Acad Sci **686**(1): 140-60.

Kawachi, I., G. A. Colditz, et al. (1993). "Smoking cessation and decreased risk of stroke in women." Jama **269**(2): 232-6.

Knekt, P. (1993). "Vitamin E and smoking and the risk of lung cancer." Ann N Y Acad Sci **686**(1): 280-7.

Lee, E. W. and G. E. D'Alonzo (1993). "Cigarette smoking, nicotine addiction, and its pharmacologic treatment." Arch Intern Med **153**(1): 34-48.

Leone, A. (1993). "Cardiovascular damage from smoking: a fact or belief?" Int J Cardiol **38**(2): 113-7.

Niki, E., S. Minamisawa, et al. (1993). "Membrane damage from lipid oxidation induced by free radicals and cigarette smoke." Ann N Y Acad Sci **686**(1): 29-37.

Rimm, E. and G. Colditz (1993). "Smoking, alcohol, and plasma levels of carotenes and vitamin E." Ann N Y Acad Sci **686**(1): 323-33.

Rimm, E. B., J. E. Manson, et al. (1993). "Cigarette smoking and the risk of diabetes in women." Am J Public Health **83**(2): 211-4.

Schectman, G. (1993). "Estimating ascorbic acid requirements for cigarette smokers." Ann N Y Acad Sci **686**(1): 335-45.

Sugiishi, M. and F. Takatsu (1993). "Cigarette smoking is a major risk factor for coronary spasm." Circulation **87**(1): 76-9.

van Antwerpen, L., A. J. Theron, et al. (1993). "Cigarette smoke-mediated oxidant stress, phagocytes, vitamin C, vitamin E, and tissue injury." Ann N Y Acad Sci **686**(1): 53-65.

van Poppel, G., S. Spanhaak, et al. (1993). "Effect of beta-carotene on immunological indexes in healthy male smokers." Am J Clin Nutr **57**(3): 402-7.

Smoke, Passive/Environmental

Zhu, B. Q., Y. P. Sun, et al. (1993). "Passive smoking increases experimental atherosclerosis in cholesterol-fed rabbits." J Am Coll Cardiol **21**(1): 225-32.

Brownson, R. C., M. C. Alavanja, et al. (1992). "Passive smoking and lung cancer in nonsmoking women." Am J Public Health **82**(11): 1525-30.

Glantz, S. A. and W. W. Parmley (1992). "Passive smoking causes heart disease and lung cancer." J Clin Epidemiol **45**(8): 815-9.

Gray, N. (1992). "Active and passive smoking [editorial]." Med J Aust **156**(12): 826-7.

Scherer, G., C. Conze, et al. (1992). "Uptake of tobacco smoke constituents on exposure to environmental tobacco smoke (ETS)." Clin Investig **70**(3-4): 352-67.

Steenland, K. (1992). "Passive smoking and the risk of heart disease [see comments]." Jama **267**(1): 94-9.

Taylor, A. E., D. C. Johnson, et al. (1992). "Environmental tobacco smoke and cardiovascular disease. A position paper from the Council on Cardiopulmonary and Critical Care, American Heart Association." Circulation **86**(2): 699-702.

Whig, J., C. B. Singh, et al. (1992). "Serum lipids & lipoprotein profiles of cigarette smokers & passive smokers." Indian J Med Res **96**(1): 282-7.

Dobson, A. J., H. M. Alexander, et al. (1991). "Passive smoking and the risk of heart attack or coronary death." Med J Aust **154**(12): 793-7.

Glantz, S. A. and W. W. Parmley (1991). "Passive smoking and heart disease. Epidemiology, physiology, and biochemistry [see comments]." Circulation **83**(1): 1-12.

Soy

Kanazawa, T., M. Tanaka, et al. (1993). "Anti-atherogenicity of soybean protein." Ann N Y Acad Sci **676**(1): 202-14.

O'Brien, B. C. and V. G. Andrews (1993). "Influence of dietary egg and soybean phospholipids and triacylglycerols on human serum lipoproteins." Lipids **28**(1): 7-12.

Sirtori, C. R., R. Even, et al. (1993). "Soybean protein diet and plasma cholesterol: from therapy to molecular mechanisms." Ann N Y Acad Sci **676**(1): 188-201.

Jacques, H., D. Laurin, et al. (1992). "Influence of diets containing cow's milk or soy protein beverage on plasma lipids in children with familial hypercholesterolemia." J Am Coll Nutr **11**(1): 69S-73S.

Santiago, L. A., M. Hiramatsu, et al. (1992). "Japanese soybean paste miso scavenges free radicals and inhibits lipid peroxidation." J Nutr Sci Vitaminol **38**(3): 297-304.

Carroll, K. K. (1991). "Review of clinical studies on cholesterol-lowering response to soy protein." J Am Diet Assoc **91**(7): 820-7.

Gaddi, A., A. Ciarrocchi, et al. (1991). "Dietary treatment for familial hypercholesterolemia—differential effects of dietary soy protein according to the apolipoprotein E phenotypes." Am J Clin Nutr **53**(5): 1191-6.

Laurin, D., H. Jacques, et al. (1991). "Effects of a soy-protein beverage on plasma lipoproteins in children with familial hypercholesterolemia." Am J Clin Nutr **54**(1): 98-103.

Messina, M. and S. Barnes (1991). "The role of soy products in reducing risk of cancer." J Natl Cancer Inst **83**(8): 541-6.

Meydani, S. N., A. H. Lichtenstein, et al. (1991). "Food use and health effects of soybean and sunflower oils." J Am Coll Nutr **10**(5): 406-28.

Slavin, J. (1991). "Nutritional benefits of soy protein and soy fiber." J Am Diet Assoc **91**(7): 816-9.

Sudden Death

(1992). "Current perspectives on the problem of sudden cardiac death. Dallas, Texas, September 24-25, 1990." Circulation **85**(1 Suppl): I1-166.

Eisenberg, M. J. (1992). "Magnesium deficiency and sudden death [editorial]." Am Heart J **124**(2): 544-9.

Kohl, H. 3., K. E. Powell, et al. (1992). "Physical activity, physical fitness, and sudden cardiac death." Epidemiol Rev **14**(1): 37-58.

Moss, A. J. (1992). "Prevention of sudden cardiac death." Hosp Pract **27**(11): 165-8.

Myerburg, R. J., K. M. Kessler, et al. (1992). "Sudden cardiac death. Structure, function, and time-dependence of risk." Circulation **85**(1 Suppl): I2-10.

Pitt, B. (1992). "The role of beta-adrenergic blocking agents in preventing sudden cardiac death." Circulation **85**(1 Suppl): I107-11.

Stendig-Lindberg, G. (1992). "Sudden death of athletes: is it due to long-term changes in serum magnesium, lipids and blood sugar?" J Basic Clin Physiol Pharmacol **3**(2): 153-64.

Willich, S. N., R. J. Goldberg, et al. (1992). "Increased onset of sudden cardiac death in the first three hours after awakening." Am J Cardiol **70**(1): 65-8.

Ciampricotti, R., R. Taverne, et al. (1991). "Clinical and angiographic observations on resuscitated victims of exercise-related sudden ischemic death." Am J Cardiol **68**(1): 47-50.

Drory, Y., Y. Turetz, et al. (1991). "Sudden unexpected death in persons less than 40 years of age." Am J Cardiol **68**(13): 1388-92.

Olsson, G. and L. Ryden (1991). "Prevention of sudden death using beta-blockers. Review of possible contributory actions." Circulation **84**(6 Suppl): VI33-7.

Shen, W. K. and S. C. Hammill (1991). "Survivors of acute myocardial infarction: who is at risk for sudden cardiac death?" Mayo Clin Proc **66**(9): 950-62.

Ciampricotti, R., M. el-Gamal, et al. (1990). "Clinical characteristics and coronary angiographic findings of patients with unstable angina, acute myocardial infarction, and survivors of sudden ischemic death occurring during and after sport." Am Heart J **120**(6 (Pt 1): 1267-78.

Davies, M. J. and A. C. Thomas (1985). "Plaque fissuring—the cause of acute myocardial infarction, sudden ischaemic death, and crescendo angina." Br Heart J **53**(4): 363-73.

Sugar

Bantle, J. P., J. E. Swanson, et al. (1992). "Metabolic effects of dietary fructose in diabetic subjects." Diabetes Care **15**(11): 1468-76.

Lewis, C. J., Y. K. Park, et al. (1992). "Nutrient intakes and body weights of persons consuming high and moderate levels of added sugars." J Am Diet Assoc **92**(6): 708-13.

Preuss, H. G., J. J. Knapka, et al. (1992). "High sucrose diets increase blood pressure of both salt-sensitive and salt-resistant rats." Am J Hypertens **5**(9): 585-91.

Swanson, J. E., D. C. Laine, et al. (1992). "Metabolic effects of dietary fructose in healthy subjects." Am J Clin Nutr **55**(4): 851-6.

Pivonka, E. E. and K. K. Grunewald (1990). "Aspartame- or sugar-sweetened beverages: effects on mood in young women." J Am Diet Assoc **90**(2): 250-4.

Bantle, J. P. (1989). "Clinical aspects of sucrose and fructose metabolism." Diabetes Care **12**(1): 56-61.

Colagiuri, S., J. J. Miller, et al. (1989). "Metabolic effects of adding sucrose and aspartame to the diet of subjects with noninsulin-dependent diabetes mellitus." Am J Clin Nutr **50**(3): 474-8.

Kozlovsky, A. S., P. B. Moser, et al. (1986). "Effects of diets high in simple sugars on urinary chromium losses." Metabolism **35**(6): 515-8.

Syndrome X/Insulin Resistance

Jiang, X., S. R. Srinivasan, et al. (1993). "Association of fasting insulin with blood pressure in young individuals. The Bogalusa Heart Study [see comments]." Arch Intern Med **153**(3): 323-8.

McKeigue, P. M., J. E. Ferrie, et al. (1993). "Association of early-onset coronary heart disease in South Asian men with glucose intolerance and hyperinsulinemia." Circulation **87**(1): 152-61.

Nadler, J. L., T. Buchanan, et al. (1993). "Magnesium deficiency produces insulin resistance and increased thromboxane synthesis." Hypertension **21**: 1024-1029.

Paolisso, G., A. D'Amore, et al. (1993). "Pharmacologic doses of vitamin E improve insulin action in healthy subjects and non-insulin-dependent diabetic patients." Am J Clin Nutr **57**(5): 650-6.

De Fronzo, R. A. (1992). "Insulin resistance, hyperinsulinemia, and coronary artery disease: a complex metabolic web." J Cardiovasc Pharmacol **20**(1): S1-16.

Durrington, P. N. (1992). "Is insulin atherogenic?" Diabet Med **9**(7): 597-600.

Enas, E. A., S. Yusuf, et al. (1992). "Prevalence of coronary artery disease in Asian Indians [editorial]." Am J Cardiol **70**(9): 945-9.

Haffner, S. M., R. A. Valdez, et al. (1992). "Prospective analysis of the insulin-resistance syndrome (syndrome X)." Diabetes **41**(6): 715-22.

Hjermann, I. (1992). "The metabolic cardiovascular syndrome: syndrome X, Reaven's syndrome, insulin resistance syndrome, atherothrombogenic syndrome." J Cardiovasc Pharmacol **20**(1): S5-10.

Kaplan, N. M. (1992). "Effects of antihypertensive therapy on insulin resistance." Hypertension **19**(1 Suppl): I116-8.

Kaplan, N. M. (1992). "Syndromes X: two too many [editorial]." Am J Cardiol **69**(19): 1643-4.

Karam, J. H. (1992). "Type II diabetes and syndrome X. Pathogenesis and glycemic management." Endocrinol Metab Clin North Am **21**(2): 329-50.

Laakso, M. (1992). "Dyslipidaemias, insulin resistance and atherosclerosis." Ann Med **24**(6): 505-9.

Landin, K., G. Holm, et al. (1992). "Guar gum improves insulin sensitivity, blood lipids, blood pressure, and fibrinolysis in healthy men." Am J Clin Nutr **56**(6): 1061-5.

Laws, A. and G. M. Reaven (1992). "Evidence for an independent relationship between insulin resistance and fasting plasma HDL-cholesterol, triglyceride and insulin concentrations." J Intern Med **231**(1): 25-30.

Mark, A. L. (1992). "Syndrome X: a cause of hypertension? Negative [comment]." Hosp Pract **27**(1): 41-4.

Morris, B. W., A. Blumsohn, et al. (1992). "The trace element chromium—a role in glucose homeostasis." Am J Clin Nutr **55**(5): 989-91.

Paolisso, G., E. Ferrannini, et al. (1992). "Hyperinsulinemia in patients with hypercholesterolemia." J Clin Endocrinol Metab **75**(6): 1409-12.

Paolisso, G., S. Sgambato, et al. (1992). "Daily magnesium supplements improve glucose handling in elderly subjects." Am J Clin Nutr **55**(6): 1161-7.

Parillo, M., A. A. Rivellese, et al. (1992). "A high-monounsaturated-fat/low-carbohydrate diet improves peripheral insulin sensitivity in non-insulin-dependent diabetic patients." Metabolism **41**(12): 1373-8.

Resnick, L. M. (1992). "Cellular calcium and magnesium metabolism in the pathophysiology and treatment of hypertension and related metabolic disorders." Am J Med **93**(2A): 11S-20S.

Resnick, L. M. (1992). "Cellular ions in hypertension, insulin resistance, obesity, and diabetes: a unifying theme." J Am Soc Nephrol **3**(4 Suppl): S78-85.

Rett, K., M. Wicklmayr, et al. (1992). "What is the clinical significance of insulin resistance?" J Cardiovasc Pharmacol **20**(1): S22-6.

Ruderman, N. B. and S. H. Schneider (1992). "Diabetes, exercise, and atherosclerosis." Diabetes Care **15**(11): 1787-93.

Rupp, H. (1992). "Insulin resistance, hyperinsulinemia, and cardiovascular disease. The need for novel dietary prevention strategies [editorial]." Basic Res Cardiol **87**(2): 99-105.

Sowers, J. R. (1992). "Insulin resistance, hyperinsulinemia, dyslipidemia, hypertension, and accelerated atherosclerosis." J Clin Pharmacol **32**(6): 529-35.

Stern, M. P. (1992). "'Syndrome X': is it a significant cause of hypertension? Affirmative [see comments]." Hosp Pract **27**(1): 37-40.

Vaaler, S. (1992). "Carbohydrate metabolism, insulin resistance, and metabolic cardiovascular syndrome." J Cardiovasc Pharmacol **20**(1): S11-4.

Westheim, A. and I. Os (1992). "Physical activity and the metabolic cardiovascular syndrome." J Cardiovasc Pharmacol **20**(1): S49-53.

De Fronzo, R. A. and E. Ferrannini (1991). "Insulin resistance. A multifaceted syndrome responsible for NIDDM, obesity, hypertension, dyslipidemia, and atherosclerotic cardiovascular disease." Diabetes Care **14**(3): 173-94.

Ferrannini, E., S. M. Haffner, et al. (1991). "Hyperinsulinaemia: the key feature of a cardiovascular and metabolic syndrome." Diabetologia **34**(6): 416-22.

Ferrannini, E. and A. Natali (1991). "Essential hypertension, metabolic disorders, and insulin resistance." Am Heart J **121**(4 Pt 2): 1274-82.

Gwinup, G. and A. N. Elias (1991). "Hypothesis: insulin is responsible for the vascular complications of diabetes." Med Hypotheses **34**(1): 1-6.

Kaplan, N. M. (1991). "Hypertension and hyperinsulinemia." Prim Care **18**(3): 483-94.

Laakso, M., H. Sarlund, et al. (1991). "Asymptomatic atherosclerosis and insulin resistance." Arterioscler Thromb **11**(4): 1068-76.

Laws, A., A. C. King, et al. (1991). "Relation of fasting plasma insulin concentration to high density lipoprotein cholesterol and triglyceride concentrations in men." Arterioscler Thromb **11**(6): 1636-42.

Maron, D. J., J. M. Fair, et al. (1991). "Saturated fat intake and insulin resistance in men with coronary artery disease. The Stanford Coronary Risk Intervention Project Investigators and Staff." Circulation **84**(5): 2020-7.

Modan, M., J. Or, et al. (1991). "Hyperinsulinemia, sex, and risk of atherosclerotic cardiovascular disease [see comments]." Circulation **84**(3): 1165-75.

Pyorala, K. (1991). "Hyperinsulinaemia as predictor of atherosclerotic vascular disease: epidemiological evidence." Diabete Metab **17**(1 Pt 2): 87-92.

Reaven, G. M. (1991). "Insulin resistance, hyperinsulinemia, and hypertriglyceridemia in the etiology and clinical course of hypertension." Am J Med **90**(2A): 7S-12S.

Reaven, G. M. (1991). "Relationship between insulin resistance and hypertension." Diabetes Care **14**(1): 33-8.

Reaven, G. M. (1991). "Resistance to insulin-stimulated glucose uptake and hyperinsulinemia: role in non-insulin-dependent diabetes, high blood pressure, dyslipidemia and coronary heart disease." Diabete Metab **17**(1 Pt 2): 78-86.

Resnick, L. M. (1991). "Calcium metabolism in hypertension and allied metabolic disorders." Diabetes Care **14**(6): 505-20.

Singh, R. B. and H. Mori (1991). "Can nutritional factors enhance hyperinsulinemia leading to coronary heart disease? [letter]." Cardiovasc Drugs Ther **5**(6): 1045-6.

Foster, D. W. (1989). "Insulin resistance—a secret killer? [editorial]." N Engl J Med **320**(11): 733-4.

Simonoff, M. (1984). "Chromium deficiency and cardiovascular risk." Cardiovasc Res **18**(10): 591-6.

Tea

Yang, C. S. and Z. Y. Wang (1993). "Tea and cancer." J Natl Cancer Inst **85**(13): 1038-49.

Green, M. S. and G. Harari (1992). "Association of serum lipoproteins and health-related habits with coffee and tea consumption in free-living subjects examined in the Israeli CORDIS Study." Prev Med **21**(4): 532-45.

Ho, C. T., Q. Chen, et al. (1992). "Antioxidative effect of polyphenol extract prepared from various Chinese teas." Prev Med **21**(4): 520-5.

Stensvold, I., A. Tverdal, et al. (1992). "Tea consumption. relationship to cholesterol, blood pressure, and coronary and total mortality." Prev Med **21**(4): 546-53.

Stich, H. F. (1992). "Teas and tea components as inhibitors of carcinogen formation in model systems and man." Prev Med **21**(3): 377-84.

Tea—Green

Chung, F. L., M. A. Morse, et al. (1993). "Inhibition of tobacco-specific nitrosamine-induced lung tumorigenesis by compounds derived from cruciferous vegetables and green tea." Ann N Y Acad Sci **686**(1): 186-201.

Yang, C. S. and Z. Y. Wang (1993). "Tea and cancer." J Natl Cancer Inst **85**(13): 1038-49.

Chen, J. (1992). "The antimutagenic and anticarcinogenic effects of tea, garlic and other natural foods in China: a review." Biomed Environ Sci **5**(1): 1-17.

Conney, A. H., Z. Y. Wang, et al. (1992). "Inhibitory effect of green tea on tumorigenesis by chemicals and ultraviolet light." Prev Med **21**(3): 361-9.

Graham, H. N. (1992). "Green tea composition, consumption, and polyphenol chemistry." Prev Med **21**(3): 334-50.

Ho, C. T., Q. Chen, et al. (1992). "Antioxidative effect of polyphenol extract prepared from various Chinese teas." Prev Med **21**(4): 520-5.

Ikeda, I., Y. Imasato, et al. (1992). "Tea catechins decrease micellar solubility and intestinal absorption of cholesterol in rats." Biochim Biophys Acta **1127**(2): 141-6.

Khan, S. G., S. K. Katiyar, et al. (1992). "Enhancement of antioxidant and phase II enzymes by oral feeding of green tea polyphenols in drinking water to SKH-1 hairless mice: possible role in cancer chemoprevention." Cancer Res **52**(14): 4050-2.

Klaunig, J. E. (1992). "Chemopreventive effects of green tea components on hepatic carcinogenesis." Prev Med **21**(4): 510-9.

Kono, S., K. Shinchi, et al. (1992). "Green tea consumption and serum lipid profiles: a cross-sectional study in northern Kyushu, Japan." Prev Med **21**(4): 526-31.

Luo, D. and Y. Li (1992). "[Preventive effect of green tea on MNNG-induced lung cancers and precancerous lesions in LACA mice]." Hua Hsi I Ko Ta Hsueh Hsueh Pao **23**(4): 433-7.

Mukhtar, H., Z. Y. Wang, et al. (1992). "Tea components: antimutagenic and anticarcinogenic effects." Prev Med **21**(3): 351-60.

Sadakata, S., A. Fukao, et al. (1992). "Mortality among female practitioners of Chanoyu (Japanese "tea-ceremony")." Tohoku J Exp Med **166**(4): 475-7.

Stich, H. F. (1992). "Teas and tea components as inhibitors of carcinogen formation in model systems and man." Prev Med **21**(3): 377-84.

Taniguchi, S., H. Fujiki, et al. (1992). "Effect of (-)-epigallocatechin gallate, the main constituent of green tea, on lung metastasis with mouse B16 melanoma cell lines." Cancer Lett **65**(1): 51-4.

Cheng, S., L. Ding, et al. (1991). "Progress in studies on the antimutagenicity and anticarcinogenicity of green tea epicatechins." Chin Med Sci J **6**(4): 233-8.

Horiba, N., Y. Maekawa, et al. (1991). "A pilot study of Japanese green tea as a medicament: antibacterial and bactericidal effects." J Endod **17**(3): 122-4.

Yamaguchi, Y., M. Hayashi, et al. (1991). "[Preventive effects of green tea extract on lipid abnormalities in serum, liver and aorta of mice fed a atherogenic diet]." Nippon Yakurigaku Zasshi **97**(6): 329-37.

Trans-fatty Acids

Lichtenstein, A. H., L. M. Ausman, et al. (1993). "Hydrogenation impairs the hypolipidemic effect of corn oil in humans. Hydrogenation, trans fatty acids, and plasma lipids." Arterioscler Thromb **13**(2): 154-61.

Siguel, E. N. and R. H. Lerman (1993). "Trans-fatty acid patterns in patients with angiographically documented coronary artery disease." Am J Cardiol **71**(April 15): 916-920.

Willett, W. C., M. J. Stampfer, et al. (1993). "Intake of trans fatty acids and risk of coronary heart disease among women." Lancet **341**(8845): 581-5.

Wood, R., K. Kubena, et al. (1993). "Effect of butter, mono- and polyunsaturated fatty acid-enriched butter, trans fatty acid margarine, and zero trans fatty acid margarine on serum lipids and lipoproteins in healthy men." J Lipid Res **34**(1): 1-11.

Mensink, R. P., P. L. Zock, et al. (1992). "Effect of dietary cis and trans fatty acids on serum lipoprotein[a] levels in humans." J Lipid Res **33**(10): 1493-501.

Nestel, P., M. Noakes, et al. (1992). "Plasma lipoprotein lipid and Lp[a] changes with substitution of elaidic acid for oleic acid in the diet." J Lipid Res **33**(7): 1029-36.

Nestel, P. J., M. Noakes, et al. (1992). "Plasma cholesterol-lowering potential of edible-oil blends suitable for commercial use." Am J Clin Nutr **55**(1): 46-50.

Troisi, R., W. C. Willett, et al. (1992). "Trans-fatty acid intake in relation to serum lipid concentrations in adult men." Am J Clin Nutr **56**(6): 1019-24.

Zock, P. L. and M. B. Katan (1992). "Hydrogenation alternatives: effects of trans fatty acids and stearic acid versus linoleic acid on serum lipids and lipoproteins in humans." J Lipid Res **33**(3): 399-410.

Chiang, M. T., M. I. Otomo, et al. (1991). "Effect of trans fatty acids on plasma lipids, platelet function and systolic blood pressure in stroke-prone spontaneously hypertensive rats." Lipids **26**(1): 46-52.

Dupont, J., P. J. White, et al. (1991). "Saturated and hydrogenated fats in food in relation to health [see comments]." J Am Coll Nutr **10**(6): 577-92.

Mensink, R. P., M. H. de Louw, et al. (1991). "Effects of dietary trans fatty acids on blood pressure in normotensive subjects." Eur J Clin Nutr **45**(8): 375-82.

Mensink, R. P. and M. B. Katan (1990). "Effect of dietary trans fatty acids on high-density and low-density lipoprotein cholesterol levels in healthy subjects [see comments]." N Engl J Med **323**(7): 439-45.

Triglycerides

(1993). "NIH Consensus conference. Triglyceride, high-density lipoprotein, and coronary heart disease. NIH Consensus Development Panel on Triglyceride, High-Density Lipoprotein, and Coronary Heart Disease." Jama **269**(4): 505-10.

Elwood, P. C., J. W. Yarnell, et al. (1993). "Exercise, fibrinogen, and other risk factors for ischaemic heart disease. Caerphilly Prospective Heart Disease Study." Br Heart J **69**(2): 183-7.

Franceschini, G. and R. Paoletti (1993). "Drugs controlling triglyceride metabolism." Med Res Rev **13**(2): 125-38.

Karpe, F., G. Steiner, et al. (1993). "Metabolism of triglyceride-rich lipoproteins during alimentary lipemia." J Clin Invest **91**(3): 748-58.

(1992). "Triglyceride, high density lipoprotein, and coronary heart disease." Consens Statement **10**(2): 1-28.

Assmann, G. and H. Schulte (1992). "The importance of triglycerides: results from the Prospective Cardiovascular Munster (PROCAM) Study." Eur J Epidemiol **8**(1): 99-103.

Assmann, G. and H. Schulte (1992). "Relation of high-density lipoprotein cholesterol and triglycerides to incidence of atherosclerotic coronary artery disease (the PROCAM experience). Prospective Cardiovascular Munster study." Am J Cardiol **70**(7): 733-7.

Assmann, G. and H. Schulte (1992). "Role of triglycerides in coronary artery disease: lessons from the Prospective Cardiovascular Munster Study." Am J Cardiol **70**(19): 10H-13H.

Bainton, D., N. E. Miller, et al. (1992). "Plasma triglyceride and high density lipoprotein cholesterol as predictors of ischaemic heart disease in British men. The Caerphilly and Speedwell Collaborative Heart Disease Studies." Br Heart J **68**(1): 60-6.

Castelli, W. P. (1992). "Epidemiology of triglycerides: a view from Framingham." Am J Cardiol **70**(19): 3H-9H.

Coniglio, J. G. (1992). "How does fish oil lower plasma triglycerides?" Nutr Rev **50**(7): 195-7.

Ding, Y. A. (1992). "Plasma triglycerides: a cardiovascular risk factor?" Chung Hua I Hsueh Tsa Chih **49**(5): 297-302.

Genest, J., Jr., S. S. Martin-Munley, et al. (1992). "Familial lipoprotein disorders in patients with premature coronary artery disease." Circulation **85**(6): 2025-33.

Geurian, K., J. B. Pinson, et al. (1992). "The triglyceride connection in atherosclerosis." Ann Pharmacother **26**(9): 1109-17.

Gotto, A., Jr. (1992). "Hypertriglyceridemia: risks and perspectives." Am J Cardiol **70**(19): 19H-25H.

Grundy, S. M. and G. L. Vega (1992). "Two different views of the relationship of hypertriglyceridemia to coronary heart disease. Implications for treatment." Arch Intern Med **152**(1): 28-34.

Johansson, J., G. Walldius, et al. (1992). "Close correlation between high-density lipoprotein and triglycerides in normotriglyceridaemia." J Intern Med **232**(1): 43-51.

Laws, A. and G. M. Reaven (1992). "Evidence for an independent relationship between insulin resistance and fasting plasma HDL-cholesterol, triglyceride and insulin concentrations." J Intern Med **231**(1): 25-30.

Manninen, V., L. Tenkanen, et al. (1992). "Joint effects of serum triglyceride and LDL cholesterol and HDL cholesterol concentrations on coronary heart disease risk in the Helsinki Heart Study. Implications for treatment [see comments]." Circulation **85**(1): 37-45.

Mitropoulos, K. A., G. J. Miller, et al. (1992). "Lipolysis of triglyceride-rich lipoproteins activates coagulant factor XII: a study in familial lipoprotein-lipase deficiency." Atherosclerosis **95**(2-3): 119-25.

Rotzsch, W., V. Richter, et al. (1992). "[Postprandial lipemia under treatment with Allium sativum. Controlled double-blind study of subjects with reduced HDL2-cholesterol]." Arzneimittelforschung **42**(10): 1223-7.

Simons, L. A. (1992). "Triglyceride levels and the risk of coronary artery disease: a view from Australia." Am J Cardiol **70**(19): 14H-18H.

Stein, Y. and A. Gotto Jr. (1992). "A symposium: triglycerides as a vascular risk factor: a global forum. Introduction." Am J Cardiol **70**(19): 1H-2H.

Sum, C. F., C. E. Tan, et al. (1992). "Triglycerides and coronary artery disease [editorial]." Singapore Med J **33**(5): 443-5.

Superko, H. R. (1992). "Effects of acute and chronic alcohol consumption on postprandial lipemia in healthy normotriglyceridemic men." Am J Cardiol **69**(6): 701-4.

Vegetarian Diet

Draper, A., J. Lewis, et al. (1993). "The energy and nutrient intakes of different types of vegetarians: a case for supplements?" Br J Nutr **69**(1): 3-19.

Chang-Claude, J., R. Frentzel-Beyme, et al. (1992). "Mortality pattern of German vegetarians after 11 years of follow-up [see comments]." Epidemiology **3**(5): 395-401.

McMichael, A. J. (1992). "Vegetarians and longevity: imagining a wider reference population [editorial; comment]." Epidemiology **3**(5): 389-91.

Pronczuk, A., Y. Kipervarg, et al. (1992). "Vegetarians have higher plasma alpha-tocopherol relative to cholesterol than do nonvegetarians." J Am Coll Nutr **11**(1): 50-5.

McMurry, M. P., M. T. Cerqueira, et al. (1991). "Changes in lipid and lipoprotein levels and body weight in Tarahumara Indians after consumption of an affluent diet [see comments]." N Engl J Med **325**(24): 1704-8.

Negri, E., C. La Vecchia, et al. (1991). "Vegetable and fruit consumption and cancer risk." Int J Cancer **48**(3): 350-4.

Resnicow, K., J. Barone, et al. (1991). "Diet and serum lipids in vegan vegetarians: a model for risk reduction [published erratum appears in J Am Diet Assoc 1991 Jun; 91(6):655]." J Am Diet Assoc **91**(4): 447-53.

Thorogood, M., R. Carter, et al. (1987). "Plasma lipids and lipoprotein cholesterol concentrations in people with different diets in Britain." Br Med J **295**(6594): 351-3.

Vitamin A

Hunter, D. J., J. E. Manson, et al. (1993). "A prospective study of the intake of vitamins C, E, and A and the risk of breast cancer." N Engl J Med **329**(4): 234-40.

Pastorino, U., M. Infante, et al. (1993). "Adjuvant treatment of stage I lung cancer with high-dose vitamin A [see comments]." J Clin Oncol **11**(7): 1216-22.

Rohan, T. E., G. R. Howe, et al. (1993). "Dietary fiber, vitamins A, C, and E, and risk of breast cancer: a cohort study." Cancer Causes Control **4**(1): 29-37.

Comstock, G. W., T. L. Bush, et al. (1992). "Serum retinol, beta-carotene, vitamin E, and selenium as related to subsequent cancer of specific sites." Am J Epidemiol **135**(2): 115-21.

De Keyser, J., N. De Klippel, et al. (1992). "Serum concentrations of vitamins A and E and early outcome after ischaemic stroke." Lancet **339**(8809): 1562-5.

Goodman, G. E. and G. S. Omenn (1992). "Carotene and retinol efficacy trial: lung cancer chemoprevention trial in heavy cigarette smokers and asbestos-exposed workers. CARET Coinvestigators and Staff." Adv Exp Med Biol **320**(1): 137-40.

Paganelli, G. M., G. Biasco, et al. (1992). "Effect of vitamin A, C, and E supplementation on rectal cell proliferation in patients with colorectal adenomas." J Natl Cancer Inst **84**(1): 47-51.

Tee, E. S. (1992). "Carotenoids and retinoids in human nutrition." Crit Rev Food Sci Nutr **31**(1-2): 103-63.

Tominaga, K., Y. Saito, et al. (1992). "An evaluation of serum microelement concentrations in lung cancer and matched non-cancer patients to determine the risk of developing lung cancer: a preliminary study." Jpn J Clin Oncol **22**(2): 96-101.

Weiser, H., H. P. Probst, et al. (1992). "Vitamin E prevents side effects of high doses of vitamin A in chicks." Ann N Y Acad Sci **669**(1): 396-8.

Krempf, M., S. Ranganathan, et al. (1991). "Plasma vitamin A and E in type 1 (insulin-dependent) and type 2 (non-insulin-dependent) adult diabetic patients." Int J Vitam Nutr Res **61**(1): 38-42.

Riemersma, R. A., D. A. Wood, et al. (1991). "Risk of angina pectoris and plasma concentrations of vitamins A, C, and E and carotene [see comments]." Lancet **337**(8732): 1-5.

Willett, W. C. (1990). "Vitamin A and lung cancer." Nutr Rev **48**(5): 201-11.

Vitamin B6

Folkers, K., M. Morita, et al. (1993). "The activities of coenzyme Q10 and vitamin B6 for immune responses." Biochem Biophys Res Commun **193**(1): 88-92.

Ubbink, J. B., W. J. Vermaak, et al. (1993). "Vitamin B-12, vitamin B-6, and folate nutritional status in men with hyperhomocysteinemia." Am J Clin Nutr **57**(1): 47-53.

Leklem, J. E. (1992). "Vitamin B6. Reservoirs, receptors, and red-cell reactions." Ann N Y Acad Sci **669**(1): 34-41.

Mason, J. B. and J. W. Miller (1992). "The effects of vitamins B12, B6, and folate on blood homocysteine levels." Ann N Y Acad Sci **669**(1): 197-203.

Meydani, S. N., M. Hayek, et al. (1992). "Influence of vitamins E and B6 on immune response." Ann N Y Acad Sci **669**(1): 125-39.

Miller, J. W., M. J. Ribaya, et al. (1992). "Effect of vitamin B-6 deficiency on fasting plasma homocysteine concentrations." Am J Clin Nutr **55**(6): 1154-60.

Meydani, S. N., J. D. Ribaya-Mercado, et al. (1991). "Vitamin B-6 deficiency impairs interleukin 2 production and lymphocyte proliferation in elderly adults." Am J Clin Nutr **53**(5): 1275-80.

Vermaak, W. J., J. B. Ubbink, et al. (1990). "Vitamin B-6 nutrition status and cigarette smoking." Am J Clin Nutr **51**(6): 1058-61.

Serfontein, W. J., J. B. Ubbink, et al. (1985). "Plasma pyridoxal-5-phosphate level as risk index for coronary artery disease." Atherosclerosis **55**(3): 357-61.

Vitamin B_{12}

Ubbink, J. B., W. J. Vermaak, et al. (1993). "Vitamin B-12, vitamin B-6, and folate nutritional status in men with hyperhomocysteinemia." Am J Clin Nutr **57**(1): 47-53.

Mason, J. B. and J. W. Miller (1992). "The effects of vitamins B12, B6, and folate on blood homocysteine levels." Ann N Y Acad Sci **669**(1): 197-203.

Pennypacker, L. C., R. H. Allen, et al. (1992). "High prevalence of cobalamin deficiency in elderly outpatients." J Am Geriatr Soc **40**(12): 1197-204.

Vitamin C

Buettner, G. R. (1993). "The pecking order of free radicals and antioxidants: lipid peroxidation, alpha-tocopherol, and ascorbate." Arch Biochem Biophys **300**(2): 535-43.

Constantinescu, A., D. Han, et al. (1993). "Vitamin E recycling in human erythrocyte membranes." J Biol Chem **268**(15): 10906-13.

Gey, K. F., U. K. Moser, et al. (1993). "Increased risk of cardiovascular disease at suboptimal plasma concentrations of essential antioxidants: an epidemiological update with special attention to carotene and vitamin C." Am J Clin Nutr **57**(5 Suppl): 787S-797S.

Gey, K. F., H. B. Stahelin, et al. (1993). "Poor plasma status of carotene and vitamin C is associated with higher mortality from ischemic heart disease and stroke: Basel Prospective Study." Clin Investig **71**(1): 3-6.

Hunter, D. J., J. E. Manson, et al. (1993). "A prospective study of the intake of vitamins C, E, and A and the risk of breast cancer." N Engl J Med **329**(4): 234-40.

Moran, J. P., L. Cohen, et al. (1993). "Plasma ascorbic acid concentrations relate inversely to blood pressure in human subjects." Am J Clin Nutr **57**(2): 213-7.

Retsky, K. L., M. W. Freeman, et al. (1993). "Ascorbic acid oxidation product(s) protect human low density lipoprotein against atherogenic modification. Anti- rather than prooxidant activity of vitamin C in the presence of transition metal ions." J Biol Chem **268**(2): 1304-9.

Rohan, T. E., G. R. Howe, et al. (1993). "Dietary fiber, vitamins A, C, and E, and risk of breast cancer: a cohort study." Cancer Causes Control **4**(1): 29-37.

Schectman, G. (1993). "Estimating ascorbic acid requirements for cigarette smokers." Ann N Y Acad Sci **686**(1): 335-45.

Sinha, R., G. Block, et al. (1993). "Problems with estimating vitamin C intakes." Am J Clin Nutr **57**(4): 547-50.

van Antwerpen, L., A. J. Theron, et al. (1993). "Cigarette smoke-mediated oxidant stress, phagocytes, vitamin C, vitamin E, and tissue injury." Ann N Y Acad Sci **686**(1): 53-65.

Block, G. (1992). "Vitamin C and reduced mortality [editorial; comment]." Epidemiology **3**(3): 189-91.

Block, G. (1992). "Vitamin C status and cancer. Epidemiologic evidence of reduced risk." Ann N Y Acad Sci **669**(1): 280-90.

Bui, M. H., A. Sauty, et al. (1992). "Dietary vitamin C intake and concentrations in the body fluids and cells of male smokers and nonsmokers." J Nutr **122**(2): 312-6.

Byers, T. and G. Perry (1992). "Dietary carotenes, vitamin C, and vitamin E as protective antioxidants in human cancers." Annu Rev Nutr **12**(1): 139-59.

Dasgupta, A. and T. Zdunek (1992). "In vitro lipid peroxidation of human serum catalyzed by cupric ion: antioxidant rather than prooxidant role of ascorbate." Life Sci **50**(12): 875-82.

Davie, S. J., B. J. Gould, et al. (1992). "Effect of vitamin C on glycosylation of proteins." Diabetes **41**(2): 167-73.

Enstrom, J. E., L. E. Kanim, et al. (1992). "Vitamin C intake and mortality among a sample of the United States population [see comments]." Epidemiology **3**(3): 194-202.

Fahn, S. (1992). "A pilot trial of high-dose alpha-tocopherol and ascorbate in early Parkinson's disease." Ann Neurol **32**(1): 32.

Feldman, E. B., S. Gold, et al. (1992). "Ascorbic acid supplements and blood pressure. A four-week pilot study." Ann N Y Acad Sci **669**(1): 342-4.

Hornig, D. and F. Strolz (1992). "Recommended dietary allowance: support from recent research." J Nutr Sci Vitaminol **1**(6): 173-6.

Hunt, J. V., M. A. Bottoms, et al. (1992). "Ascorbic acid oxidation: a potential cause of the elevated severity of atherosclerosis in diabetes mellitus?" Febs Lett **311**(2): 161-4.

Jacques, P. F. (1992). "A cross-sectional study of vitamin C intake and blood pressure in the elderly." Int J Vitam Nutr Res **62**(3): 252-5.

Jacques, P. F. (1992). "Effects of vitamin C on high-density lipoprotein cholesterol and blood pressure." J Am Coll Nutr **11**(2): 139-44.

Jacques, P. F. (1992). "Relationship of vitamin C status to cholesterol and blood pressure." Ann N Y Acad Sci **669**(1): 205-13.

Kalyanaraman, B., U. V. Darley, et al. (1992). "Synergistic interaction between the probucol phenoxyl radical and ascorbic acid in inhibiting the oxidation of low density lipoprotein." J Biol Chem **267**(10): 6789-95.

Nishinaka, Y., S. Sugiyama, et al. (1992). "The effects of a high dose of ascorbate on ischemia-reperfusion-induced mitochondrial dysfunction in canine hearts." Heart Vessels **7**(1): 18-23.

Paganelli, G. M., G. Biasco, et al. (1992). "Effect of vitamin A, C, and E supplementation on rectal cell proliferation in patients with colorectal adenomas." J Natl Cancer Inst **84**(1): 47-51.

Sies, H., W. Stahl, et al. (1992). "Antioxidant functions of vitamins. Vitamins E and C, beta-carotene, and other carotenoids." Ann N Y Acad Sci **669**(1): 7-20.

Simon, J. A. (1992). "Vitamin C and cardiovascular disease: a review." J Am Coll Nutr **11**(2): 107-25.

Strain, J. J. and C. W. Mulholland (1992). "Vitamin C and vitamin E—synergistic interactions in vivo?" Exs **62**(1): 419-22.

Urivetzky, M., D. Kessaris, et al. (1992). "Ascorbic acid overdosing: a risk factor for calcium oxalate nephrolithiasis." J Urol **147**(5): 1215-8.

(1991). "Vitamin C: biologic functions and relation to cancer. September 10-12, 1990, Bethesda, Maryland. Abstracts." Nutr Cancer **15**(3-4): 249-80.

Barinaga, M. (1991). "Vitamin C gets a little respect [news]." Science **254**(5030): 374-6.

Behrens, W. A. and R. Madere (1991). "Vitamin C and vitamin E status in the spontaneously diabetic BB rat before the onset of diabetes." Metabolism **40**(1): 72-6.

Block, G. (1991). "Epidemiologic evidence regarding vitamin C and cancer." Am J Clin Nutr **54**(6 Suppl): 1310S-1314S.

Block, G. (1991). "Vitamin C and cancer prevention: the epidemiologic evidence." Am J Clin Nutr **53**(1 Suppl): 270S-282S.

Block, G., D. E. Henson, et al. (1991). "Vitamin C: a new look [editorial]." Ann Intern Med **114**(10): 909-10.

Devamanoharan, P. S., M. Henein, et al. (1991). "Prevention of selenite cataract by vitamin C." Exp Eye Res **52**(5): 563-8.

Frei, B. (1991). "Ascorbic acid protects lipids in human plasma and low-density lipoprotein against oxidative damage." Am J Clin Nutr **54**(6 Suppl): 1113S-1118S.

Frei, B., T. M. Forte, et al. (1991). "Gas phase oxidants of cigarette smoke induce lipid peroxidation and changes in lipoprotein properties in human blood plasma. Protective effects of ascorbic acid." Biochem J **277**(Pt 1): 133-8.

Fujimura, I., S. M. Geraldes, et al. (1991). "[Correlation between hypercholesterolemia and vitamin C deficient diet]." Rev Hosp Clin Fac Med Sao Paulo **46**(1): 14-8.

Helmrich, S. P., D. R. Ragland, et al. (1991). "Physical activity and reduced occurrence of non-insulin-dependent diabetes mellitus [see comments]." N Engl J Med **325**(3): 147-52.

Hemila, H. (1991). "Vitamin C and lowering of blood pressure: need for intervention trials? [letter; comment]." J Hypertens **9**(11): 1076-8.

Henning, S. M., J. Z. Zhang, et al. (1991). "Glutathione blood levels and other oxidant defense indices in men fed diets low in vitamin C." J Nutr **121**(12): 1969-75.

Henson, D. E., G. Block, et al. (1991). "Ascorbic acid: biologic functions and relation to cancer." J Natl Cancer Inst **83**(8): 547-50.

Jacob, R. A., D. S. Kelley, et al. (1991). "Immunocompetence and oxidant defense during ascorbate depletion of healthy men." Am J Clin Nutr **54**(6 Suppl): 1302S-1309S.

Jialal, I. and S. M. Grundy (1991). "Preservation of the endogenous antioxidants in low density lipoprotein by ascorbate but not probucol during oxidative modification." J Clin Invest **87**(2): 597-601.

Niki, E. (1991). "Action of ascorbic acid as a scavenger of active and stable oxygen radicals." Am J Clin Nutr **54**(6 Suppl): 1119S-1124S.

Padh, H. (1991). "Vitamin C: newer insights into its biochemical functions." Nutr Rev **49**(3): 65-70.

Rebouche, C. J. (1991). "Ascorbic acid and carnitine biosynthesis." Am J Clin Nutr **54**(6 Suppl): 1147S-1152S.

Riemersma, R. A., D. A. Wood, et al. (1991). "Risk of angina pectoris and plasma concentrations of vitamins A, C, and E and carotene [see comments]." Lancet **337**(8732): 1-5.

Robertson, J. M., A. P. Donner, et al. (1991). "A possible role for vitamins C and E in cataract prevention." Am J Clin Nutr **53**(1 Suppl): 346S-351S.

Schectman, G., J. C. Byrd, et al. (1991). "Ascorbic acid requirements for smokers: analysis of a population survey." Am J Clin Nutr **53**(6): 1466-70.

Taylor, A., P. F. Jacques, et al. (1991). "Relationship in humans between ascorbic acid consumption and levels of total and reduced ascorbic acid in lens, aqueous humor, and plasma." Curr Eye Res **10**(8): 751-9.

Trout, D. L. (1991). "Vitamin C and cardiovascular risk factors." Am J Clin Nutr **53**(1 Suppl): 322S-325S.

Harats, D., M. Ben-Naim, et al. (1990). "Effect of vitamin C and E supplementation on susceptibility of plasma lipoproteins to peroxidation induced by acute smoking." Atherosclerosis **85**(1): 47-54.

Jialal, I., G. L. Vega, et al. (1990). "Physiologic levels of ascorbate inhibit the oxidative modification of low density lipoprotein." Atherosclerosis **82**(3): 185-91.

Riemersma, R. A., M. Oliver, et al. (1990). "Plasma antioxidants and coronary heart disease: vitamins C and E, and selenium." Eur J Clin Nutr **44**(2): 143-50.

Ginter, E. (1989). "Ascorbic acid in cholesterol metabolism and in detoxification of xenobiotic substances: problem of optimum vitamin C intake." Nutrition **5**(6): 369-74.

Vitamin E

Axford-Gately, R. A. and G. J. Wilson (1993). "Myocardial infarct size reduction by single high dose or repeated low dose vitamin E supplementation in rabbits [see comments]." Can J Cardiol **9**(1): 94-8.

Benner, S. E., R. J. Winn, et al. (1993). "Regression of oral leukoplakia with alpha-tocopherol: a community clinical oncology program chemoprevention study." J Natl Cancer Inst **85**(1): 44-7.

Buettner, G. R. (1993). "The pecking order of free radicals and antioxidants: lipid peroxidation, alpha-tocopherol, and ascorbate." Arch Biochem Biophys **300**(2): 535-43.

Constantinescu, A., D. Han, et al. (1993). "Vitamin E recycling in human erythrocyte membranes." J Biol Chem **268**(15): 10906-13.

Donnan, P. T., M. Thomson, et al. (1993). "Diet as a risk factor for peripheral arterial disease in the general population: the Edinburgh Artery Study." Am J Clin Nutr **57**(6): 917-21.

Ferns, G. A., M. Konneh, et al. (1993). "Vitamin E: the evidence for an anti-atherogenic role." Artery **20**(2): 61-94.

Gerrish, K. E. and H. L. Gensler (1993). "Prevention of photocarcinogenesis by dietary vitamin E." Nutr Cancer **19**(2): 125-33.

Gey, K. F., U. K. Moser, et al. (1993). "Increased risk of cardiovascular disease at suboptimal plasma concentrations of essential antioxidants: an epidemiological update with special attention to carotene and vitamin C." Am J Clin Nutr **57**(5 Suppl): 787S-797S.

Hennig, B., C. J. McClain, et al. (1993). "Function of vitamin E and zinc in maintaining endothelial integrity. Implications in atherosclerosis." Ann N Y Acad Sci **686**(1): 99-109.

Hunter, D. J., J. E. Manson, et al. (1993). "A prospective study of the intake of vitamins C, E, and A and the risk of breast cancer." N Engl J Med **329**(4): 234-40.

Ingold, K. U., V. W. Bowry, et al. (1993). "Autoxidation of lipids and antioxidation by alpha-tocopherol and ubiquinol in homogeneous solution and in aqueous dispersions of lipids: unrecognized consequences of lipid particle size as exemplified by oxidation of human low density lipoprotein." Proc Natl Acad Sci U S A **90**(1): 45-9.

Kahl, R. and H. Kappus (1993). "[Toxicology of the synthetic antioxidants BHA and BHT in comparison with the natural antioxidant vitamin E]." Z Lebensm Unters Forsch **196**(4): 329-38.

Knekt, P. (1993). "Vitamin E and smoking and the risk of lung cancer." Ann N Y Acad Sci **686**(1): 280-7.

McIntosh, M. K., A. H. Goldfarb, et al. (1993). "Vitamin E alters hepatic antioxidant enzymes in rats treated with dehydroepiandrosterone (DHEA)." J Nutr **123**(2): 216-24.

Meydani, M., W. J. Evans, et al. (1993). "Protective effect of vitamin E on exercise-induced oxidative damage in young and older adults." Am J Physiol **264**(5 Pt 2): R992-8.

Mickle, D. A. and R. D. Weisel (1993). "Future directions of vitamin E and its analogues in minimizing myocardial ischemia-reperfusion injury [see comments]." Can J Cardiol **9**(1): 89-93.

Mitchel, R. E. and R. McCann (1993). "Vitamin E is a complete tumor promoter in mouse skin (repeated topical exposure)." Carcinogenesis **14**(4): 659-62.

Nakamura, H. and M. Suzukawa (1993). "[Atherosclerosis, with special reference to vitamin E]." Nippon Rinsho **51**(4): 997-1003.

Ozer, N. K., P. Palozza, et al. (1993). "d-alpha-Tocopherol inhibits low density lipoprotein induced proliferation and protein kinase C activity in vascular smooth muscle cells." Febs Lett **322**(3): 307-10.

Paolisso, G., A. D'Amore, et al. (1993). "Pharmacologic doses of vitamin E improve insulin action in healthy subjects and non-insulin-dependent diabetic patients." Am J Clin Nutr **57**(5): 650-6.

Prasad, K. and J. Kalra (1993). "Oxygen free radicals and hypercholesterolemic atherosclerosis: effect of vitamin E." Am Heart J **125**(4): 958-73.

Reaven, P. D., A. Khouw, et al. (1993). "Effect of dietary antioxidant combinations in humans. Protection of LDL by vitamin E but not by beta-carotene." Arterioscler Thromb **13**(4): 590-600.

Reaven, P. D. and J. L. Witztum (1993). "Comparison of supplementation of RRR-alpha-tocopherol and racemic alpha-tocopherol in humans. Effects on lipid levels and lipoprotein susceptibility to oxidation." Arterioscler Thromb **13**(4): 601-8.

Rimm, E. and G. Colditz (1993). "Smoking, alcohol, and plasma levels of carotenes and vitamin E." Ann N Y Acad Sci **686**(1): 323-33.

Rimm, E. B., M. J. Stampfer, et al. (1993). "Vitamin E consumption and the risk of coronary heart disease in men [see comments]." N Engl J Med **328**(20): 1450-6.

Rohan, T. E., G. R. Howe, et al. (1993). "Dietary fiber, vitamins A, C, and E, and risk of breast cancer: a cohort study." Cancer Causes Control **4**(1): 29-37.

Sheehy, P. J., P. A. Morrissey, et al. (1993). "Influence of heated vegetable oils and alpha-tocopheryl acetate supplementation on alpha-tocopherol, fatty acids and lipid peroxidation in chicken muscle." Br Poult Sci **34**(2): 367-81.

Smith, D., V. J. O'Leary, et al. (1993). "The role of alpha-tocopherol as a peroxyl radical scavenger in human low density lipoprotein." Biochem Pharmacol **45**(11): 2195-201.

Stampfer, M. J., C. H. Hennekens, et al. (1993). "Vitamin E consumption and the risk of coronary disease in women [see comments]." N Engl J Med **328**(20): 1444-9.

Steiner, M. (1993). "Vitamin E: more than an antioxidant." Clin Cardiol **16**(4 Suppl 1): I16-8.

van Antwerpen, L., A. J. Theron, et al. (1993). "Cigarette smoke-mediated oxidant stress, phagocytes, vitamin C, vitamin E, and tissue injury." Ann N Y Acad Sci **686**(1): 53-65.

Yano, T., G. Ishikawa, et al. (1993). "Is vitamin E a useful agent to protect against oxy radical-promoted lung tumorigenesis in ddY mice?" Carcinogenesis **14**(6): 1133-6.

Zheng, W., W. J. Blot, et al. (1993). "Serum micronutrients and the subsequent risk of oral and pharyngeal cancer." Cancer Res **53**(4): 795-8.

Ascherio, A., M. J. Stampfer, et al. (1992). "Correlations of vitamin A and E intakes with the plasma concentrations of carotenoids and tocopherols among American men and women." J Nutr **122**(9): 1792-801.

Barsacchi, R., G. Pelosi, et al. (1992). "Myocardial vitamin E is consumed during cardiopulmonary bypass: indirect evidence of free radical generation in human ischemic heart." Int J Cardiol **37**(3): 339-43.

Bendich, A. (1992). "Vitamin E status of US children." J Am Coll Nutr **11**(4): 441-4.

Bierenbaum, M. L., R. P. Reichstein, et al. (1992). "Relationship between serum lipid peroxidation products in hypercholesterolemic subjects and vitamin E status." Biochem Int **28**(1): 57-66.

Bowry, V. W., K. U. Ingold, et al. (1992). "Vitamin E in human low-density lipoprotein. When and how this antioxidant becomes a pro-oxidant." Biochem J **288**(Pt 2): 341-4.

Byers, T. and G. Perry (1992). "Dietary carotenes, vitamin C, and vitamin E as protective antioxidants in human cancers." Annu Rev Nutr **12**(1): 139-59.

Comstock, G. W., T. L. Bush, et al. (1992). "Serum retinol, beta-carotene, vitamin E, and selenium as related to subsequent cancer of specific sites." Am J Epidemiol **135**(2): 115-21.

De Keyser, J., N. De Klippel, et al. (1992). "Serum concentrations of vitamins A and E and early outcome after ischaemic stroke." Lancet **339**(8809): 1562-5.

De Maio, S. J., S. 3. King, et al. (1992). "Vitamin E supplementation, plasma lipids and incidence of restenosis after percutaneous transluminal coronary angioplasty (PTCA)." J Am Coll Nutr **11**(1): 68-73.

Ernster, L., P. Forsmark, et al. (1992). "The mode of action of lipid-soluble antioxidants in biological membranes. Relationship between the effects of ubiquinol and vitamin E as inhibitors of lipid peroxidation in submitochondrial particles." J Nutr Sci Vitaminol **1**(51): 548-51.

Ernster, L., P. Forsmark, et al. (1992). "The mode of action of lipid-soluble antioxidants in biological membranes: relationship between the effects of ubiquinol and vitamin E as inhibitors of lipid peroxidation in submitochondrial particles." Biofactors **3**(4): 241-8.

Esterbauer, H., H. Puhl, et al. (1992). "Vitamin E and atherosclerosis: an overview." J Nutr Sci Vitaminol **1**(82): 177-82.

Fahn, S. (1992). "A pilot trial of high-dose alpha-tocopherol and ascorbate in early Parkinson's disease." Ann Neurol **32**(1): 32.

Fernandez-Calle, P., J. A. Molina, et al. (1992). "Serum levels of alpha-tocopherol (vitamin E) in Parkinson's disease." Neurology **42**(5): 1064-6.

Gridley, G., J. K. McLaughlin, et al. (1992). "Vitamin supplement use and reduced risk of oral and pharyngeal cancer." Am J Epidemiol **135**(10): 1083-92.

Jialal, I. and S. M. Grundy (1992). "Effect of dietary supplementation with alpha-tocopherol on the oxidative modification of low density lipoprotein." J Lipid Res **33**(6): 899-906.

Kagan, V. E., E. A. Serbinova, et al. (1992). "Recycling of vitamin E in human low density lipoproteins." J Lipid Res **33**(3): 385-97.

Kappus, H. and A. T. Diplock (1992). "Tolerance and safety of vitamin E: a toxicological position report." Free Radic Biol Med **13**(1): 55-74.

Karlsson, J., B. Diamant, et al. (1992). "Plasma ubiquinone, alpha-tocopherol and cholesterol in man." Int J Vitam Nutr Res **62**(2): 160-4.

Kowdley, K. V., J. B. Mason, et al. (1992). "Vitamin E deficiency and impaired cellular immunity related to intestinal fat malabsorption." Gastroenterology **102**(6): 2139-42.

Kumar, C. T., V. K. Reddy, et al. (1992). "Dietary supplementation of vitamin E protects heart tissue from exercise-induced oxidant stress." Mol Cell Biochem **111**(1-2): 109-15.

Kunisaki, M., F. Umeda, et al. (1992). "Vitamin E binds to specific binding sites and enhances prostacyclin production by cultured aortic endothelial cells." Thromb Haemost **68**(6): 744-51.

Kunisaki, M., F. Umeda, et al. (1992). "Vitamin E restores reduced prostacyclin synthesis in aortic endothelial cells cultured with a high concentration of glucose." Metabolism **41**(6): 613-21.

Longnecker, M. P., J. M. Martin-Moreno, et al. (1992). "Serum alpha-tocopherol concentration in relation to subsequent colorectal cancer: pooled data from five cohorts." J Natl Cancer Inst **84**(6): 430-5.

Meydani, M. (1992). "Modulation of the platelet thromboxane A2 and aortic prostacyclin synthesis by dietary selenium and vitamin E." Biol Trace Elem Res **33**(1): 79-86.

Meydani, M. (1992). "Vitamin E requirement in relation to dietary fish oil and oxidative stress in elderly." Exs **62**(1): 411-8.

Meydani, M., W. Evans, et al. (1992). "Antioxidant response to exercise-induced oxidative stress and protection by vitamin E." Ann N Y Acad Sci **669**(1): 363-4.

Meydani, S. N., M. Hayek, et al. (1992). "Influence of vitamins E and B6 on immune response." Ann N Y Acad Sci **669**(1): 125-39.

Meydani, S. N., A. C. Shapiro, et al. (1992). "Lung eicosanoid synthesis is affected by age, dietary fat and vitamin E." J Nutr **122**(8): 1627-33.

Murphy, M. E., R. Kolvenbach, et al. (1992). "Antioxidant depletion in aortic crossclamping ischemia: increase of the plasma alpha-tocopheryl quinone/alpha-tocopherol ratio." Free Radic Biol Med **13**(2): 95-100.

Musial, J., T. B. Domagala, et al. (1992). "Lipid peroxidation, vitamin E, and cardiovascular disease." J Nutr Sci Vitaminol **1**(3): 200-3.

Odeleye, O. E., C. D. Eskelson, et al. (1992). "Vitamin E inhibition of lipid peroxidation and ethanol-mediated promotion of esophageal tumorigenesis." Nutr Cancer **17**(3): 223-34.

Packer, L. (1992). "Interactions among antioxidants in health and disease: vitamin E and its redox cycle." Proc Soc Exp Biol Med **200**(2): 271-6.

Paganelli, G. M., G. Biasco, et al. (1992). "Effect of vitamin A, C, and E supplementation on rectal cell proliferation in patients with colorectal adenomas." J Natl Cancer Inst **84**(1): 47-51.

Palozza, P. and N. I. Krinsky (1992). "beta-Carotene and alpha-tocopherol are synergistic antioxidants." Arch Biochem Biophys **297**(1): 184-7.

Panemangalore, M. and C. J. Lee (1992). "Evaluation of the indices of retinol and alpha-tocopherol status in free-living elderly." J Gerontol **47**(3): b98-104.

Pearce, B. C., R. A. Parker, et al. (1992). "Hypocholesterolemic activity of synthetic and natural tocotrienols." J Med Chem **35**(20): 3595-606.

Prasad, K. N. and J. Edwards-Prasad (1992). "Vitamin E and cancer prevention: recent advances and future potentials." J Am Coll Nutr **11**(5): 487-500.

Princen, H. M., P. G. van, et al. (1992). "Supplementation with vitamin E but not beta-carotene in vivo protects low density lipoprotein from lipid peroxidation in vitro. Effect of cigarette smoking." Arterioscler Thromb **12**(5): 554-62.

Pronczuk, A., Y. Kipervarg, et al. (1992). "Vegetarians have higher plasma alpha-tocopherol relative to cholesterol than do nonvegetarians." J Am Coll Nutr **11**(1): 50-5.

Reznick, A. Z., E. Witt, et al. (1992). "Vitamin E inhibits protein oxidation in skeletal muscle of resting and exercised rats." Biochem Biophys Res Commun **189**(2): 801-6.

Sanders, T. A. and A. Hinds (1992). "The influence of a fish oil high in docosahexaenoic acid on plasma lipoprotein and vitamin E concentrations and haemostatic function in healthy male volunteers." Br J Nutr **68**(1): 163-73.

Sies, H. (1992). "Carotenoids and tocopherols as antioxidants and singlet oxygen quenchers." J Nutr Sci Vitaminol **1**(33): 27-33.

Sies, H., W. Stahl, et al. (1992). "Antioxidant functions of vitamins. Vitamins E and C, beta-carotene, and other carotenoids." Ann N Y Acad Sci **669**(1): 7-20.

Smigel, K. (1992). "Vitamin E moves on stage in cancer prevention studies [news] [published erratum appears in J Natl Cancer Inst 1992 Aug 19; 84(16):1237]." J Natl Cancer Inst **84**(13): 996-7.

Steiner, M. (1992). "Alpha-tocopherol: a potent inhibitor of platelet adhesion." J Nutr Sci Vitaminol **1**(5): 191-5.

Strain, J. J. and C. W. Mulholland (1992). "Vitamin C and vitamin E—synergistic interactions in vivo?" Exs **62**(1): 419-22.

Tanaka, M., A. Sotomatsu, et al. (1992). "Aging of the brain and vitamin E." J Nutr Sci Vitaminol **1**(3): 240-3.

Tominaga, K., Y. Saito, et al. (1992). "An evaluation of serum microelement concentrations in lung cancer and matched non-cancer patients to determine the risk of developing lung cancer: a preliminary study." Jpn J Clin Oncol **22**(2): 96-101.

Van Vleet, J. F. and V. J. Ferrans (1992). "Etiologic factors and pathologic alterations in selenium-vitamin E deficiency and excess in animals and humans." Biol Trace Elem Res **33**(1): 1-21.

Vatassery, G. T. (1992). "Vitamin E. Neurochemistry and implications for neurodegeneration in Parkinson's disease." Ann N Y Acad Sci **669**(1): 97-109.

Veera Reddy, K., T. Charles Kumar, et al. (1992). "Exercise-induced oxidant stress in the lung tissue: role of dietary supplementation of vitamin E and selenium." Biochem Int **26**(5): 863-71.

Verlangieri, A. J. and M. J. Bush (1992). "Effects of d-alpha-tocopherol supplementation on experimentally induced primate atherosclerosis." J Am Coll Nutr **11**(2): 131-8.

Wadleigh, R. G., R. S. Redman, et al. (1992). "Vitamin E in the treatment of chemotherapy-induced mucositis." Am J Med **92**(5): 481-4.

Weiser, H., H. P. Probst, et al. (1992). "Vitamin E prevents side effects of high doses of vitamin A in chicks." Ann N Y Acad Sci **669**(1): 396-8.

Williams, R. J., J. M. Motteram, et al. (1992). "Dietary vitamin E and the attenuation of early lesion development in modified Watanabe rabbits." Atherosclerosis **94**(2-3): 153-9.

Wu, H. P., T. Y. Tai, et al. (1992). "Effect of tocopherol on platelet aggregation in non-insulin-dependent diabetes mellitus: ex vivo and in vitro studies." Taiwan I Hsueh Hui Tsa Chih **91**(3): 270-5.

Axford-Gatley, R. A. and G. J. Wilson (1991). "Reduction of experimental myocardial infarct size by oral administration of alpha tocopherol." Cardiovasc Res **25**(2): 89-92.

Behrens, W. A. and R. Madere (1991). "Vitamin C and vitamin E status in the spontaneously diabetic BB rat before the onset of diabetes." Metabolism **40**(1): 72-6.

Cabrini, L., C. Stefanelli, et al. (1991). "Ubiquinol prevents alpha-tocopherol consumption during liposome peroxidation." Biochem Int **23**(4): 743-9.

Ceriello, A., D. Giugliano, et al. (1991). "Vitamin E reduction of protein glycosylation in diabetes. New prospect for prevention of diabetic complications?" Diabetes Care **14**(1): 68-72.

Chan, A. C., K. Tran, et al. (1991). "Regeneration of vitamin E in human platelets." J Biol Chem **266**(26): 17290-5.

Chow, C. K. (1991). "Vitamin E and oxidative stress." Free Radic Biol Med **11**(2): 215-32.

Clausen, J. (1991). "The influence of selenium and vitamin E on the enhanced respiratory burst reaction in smokers." Biol Trace Elem Res **31**(3): 281-91.

Comstock, G. W., K. J. Helzlsouer, et al. (1991). "Prediagnostic serum levels of carotenoids and vitamin E as related to subsequent cancer in Washington County, Maryland." Am J Clin Nutr **53**(1 Suppl): 260S-264S.

Di Mascio, P., M. E. Murphy, et al. (1991). "Antioxidant defense systems: the role of carotenoids, tocopherols, and thiols." Am J Clin Nutr **53**(1 Suppl): 194S-200S.

Dieber-Rotheneder, M., H. Puhl, et al. (1991). "Effect of oral supplementation with D-alpha-tocopherol on the vitamin E content of human low density lipoproteins and resistance to oxidation." J Lipid Res **32**(8): 1325-32.

Dimitrov, N. V., C. Meyer, et al. (1991). "Plasma tocopherol concentrations in response to supplemental vitamin E." Am J Clin Nutr **53**(3): 723-9.

Drevon, C. A. (1991). "Absorption, transport and metabolism of vitamin E." Free Radic Res Commun **14**(4): 229-46.

Duthie, G. G., J. R. Arthur, et al. (1991). "Effects of smoking and vitamin E on blood antioxidant status." Am J Clin Nutr **53**(4 Suppl): 1061S-1063S.

Esterbauer, H., M. Dieber-Rotheneder, et al. (1991). "Role of vitamin E in preventing the oxidation of low-density lipoprotein." Am J Clin Nutr **53**(1 Suppl): 314S-321S.

Gey, K. F., P. Puska, et al. (1991). "Inverse correlation between plasma vitamin E and mortality from ischemic heart disease in cross-cultural epidemiology." Am J Clin Nutr **53**(1 Suppl): 326S-334S.

Haglund, O., R. Luostarinen, et al. (1991). "The effects of fish oil on triglycerides, cholesterol, fibrinogen and malondialdehyde in humans supplemented with vitamin E." J Nutr **121**(2): 165-9.

Horwitt, M. K. (1991). "Data supporting supplementation of humans with vitamin E." J Nutr **121**(3): 424-9.

Janero, D. R. (1991). "Therapeutic potential of vitamin E against myocardial ischemic-reperfusion injury." Free Radic Biol Med **10**(5): 315-24.

Janero, D. R. (1991). "Therapeutic potential of vitamin E in the pathogenesis of spontaneous atherosclerosis." Free Radic Biol Med **11**(1): 129-44.

Johansen, K., H. Theorell, et al. (1991). "Coenzyme Q10, alpha-tocopherol and free cholesterol in HDL and LDL fractions." Ann Med **23**(6): 649-56.

Knekt, P. (1991). "Role of vitamin E in the prophylaxis of cancer." Ann Med **23**(1): 3-12.

Knekt, P., A. Aromaa, et al. (1991). "Vitamin E and cancer prevention." Am J Clin Nutr **53**(1 Suppl): 283S-286S.

Kokoglu, E. and E. Ulakoglu (1991). "The transport of vitamin E in plasma and its correlation to plasma lipoproteins in non-insulin-dependent diabetes mellitus." Diabetes Res Clin Pract **14**(3): 175-81.

Kramer, T. R., N. Schoene, et al. (1991). "Increased vitamin E intake restores fish-oil-induced suppressed blastogenesis of mitogen-stimulated T lymphocytes." Am J Clin Nutr **54**(5): 896-902.

Krempf, M., S. Ranganathan, et al. (1991). "Plasma vitamin A and E in type 1 (insulin-dependent) and type 2 (non-insulin-dependent) adult diabetic patients." Int J Vitam Nutr Res **61**(1): 38-42.

Lenz, P. H., T. Watkins, et al. (1991). "Effect of dietary menhaden, Canola and partially hydrogenated soy oil supplemented with vitamin E upon plasma lipids and platelet aggregation." Thromb Res **61**(3): 213-24.

Meydani, M., F. Natiello, et al. (1991). "Effect of long-term fish oil supplementation on vitamin E status and lipid peroxidation in women." J Nutr **121**(4): 484-91.

Packer, L. (1991). "Protective role of vitamin E in biological systems." Am J Clin Nutr **53**(4 Suppl): 1050S-1055S.

Pryor, W. A. (1991). "Can vitamin E protect humans against the pathological effects of ozone in smog?" Am J Clin Nutr **53**(3): 702-22.

Riemersma, R. A., D. A. Wood, et al. (1991). "Risk of angina pectoris and plasma concentrations of vitamins A, C, and E and carotene [see comments]." Lancet **337**(8732): 1-5.

Robertson, J. M., A. P. Donner, et al. (1991). "A possible role for vitamins C and E in cataract prevention." Am J Clin Nutr **53**(1 Suppl): 346S-351S.

Rozewicka, L., W. B. Barcew, et al. (1991). "Protective effect of selenium and vitamin E against changes induced in heart vessels of rabbits fed chronically on a high-fat diet." Kitasato Arch Exp Med **64**(4): 183-92.

Sies, H. and M. E. Murphy (1991). "Role of tocopherols in the protection of biological systems against oxidative damage." J Photochem Photobiol B **8**(2): 211-8.

Steiner, M. (1991). "Influence of vitamin E on platelet function in humans." J Am Coll Nutr **10**(5): 466-73.

Urano, S., M. Hoshi-Hashizume, et al. (1991). "Vitamin E and the susceptibility of erythrocytes and reconstituted liposomes to oxidative stress in aged diabetics." Lipids **26**(1): 58-61.

Wiklund, O., L. Mattsson, et al. (1991). "Uptake and degradation of low density lipoproteins in atherosclerotic rabbit aorta: role of local LDL modification." J Lipid Res **32**(1): 55-62.

Wojcicki, J., L. Rozewicka, et al. (1991). "Effect of selenium and vitamin E on the development of experimental atherosclerosis in rabbits." Atherosclerosis **87**(1): 9-16.

Yoshizawa, Y., T. Miki, et al. (1991). "Effects of vitamin E-enriched egg yolk on lipid peroxidation, hemolysis and serum lipid concentration in young and old rats." J Nutr Sci Vitaminol **37**(3): 213-27.

Zamora, R., F. J. Hidalgo, et al. (1991). "Comparative antioxidant effectiveness of dietary beta-carotene, vitamin E, selenium and coenzyme Q10 in rat erythrocytes and plasma." J Nutr **121**(1): 50-6.

Babiy, A. V., J. M. Gebicki, et al. (1990). "Vitamin E content and low density lipoprotein oxidizability induced by free radicals." Atherosclerosis **81**(3): 175-82.

Harats, D., M. Ben-Naim, et al. (1990). "Effect of vitamin C and E supplementation on susceptibility of plasma lipoproteins to peroxidation induced by acute smoking." Atherosclerosis **85**(1): 47-54.

Hoshino, E., R. Shariff, et al. (1990). "Vitamin E suppresses increased lipid peroxidation in cigarette smokers." Jpen J Parenter Enteral Nutr **14**(3): 300-5.

Leibovitz, B., M. L. Hu, et al. (1990). "Dietary supplements of vitamin E, beta-carotene, coenzyme Q10 and selenium protect tissues against lipid peroxidation in rat tissue slices." J Nutr **120**(1): 97-104.

Meydani, S. N., M. P. Barklund, et al. (1990). "Vitamin E supplementation enhances cell-mediated immunity in healthy elderly subjects [see comments]." Am J Clin Nutr **52**(3): 557-63.

Noma, A., S. Maeda, et al. (1990). "Reduction of serum lipoprotein(a) levels in hyperlipidaemic patients with alpha-tocopheryl nicotinate." Atherosclerosis **84**(2-3): 213-7.

Riemersma, R. A., M. Oliver, et al. (1990). "Plasma antioxidants and coronary heart disease: vitamins C and E, and selenium." Eur J Clin Nutr **44**(2): 143-50.

Violi, F., D. Pratico, et al. (1990). "Inhibition of cyclooxygenase-independent platelet aggregation by low vitamin E concentration." Atherosclerosis **82**(3): 247-52.

Jandak, J., M. Steiner, et al. (1989). "Alpha-tocopherol, an effective inhibitor of platelet adhesion." Blood **73**(1): 141-9.

Muckle, T. J. and D. J. Nazir (1989). "Variation in human blood high-density lipoprotein response to oral vitamin E megadosage." Am J Clin Pathol **91**(2): 165-71.

Rubba, P., M. Mancini, et al. (1989). "Plasma vitamin E, apolipoprotein B and HDL-cholesterol in middle-aged men from southern Italy." Atherosclerosis **77**(1): 25-9.

Bendich, A. and L. J. Machlin (1988). "Safety of oral intake of vitamin E." Am J Clin Nutr **48**(3): 612-9.

Gisinger, C., J. Jeremy, et al. (1988). "Effect of vitamin E supplementation on platelet thromboxane A2 production in type I diabetic patients. Double-blind crossover trial." Diabetes **37**(9): 1260-4.

Vitamin Supplements

(1993). "Mighty vitamins. Vitamins emerging as disease fighters, not just supplements. (Cover story)." Medical World News **34**(1): 24-32.

Bates, C. J. (1993). "Vitamin undernutrition." Proc Nutr Soc **52**(1): 143-54.

Block, G. (1993). "Micronutrients and cancer: time for action? [editorial; comment]." J Natl Cancer Inst **85**(11): 846-8.

Draper, A., J. Lewis, et al. (1993). "The energy and nutrient intakes of different types of vegetarians: a case for supplements?" Br J Nutr **69**(1): 3-19.

Kim, I., D. F. Williamson, et al. (1993). "Vitamin and mineral supplement use and mortality in a US cohort (no benefit)." Am J Public Health **83**(4): 546-50.

Krinsky, N. I. (1993). "Micronutrients and their influence on mutagenicity and malignant transformation." Ann N Y Acad Sci **686**(1): 229-42.

Russell, R. M. and P. M. Suter (1993). "Vitamin requirements of elderly people: an update." Am J Clin Nutr **58**(1): 4-14.

Tanaka, N., K. Ochi, et al. (1993). "[Clinical application of vitamin A, D and E against malignant tumor in humans]." Nippon Rinsho **51**(4): 989-96.

Zifferblatt, S. M. (1993). "Nutrition and fitness recommendations when science is in transition. Vitamin and mineral supplementation: a case in point." World Rev Nutr Diet **72**(1): 177-89.

(1992). "Vitamin supplements win new-found respect: Skeptics are changing their minds over the value of these compounds." Modern Medicine **60**: 15-18.

Baker, D. E. and R. K. Campbell (1992). "Vitamin and mineral supplementation in patients with diabetes mellitus." Diabetes Educ **18**(5): 420-7.

Barone, J., E. Taioli, et al. (1992). "Vitamin supplement use and risk for oral and esophageal cancer." Nutr Cancer **18**(1): 31-41.

Bender, M. M., A. S. Levy, et al. (1992). "Trends in prevalence and magnitude of vitamin and mineral supplement usage and correlation with health status." J Am Diet Assoc **92**(9): 1096-101.

Chandra, R. K. (1992). "Effect of vitamin and trace-element supplementation on immune responses and infection in elderly subjects." Lancet **340**(8828): 1124-7.

Gridley, G., J. K. McLaughlin, et al. (1992). "Vitamin supplement use and reduced risk of oral and pharyngeal cancer." Am J Epidemiol **135**(10): 1083-92.

Hornig, D. and F. Strolz (1992). "Recommended dietary allowance: support from recent research." J Nutr Sci Vitaminol **1**(6): 173-6.

Johnson, K. and E. W. Kligman (1992). "Preventive nutrition: disease-specific dietary interventions for older adults." Geriatrics **47**(11): 39-40.

Machlin, L. J. (1992). "Beyond deficiency. New views on the function and health effects of vitamins. Introduction." Ann N Y Acad Sci **669**(1): 1-6.

Paganelli, G. M., G. Biasco, et al. (1992). "Effect of vitamin A, C, and E supplementation on rectal cell proliferation in patients with colorectal adenomas." J Natl Cancer Inst **84**(1): 47-51.

Shibata, A., A. Paganini-Hill, et al. (1992). "Intake of vegetables, fruits, beta-carotene, vitamin C and vitamin supplements and cancer incidence among the elderly: a prospective study." Br J Cancer **66**(4): 673-9.

Toufexis, A. (1992). The new scoop on vitamins. The real power of vitamins. New research shows they may help fight cancer, heart disease, and the ravages of aging. (Cover story). Time. 54-59.

Havivi, E., H. Bar On, et al. (1991). "Vitamins and trace metals status in non insulin dependent diabetes mellitus." Int J Vitam Nutr Res **61**(4): 328-33.

Park, Y. K., I. Kim, et al. (1991). "Characteristics of vitamin and mineral supplement products in the United States." Am J Clin Nutr **54**(4): 750-9.

Weisburger, J. H. (1991). "Nutritional approach to cancer prevention with emphasis on vitamins, antioxidants, and carotenoids." Am J Clin Nutr **53**(1 Suppl):

Wheat Germ

Cara, L., M. Armand, et al. (1992). "Long-term wheat germ intake beneficially affects plasma lipids and lipoproteins in hypercholesterolemic human subjects." J Nutr **122**(2): 317-26.

Cara, L., C. Dubois, et al. (1992). "Effects of oat bran, rice bran, wheat fiber, and wheat germ on postprandial lipemia in healthy adults." Am J Clin Nutr **55**(1): 81-8.

Women/Estrogen

Boyden, T. W., R. W. Pamenter, et al. (1993). "Resistance exercise training is associated with decreases in serum low-density lipoprotein cholesterol levels in premenopausal women." Arch Intern Med **153**(1): 97-100.

Bunce, G. E. (1993). "Antioxidant nutrition and cataract in women: a prospective study." Nutr Rev **51**(3): 84-6.

Colditz, G. A. (1993). "Epidemiology of breast cancer. Findings from the nurses' health study." Cancer **71**(4 Suppl): 1480-9.

Demirovic, J., H. Blackburn, et al. (1993). "Sex differences in coronary heart disease mortality trends: the Minnesota Heart Survey, 1970-1988." Epidemiology **4**(1): 79-82.

Finucane, F. F., J. H. Madans, et al. (1993). "Decreased risk of stroke among postmenopausal hormone users. Results from a national cohort." Arch Intern Med **153**(1): 73-9.

Garg, R., D. K. Wagener, et al. (1993). "Alcohol consumption and risk of ischemic heart disease in women." Arch Int Med **153**: 1211-1216.

Green, A. and C. Bain (1993). "Epidemiological overview of oestrogen replacement and cardiovascular disease." Baillieres Clin Endocrinol Metab **7**(1): 95-112.

Harlan, L. C., R. J. Coates, et al. (1993). "Estrogen receptor status and dietary intakes in breast cancer patients." Epidemiology **4**(1): 25-31.

Jenner, J. L., J. M. Ordovas, et al. (1993). "Effects of age, sex, and menopausal status on plasma lipoprotein(a) levels. The Framingham offspring study." Circulation **87**: 1135-1141.

Kanaley, J. A., M. L. Andresen-Reid, et al. (1993). "Differential health benefits of weight loss in upper-body and lower-body obese women." Am J Clin Nutr **57**(1): 20-6.

Kawachi, I., G. A. Colditz, et al. (1993). "Smoking cessation and decreased risk of stroke in women." Jama **269**(2): 232-6.

Martin, K. A. and M. W. Freeman (1993). "Postmenopausal hormone-replacement therapy [editorial; comment]." N Engl J Med **328**(15): 1115-7.

Nabulsi, A. A., A. R. Folsom, et al. (1993). "Association of hormone-replacement therapy with various cardiovascular risk factors in postmenopausal women. The Atherosclerosis Risk in Communities Study Investigators [see comments]." N Engl J Med **328**(15): 1069-75.

Nichols, J. F., D. K. Omizo, et al. (1993). "Efficacy of heavy-resistance training for active women over sixty: muscular strength, body composition, and program adherence." J Am Geriatr Soc **41**(3): 205-10.

Posner, B. M., L. A. Cupples, et al. (1993). "Diet, menopause, and serum cholesterol levels in women: the Framingham Study." Am Heart J **125**(2 Pt 1): 483-9.

Reichman, M. E., J. T. Judd, et al. (1993). "Effects of alcohol consumption on plasma and urinary hormone concentrations in premenopausal women." J Natl Cancer Inst **9**: 722-726.

Rimm, E. B., J. E. Manson, et al. (1993). "Cigarette smoking and the risk of diabetes in women." Am J Public Health **83**(2): 211-4.

Stampfer, M. J., C. H. Hennekens, et al. (1993). "Vitamin E consumption and the risk of coronary disease in women [see comments]." N Engl J Med **328**(20): 1444-9.

Taylor, P. A. and A. Ward (1993). "Women, high-density lipoprotein cholesterol, and exercise." Arch Intern Med **153**(10): 1178-84.

Taylor, P. A. and A. Ward (1993). "Women, High-density lipoprotein cholesterol, and exercise." Arch Intern Med **153**: 1178-1184.

Willett, W. C., M. J. Stampfer, et al. (1993). "Intake of trans fatty acids and risk of coronary heart disease among women." Lancet **341**(8845): 581-5.

Zinc and Copper

Chevion, M., Y. Jiang, et al. (1993). "Copper and iron are mobilized following myocardial ischemia: possible predictive criteria for tissue injury." Proc Natl Acad Sci U S A **90**(3): 1102-6.

Hennig, B., C. J. McClain, et al. (1993). "Function of vitamin E and zinc in maintaining endothelial integrity. Implications in atherosclerosis." Ann N Y Acad Sci **686**(1): 99-109.

Dasgupta, A. and T. Zdunek (1992). "In vitro lipid peroxidation of human serum catalyzed by cupric ion: antioxidant rather than prooxidant role of ascorbate." Life Sci **50**(12): 875-82.

Dasgupta, A., T. Zdunek, et al. (1992). "Differential effects of transition metal ions on in vitro lipid peroxidation of human serum and protein precipitated from serum." Clin Physiol Biochem **9**(1): 7-10.

He, J. A., G. S. Tell, et al. (1992). "Relation of serum zinc and copper to lipids and lipoproteins: the Yi People Study." J Am Coll Nutr **11**(1): 74-8.

Hennig, B., Y. Wang, et al. (1992). "Zinc deficiency alters barrier function of cultured porcine endothelial cells." J Nutr **122**(6): 1242-7.

Tan, I. K., K. S. Chua, et al. (1992). "Serum magnesium, copper, and zinc concentrations in acute myocardial infarction." J Clin Lab Anal **6**(5): 324-8.

Frambach, D. A. and R. E. Bendel (1991). "Zinc supplementation and anemia [letter; comment]." Jama **265**(7): 869.

Hing, S. A. and K. Y. Lei (1991). "Copper deficiency and hyperlipoproteinemia induced by a tetramine cupruretic agent in rabbits." Biol Trace Elem Res **28**(3): 195-211.

Kuzuya, M., K. Yamada, et al. (1991). "Oxidation of low-density lipoprotein by copper and iron in phosphate buffer." Biochim Biophys Acta **1084**(2): 198-201.

Lei, K. Y. (1991). "Dietary copper: cholesterol and lipoprotein metabolism." Annu Rev Nutr **11**(1): 265-83.

Maziere, C., M. Auclair, et al. (1991). "Estrogens inhibit copper and cell-mediated modification of low density lipoprotein." Atherosclerosis **89**(2-3): 175-82.

Salonen, J. T., R. Salonen, et al. (1991). "Serum copper and the risk of acute myocardial infarction: a prospective population study in men in eastern Finland [see comments]." Am J Epidemiol **134**(3): 268-76.

Salonen, J. T., R. Salonen, et al. (1991). "Interactions of serum copper, selenium, and low density lipoprotein cholesterol in atherogenesis." Bmj **302**(6779): 756-60.

Taylor, C. G. and T. M. Bray (1991). "Effect of hyperoxia on oxygen free radical defense enzymes in the lung of zinc-deficient rats." J Nutr **121**(4): 460-6.

Walter, R., Jr., J. Y. Uriu-Hare, et al. (1991). "Copper, zinc, manganese, and magnesium status and complications of diabetes mellitus." Diabetes Care **14**(11): 1050-6.

Index

C

D

G

H

I

J

N

O

P

Q

R

T

U

V

W

Y

Z

Dr. Joe D. Goldstrich is available for seminars and lectures covering the topics discussed in this book.

Additional copies of *The Cardiologist's Painless Prescription for a Healthy Heart and a Longer Life* can be ordered, using your Mastercard or Visa, by calling 1-800-9-HEART-9.